16 —

Sw

ADVANCES IN HOST DEFENSE MECHANISMS
Volume 1

PHAGOCYTIC CELLS

Advances in Host Defense Mechanisms
Volume 1

Phagocytic Cells

Editors

John I. Gallin, M.D.
Head, Bacterial Diseases Section
Laboratory of Clinical Investigation
National Institute of Allergy and Infectious
Diseases
National Institutes of Health
Bethesda, Maryland

Anthony S. Fauci, M.D.
Chief, Laboratory of Immunoregulation
National Institute of Allergy and Infectious
Diseases
National Institutes of Health
Bethesda, Maryland

Raven Press ■ New York

Raven Press, 1140 Avenue of the Americas, New York, New York 10036

Made in the United States of America

Library of Congress Cataloging in Publication Data
Main entry under title:

Phagocytic cells.

   (Advances in host defense mechanisms ; v. 1)
   Includes bibliographical references and index.
   I. Phagocytes.   2. Immunity.   I. Gallin, John I.
II. Fauci, Anthony S.   III. Series. [DNLM:
1. Phagocytes.   W1 AD636 v.1 / QW 690 P 533]
QR187.P4P485   616.07′9   82–302
ISBN 0–89004–574–7   AACR2

Preface

Although the concept of "host defenses" has been appreciated for over 100 years, there has been a virtual explosion of information during the last decade. We, in accordance with several of our colleagues interested in this area, feel that basic science and clinical investigators working in infectious diseases and related areas have not effectively pursued the possible clinical relevance of many of the rapidly emerging observations nor the potentially fruitful source for basic scientific approaches that could be drawn from clinical observations. Accordingly, we have initiated this new series to present a highly sophisticated form of science, with the prevailing theme being potential applicability to the understanding of clinically relevant host defense mechanisms.

The content of the articles in this series will vary. Some chapters will be basic science reviews; others will present recent clinical advances—all will be written to provide a forum for the exchange of information between basic science and clinical investigators. The eventual goals of the series include cross-fertilization between these groups leading to the pursuit of the basic scientific approach to clinical observations as well as the clinical application of observations made at the basic scientific level. The articles will be designed to be relevant and useful to students, fellows, basic scientists, and clinical investigators, as well as physicians in infectious diseases and related disciplines.

For our initial volume we have selected the phagocytic cells in host defense. Volume 2 will be devoted to the lymphoid system in host defense. Subsequently, other appropriate topics will be covered.

We are particularly fortunate that Dr. James G. Hirsch contributed the first chapter providing an historical perspective for modern concepts in host defenses. This elegant review of selected highlights of the careers of Pasteur, Duclaux, Metchnikoff, Koch, Löffler, Kitasato, Roux, Yersin, Nuttall, Erlich, Bordet, and others, focuses on the historic discoveries of phagocytic cells, antibodies, and complement and sets a high standard for all subsequent chapters.

Mononuclear phagocytes are well recognized to be critical in phagocytizing both foreign invaders such as pathogenic microorganisms and endogenous invaders such as neoplastic cells. Golde and Hocking review the maturation and development of monocytes into macrophages which can then perform their highly specialized functions. Recent studies have altered our viewpoint of the process of phagocytosis and the role of opsonins and receptors in phagocytosis; the chapter by Griffin emphasizes these advances and discusses the possible relevance of recent experimental observations to host defense against pathogenic microorganisms. Fever, an almost invariable accompaniment of infection, is a consequence of the macrophage product pyrogen. Pyrogen has been shown recently to have a multitude of potential roles in host defenses including modulation of neutrophil function, activation of lymphocytes, and mobilization of white cells from the bone marrow. The review by

Dinarello puts these "new" roles of pyrogen in their proper perspective and raises a number of intriguing questions about pyrogen as a mediator of host defenses.

The neutrophil is generally the first phagocytic cell to arrive at inflammatory foci. Although traditionally conceived as a cell whose role is solely to seek and destroy microorganisms, the neutrophil can no longer be considered in this light alone. As reviewed by Wright, the neutrophil appears to be an important secretory organ of host defense that modulates inflammatory responses in many ways. In addition to secreting enzymes, the neutrophil can modulate inflammation by highly reactive oxygen species generated during activation. The study of the biochemistry of production of these reactive oxygen species and appreciation of their importance in oxygen-dependent cytoxic mechanisms are gaining increasing interest and attention in this area. We believe that the lucid and comprehensive review of this complex subject by Klebanoff will serve as the classic state-of-the-art reference for students of infectious diseases.

The importance of phagocytes in clinical medicine was highlighted in 1967 by Quie and colleagues who described an abnormality in phagocyte microbicidal function against staphylococci in patients with chronic granulomatous disease of childhood. Since then, numerous clinical syndromes have been described with neutrophil dysfunction contributing to recurrent infection. The chapter by Quie summarizes disorders of neutrophil locomotion and microbicidal capacity and provides a thorough review of a group of patients with hyperimmunoglobulin E, recurrent infections, and intermittent phagocyte dysfunction.

One of the most intriguing and clinically important new areas of the study of phagocytes is neutrophil-antibiotic interaction. Yourtee and Root review the importance of antibiotic penetration into phagocytes in the elimination of certain microorganisms. The importance of selecting antibiotics that penetrate phagocytes in the treatment of certain infections is apparent, and the importance of developing new antibiotics that are concentrated in phagocyte lysosomes is clear.

The eosinophil has long been recognized as a phagocytic cell. However, there has been much debate as to whether there is a clinically relevant role for the eosinophil in host defense. The chapters by Bass and by Dessein and David review the current knowledge of eosinophil responses during acute infection. These chapters discuss recent work on the role of T-lymphocytes in the stimulation of eosinophil responses and review the mechanisms underlying the impressive blood and tissue eosinophilia following helminthic and certain protozoa infections. In addition, they summarize the evidence implicating the eosinophil in the destruction of invading larvae by antibody and/or complement dependent cytotoxicity mechanisms. The review by Ackerman, Durack, and Gleich summarizes the properties and activities of eosinophil proteins and their potential role in damaging parasites and causing diseases. These last three chapters provide an important summary of the recent findings by the current generation of investigators who are attempting to unravel the mystery of the role the eosinophil plays, if any, in host defense.

The remarkable advances in understanding the regulatory mechanisms of the physiology of phagocyte function reviewed in this volume give reality to the expectation that some of the disorders of phagocyte function may soon be treated effectively. More importantly, they provide optimism that successful manipulation of these important cells will be possible in future therapy of patients whose host defenses have been compromised by dysfunction of these cells.

John I. Gallin
Anthony S. Fauci

Acknowledgments

We would like to thank each of the contributors whose endeavors have made this first volume possible. In addition, we would like to express special thanks to Drs. Sheldon M. Wolff and James G. Hirsch for their helpful advice and encouragement in launching this new series.

Contents

Contributors

Steven J. Ackerman: *Departments of Medicine and Immunology, Mayo Medical School, Mayo Clinic and Foundation, Rochester, Minnesota 55905*

David A. Bass: *Department of Medicine, Division of Infectious Diseases and Immunology, Bowman Gray School of Medicine, Winston-Salem, North Carolina 27103*

John R. David: *The Department of Medicine, Harvard Medical School, and the Division of Rheumatology and Immunology, Brigham and Women's Hospital, Boston, Massachusetts 02115*

Alain J. Dessein: *The Department of Medicine, Harvard Medical School, and the Division of Rheumatology and Immunology, Brigham and Women's Hospital, Boston, Massachusetts 02115*

Charles A. Dinarello: *Division of Experimental Medicine, Department of Medicine, Tufts University School of Medicine, New England Medical Center, Boston, Massachusetts 02111*

David T. Durack: *Division of Infectious Diseases, Department of Medicine, Duke University Medical Center, Durham, North Carolina 27710*

Gerald J. Gleich: *Departments of Medicine and Immunology, Mayo Medical School, Mayo Clinic and Foundation, Rochester, Minnesota 55905*

David W. Golde: *Division of Hematology-Oncology, Department of Medicine, UCLA School of Medicine, Los Angeles, California 90024*

Frank W. Griffin Jr.: *Division of Infectious Diseases, Department of Medicine, University of Alabama in Birmingham, Birmingham, Alabama 35294*

James G. Hirsch: *The Rockefeller University, New York, New York 10021*

William G. Hocking: *Division of Hematology-Oncology, Department of Medicine, UCLA School of Medicine, Los Angeles, California 90024*

Seymour J. Klebanoff: *Department of Medicine, University of Washington School of Medicine, Seattle, Washington 98195*

Paul G. Quie: *University of Minnesota Medical School, Minneapolis, Minnesota 55455*

Richard K. Root: *Department of Internal Medicine, Section of Infectious Diseases, Yale University School of Medicine, New Haven, Connecticut 06510*

Daniel G. Wright: *Department of Hematology, Walter Reed Army Institute of Research, Washington, D.C. 20012, and USUHS School of Medicine, Bethesda, Maryland 20014*

Edward L. Yourtee: *Department of Internal Medicine, Section of Infectious Diseases, Yale University School of Medicine, New Haven, Connecticut 06510*

Advances in Host Defense Mechanisms, Vol. 1,
edited by John I. Gallin and Anthony S. Fauci,
Raven Press, New York © 1982.

Host Resistance to Infectious Diseases— A Centennial

James G. Hirsch

*Josiah Macy, Jr. Foundation, One Rockefeller Plaza,
New York, New York 10020*

The editors have selected a very appropriate time to launch a review series devoted to host resistance. This field of study is 100 years old, which justifies some celebration and taking of stock, and the accumulated knowledge is sufficiently extensive to warrant consideration of the various branches in review form. My purpose in this chapter is to consider the field of host resistance from a historical perspective, to emphasize its beginnings a century ago, and to place the major discoveries that launched the field in proper temporal relationships. The discussion will be confined to these early advances; more recent developments will undoubtedly be covered by the expert reviews in the chapters that follow.

Some might dispute my view that the field of host resistance or immunology is only 100 years old. It is true, as has been discussed in detail in recent reviews (1,2), that natural or acquired immunity to disease had been noted in antiquity, and throughout recorded history various examples of this phenomenon have been cited and speculations made on possible mechanisms at work. These provide an interesting historical background, but they do not really relate to the topics that will be treated in the present and future volumes of this series. These volumes will deal with mechanisms of host resistance in terms of modern medical science; and, in this arena, the beginning did occur only a century ago.

The beginning of modern immunology can be dated, in fact, to a specific experiment in which Pasteur and his colleagues discovered, largely by accident, that an attenuated culture of chicken cholera organisms would immunize against subsequent challenge with virulent organisms. Duclaux, who was working with Pasteur at the time, described the course of events in this epochal discovery as follows:

> The first experiments on chicken cholera dated from 1879. Interrupted by vacations, they had been resumed, but were upset at once by an unforseen obstacle. Almost all the cultures left in the laboratory had become sterile.
> As all these belonged to the experiments underway, an attempt was made to revive them, and with that end in view, transfers were made from them either into chicken boullion or into chickens. Many of these made no growth, and also spared and left unimpaired the animals into which they were inoculated, and we were about to throw them away, in order to begin anew, when it occurred to Pasteur to inoculate a fresh young culture into these chickens which, at least in appearance, had so well resisted the inoculations with the cultures made the preceding summer.

To the surprise of all, perhaps even of Pasteur himself, who did not expect such a success, almost all of these chickens resisted, whereas new chickens, just brought from the market, succumbed in the ordinary length of time, thus showing that the culture used for the inoculation was very active. With one blow . . . vaccination was discovered. (3)

Pasteur, then 58 years old, was Professor of Chemistry at the Sorbonne, and had many years previously achieved richly deserved fame on the basis of his work (3,4) on crystals, on fermentation and the germ theory, on wine and beer manufacture, and his studies of silkworm diseases. The experiments with chicken cholera formed the basis of studies on immunization (for review and list of original references, see reference 5) that were to occupy him for the remainder of his life. Studies followed on the use of anthrax grown at higher-than-usual temperature as a suitable attenuated and effective vaccine, on the use for immunization of a swine erysipelas culture suitably attenuated by passage in rabbits, and finally on rabies, using virus passed through monkeys, or virus attenuated by a 2-wk storage of infected rabbit spinal cords in dry, sterile air. The acclaim that came to Pasteur when he successfully used his rabies vaccine in the middle 1880s resulted in a movement to establish a research institute. The Pasteur Institute, the first institution of its kind to be established, was opened in the fall of 1888.

In the early 1880s, when Pasteur did his classical work on acquired immunity, there was no information on mechanisms that might account for the appearance and the specificity of the enhanced resistance of the vaccinated host. Pasteur speculated that it might be based on depletion of a specific nutrient required by the

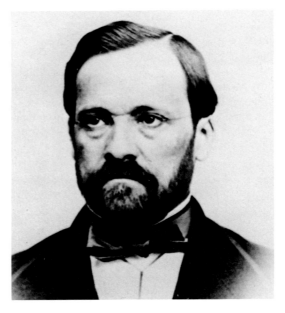

Louis Pasteur

microorganism, a nutrient not regenerated in the host. This theory, which seems far-fetched today, did provide a possible explanation for the phenomenon. It must be remembered that Pasteur's experiments were done before the protective role of phagocytic cells was recognized, and before the discovery of antibodies and complement.

The first conception of a true host-defense mechanism came in December of 1882 (6). Ilya Metchnikoff had been trained as a zoologist, and in the course of his studies of various species, mainly marine invertebrates, he noted the presence of ameboid cells, capable of locomotion and ingestion of particles, in the mesodermal tissues as well as the intestinal tract. The function of the ameboid cells in the intestinal tract was clearly a nutritional one, but the role of the tissue phagocytic cells was a puzzle. Metchnikoff, who was 34 years old in 1882, had a most unsettled early career—personal problems combined with deterioration of academic freedom at that time in Russia plagued the brilliant young scientist and led to incapacitating psychological problems and frequent job changes. In 1881, the year before his big discovery, his wife's parents died and left enough money to enable Metchnikoff to "retire" and lead the life of a gentleman scientist for the next several years. He moved to Messina in Sicily, where he had spent several summers previously doing research on sea creatures, and it was here in 1882 that the wandering, jobless zoologist conceived of the role of phagocytic cells in host defense. His own description of this conceptual breakthrough was as follows:

> One day when the family had gone to a circus to see some extraordinary performing apes, I remained alone at my microscope, observing the life in the mobile cells of a transparent starfish larva, when a new thought suddenly flashed across my brain. It struck me that similar cells might serve in the defense of the organism against intruders. Feeling that there was in this something of surpassing interest, I felt so excited that I began striding up and down the room and even went to the seashore in order to collect my thoughts.
>
> I said to myself that, if my supposition was true, a splinter introduced into the body of a starfish larva, devoid of blood vessels or of a nervous system, should soon be surrounded by mobile cells as is to be observed in a man who runs a splinter into his finger. This was no sooner said than done.
>
> There was a small garden to our dwelling, in which we had a few days previously organized a "Christmas tree" for the children on a little tangerine tree; I fetched from it a few rose thorns and introduced them at once under the skin of some beautiful starfish larvae as transparent as water.
>
> I was too excited to sleep that night in the expectation of the result of my experiment, and very early the next morning I ascertained that it had fully succeeded.
>
> That experiment formed the basis of the phagocyte theory, to the development of which I devoted the next twenty-five years of my life." (6)

How was it that Metchnikoff was the one to come up with this idea, which seems so obvious to us today? By 1880 many scientists had noted the association between bacteria and cells. For example Koch, Roser, and others had described cells filled with anthrax bacilli, but the significance of this association eluded them. What was needed was an interdisciplinary background. Metchnikoff's career as a zoologist had provided him with extensive knowledge on phagocytic cells in lower forms; this knowledge needed to be coupled with knowledge just coming to light in the newly developing field of bacteriology. As we shall discuss below, bacteriology and infectious diseases were in their infancy as scientific fields in 1882, when Metchnikoff made his breakthrough.

Metchinkoff worked alone to establish his phagocytic theory, with no facilities except for a room in his flat and his microscope, and had no academic or institutional affiliation at the time. In 1883 he conducted studies on a transparent water flea, *Daphnia*, to establish that the outcome of an infection by various strains of a fungus was correlated with the outcome of the interaction between the invading fungus and the host's phagocytes. Some strains of the fungus were engulfed and destroyed by the phagocytes, in which case no disease resulted, whereas other strains of the fungus were not attacked by the phagocytes and a disseminated fatal disease developed. Observations on phagocytic-bacterial relationships in mammalian anthrax were also in accord with an important role for these cells in host defense.

Metchnikoff's findings were the first solid scientific ones related to host-defense mechanisms, and as such they deserve a special place in the annals of modern medical science. Their historical significance is, of course, of obvious relevance to the subject of this review series. From this rather humble beginning there has emerged today a sizable scientific enterprise, as will be evident from the reviews that follow.

Obviously, knowledge of host resistance to infectious disease could hardly be expected to develop in a scientific way until the nature and causes of these diseases

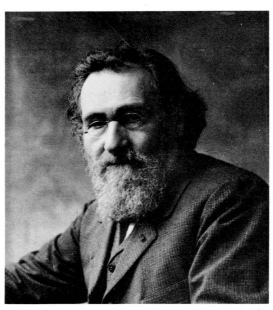

Ilya Metchnikoff

were established. Let us look briefly, then, at some of the mileposts along the road in the fields of bacteriology and infectious diseases.

Here again Pasteur played a leading role. His classical experiments in the 1860s showed clearly that microorganisms were present everywhere in the environment, and, that these tiny, invisible forms of life were responsible for various types of fermentation (3–5). In the 1870s Pasteur discovered the bacilli that cause diseases of silkworms, and he also demonstrated bacteria to be the probable cause of anthrax. Once the existence of bacteria had been established, and after Pasteur and others pointed out their likely role as agents of disease, one might assume that it should have been a simple matter to isolate the various microorganisms from human diseases and pin down their causal relationship. In fact, this was a most difficult task, because no methods or only primitive methods were available for staining bacteria in specimens, or for culturing them in pure form. Almost any material inoculated into rich culture medium grew out hordes of bacteria of several types, and it was then impossible to establish which ones were significant pathogens and which ones were contaminants. Many people tried to solve this problem with ingenious methods (5). Lister succeeded, to a degree, using a limiting dilution technique much like that used today for cloning, but it was cumbersome and impractical.

The main figure in the solution of these problems, opening the door for modern bacteriology and infectious diseases, was Robert Koch. Koch had been a field surgeon in the Franko-Prussian war of 1870 and then worked as a regional physician

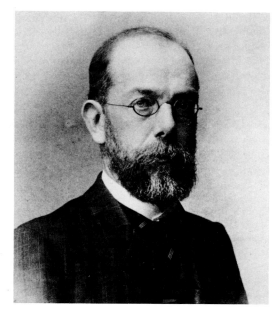

Robert Koch

in a small town in Pomerania. There, in 1876, working isolated from all academic contacts, he did his famous work establishing the life history of anthrax bacilli and their role in producing disease. In 1877 Koch devised the thinly smeared air-dried preparation and applied stains that allowed microscopic identification of bacterial forms. These methods, improved by Ehrlich in the 1880s, are basically the same as those used today. In 1881, the really important technical breakthrough occurred, which enabled bacteria to be isolated and grown in pure cultures. The method developed by Koch involved the use of transparent solid media, so that individual colonies of bacteria could be picked and grown in pure culture. Koch initially employed nutrient gelatin, which worked but tended to liquefy at body temperatures. Agar was introduced for making solid media in Koch's laboratory after the wife of one of his staff, Frau Hesse, received some agar from Batavia for use in making jelly! Various other technical refinements, such as the petri dish, pour plates, and blood agar were introduced in Koch's laboratory, and made bacterial culture and identification easy and widely available (5). From 1884 to 1886 a veritable flood of reports establishing specific strains of bacteria as causes of human disease— diphtheria, typhoid, streptococci, staphylococci, gonococci, and pneumococci— ensued.

These advances in bacteriology and infectious diseases in the middle 1880s set the stage for the next big advance in the field of immunology, namely the discovery of antibodies. The diphtheria bacillus was isolated and characterized by Löffler in 1884 (7), and Kitasato identified the tetanus bacillus in 1889 (8). In 1889 Roux and Yersin demonstrated a potent toxin in the culture fluids of diphtheria bacilli and, in the same year, Faber described tetanus toxin. The discovery of antitoxins was not long in coming. In the December 3, 1890 issue of the *Berliner klinische Wochenschrift* (9) Carl Fraenkel reported that the injection into animals of heated (65–70°C) 3-wk-old broth cultures of diphtheria bacilli produced a state of immunity to a subsequent challenge with living, virulent bacilli. The very next day the famous paper of Behring and Kitasato (10) appeared in the *Deutsche medicinische Wochenschrift*, demonstrating that the immunity of rabbits and mice treated with certain tetanus cultures was dependant on the capacity of their cell-free serum to inactivate the toxin. The following is a translation of part of that paper (10):

> Besides studies on phagocytosis, which seek an explanation [of immunity] in the vital activity of the cells, one had to consider the antibacterial action of blood and also adaptation of the animal to the toxin. . . .
>
> Now one of us (Behring) has established in studies on rats that are immune to diphtheria and on immunized guinea pigs that none of the theories mentioned above explained the immunity in these animals, and thus it became necessary to look for a different principle to explain the immunity. After many unsuccessful efforts, the direction in which to seek the basis for the resistance to diphtheria was pointed out by the finding that the blood of the immune animals had the ability to destroy the diphtheria toxin. But only in applying this concept, which we developed in studies on diphtheria to tetanus, were we able to obtain results which . . . are conclusive.

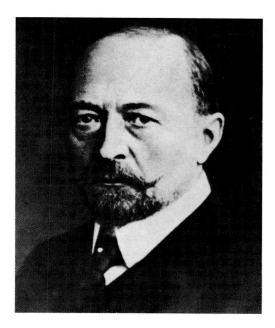

Emil Behring

A rabbit was immunized against tetanus by a method described elsewhere. In testing the degree of immunity, the animal received 10 ml of a virulent tetanus culture. 0.5 cc of such a culture would suffice to kill a normal rabbit, but the immunized rabbit remained healthy. This animal exhibited immunity not only to the living tetanus bacilli, but also to the tetanus toxin, since this animal was able to tolerate without harm 20 times as much toxin as would kill a normal rabbit.

Blood was taken from this immunized rabbit. 0.2 cc of the still liquid blood was given to one mouse intraperitoneally, 0.5 cc to another. After 24 hours both of these mice, as well as two control mice, were injected with virulent tetanus bacilli. The control animals developed tetanus within 20 hours and were dead by 36 hours, whereas the treated animals remained healthy. . . . Serum [from the same immune rabbit blood] was also given to mice: 6 mice received 0.2 cc intraperitoneally. After 24 hours the tetanus challenge was given and all six remained healthy, whereas the control mice were dead of tetanus within 48 hours.

With this serum, furthermore, one could obtain therapeutic success if the animals were first infected with tetanus and afterwards the immune serum was injected intraperitoneally.

We have done additional experiments with this serum to demonstrate its enormous toxin-destroying ability.

From a 10-day-old tetanus culture made spore-free by filtration a quantity of 0.00005 cc was enough to kill a mouse in 4 to 6 days, and 0.0001 was enough to kill a mouse in less than 2 days. We took 5 cc of serum from a tetanus-immune rabbit and mixed it with 1 cc of this culture filtrate and let it stand for 24 hours to allow the immune serum to act on the tetanus toxin contained in the filtrate. 4

mice received 0.2 cc of this mixture, i.e., 0.033 cc of the culture fluid, which is more than 300 lethal doses for mice, and all 4 mice remained healthy, whereas control mice given 0.0001 cc of the culture were all dead after 36 hours. . . .

Formerly, blood transfusions were thought to be heroic, sometimes successful therapeutic procedures, but it is now thought that the same result can be obtained with infusions of salt solutions . . .

Our experimental results lead us to be mindful [of Goethe's famous saying] that "Blood is a remarkable fluid."

A footnote in the paper suggested the name antitoxin for the material in the serum. And only one week later, on December 11, 1890, Behring published another paper on serum antitoxic immunity to diphtheria (11). These reports were immediately acclaimed. The first successful clinical use of diphtheria antitoxin was on Christmas night in 1891. However, therapy of diphtheria and tetanus with antitoxin was some time in coming. Work was required by Paul Ehrlich to establish methods for producing high-titer antisera, for measuring the antibody content, and for preserving the sera in a form suitable for treatment. Finally, in November of 1894 diphtheria antiserum became commercially available. This was a landmark event in the history of medical science, representing the first specific treatment for a human disease. Its success gave rise to hopes that all symptoms and signs of infectious diseases could be attributed to toxins, and that therapeutic antitoxins could then be made, but these hopes proved futile. Potent exotoxins were not found to be produced by most bacteria.

In relation to our topic of host resistance, Behring's discovery was the beginning of humoral immunity. Ehrlich's studies in 1891 on the plant toxins ricin and abrin (12) showed that antitoxins could be made to various protein toxins, and that these antitoxins exhibited specificity; the antiricin did not block the toxic action of abrin, and vice versa. Further work by Buchner, Metchnikoff, Roux, Salomonsen, Madsen, and Ehrlich and Morgenroth led to rapid expansion of knowledge on the specificity of antibodies and some of their actions. Much of this work was done using red blood cells as the experimental antigen (5). Agglutinating antibodies for bacteria were discovered in 1896 by Durham in London (13), Gruber and co-workers in Vienna (14), and Widal in Paris (15). Precipitins were discovered in 1897 by Kraus (16), and somewhat later came the classical studies of Landsteiner (17) on specificity of the antibody response. The role of this panoply of antibodies in host resistance and immunity was not at all clear (and still is not, in some instances). The group at the Pasteur Institute, led by Metchnikoff and Roux, stressed phagocytic cells as the mainstay of resistance, and proposed that serum factors were, in some or perhaps many instances, derived from these cells, whereas the German workers for the most part favored humoral agents as the factors primarily responsible for immunity. This humoral versus cellular polemic, which has been reviewed recently in some detail (18), was in fact something of a tempest in a teapot. It should have been obvious from the beginning, as it is now, that cellular and humoral factors are both required for efficient function of host resistance, and, furthermore, that they interact with one another at many crucial points in the immunity pathways. The Nobel committee did its best to subdue this polemic, by awarding the 1908

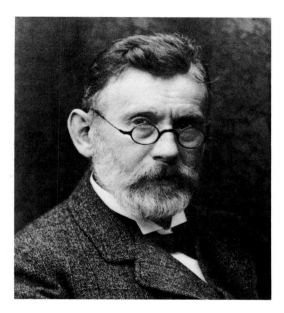

Paul Ehrlich

Prize in Medicine or Physiology jointly to Metchnikoff and Ehrlich, two of the principle protagonists in the argument.

The third great advance in the host resistance-immunity field was the discovery of complement. It is not generally recognized that observations on complement somewhat antedated those on antibody and were, in a way, connected. In 1888 Nuttall (19) demonstrated that the cell-free portion of the blood killed some bacteria *in vitro*, and that this killing power was heat labile, destroyed at 55°C. This observation was extended in 1889 by Nissen (20), who found some bacteria susceptible and others resistant, and by Buchner (21), who named this heat labile blood factor alexin. In 1890 Behring and Nissen (22) found that the fresh serum of immunized guinea pigs killed *Vibrio metchnikovi in vitro*, whereas heated serum or the serum of normal animals did not. In 1894 Pfeiffer (23) discovered that cholera vibrios were lysed in the peritoneal fluid of immunized but not normal animals. This bacteriolytic action was heat labile. In the same year Fraenkel and Sobernheim (24) found that heat-inactivated cholera-immune serum would still afford protection when transferred to normal animals, and that the bacteriolytic process was demonstrable in these recipients, thus showing that the heated immune serum, which was inactive *in vitro*, became active again *in vivo*. Finally, in 1895 Bordet (25) cleared up this rather baffling set of observations. He reported:

> Indeed it is only necessary to add to nonimmune serum, which is weakly bactericidal, a small quantity of anticholera serum, unheated or previously heated to 60°C, to induce in it a very marked bactericidal power. Thus two fluids, weakly bactericidal when separated, form together a mixture which is strongly antiseptic.

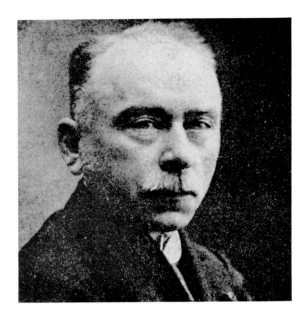

Jules Bordet

> This antiseptic power, as we shall see later, is specific. It is only manifested against the species of vibrio which was used to vaccinate the animal from which the immune serum was taken. The bactericidal power can be observed just as well whether or not the serum contains cellular elements or has been deprived of these elements. . . . (25)

Therefore, two factors were at work, one of which was thermostable and present in immune but not normal serum, the other of which was thermolabile and present in both normal and immune fresh serum. This crucial observation was rapidly confirmed and extended to hemolytic as well as bacteriolytic responses (26). Ehrlich and Morgenroth subsequently worked out the nature of the heat labile factor, which they called complement (27) rather than alexin or addiment, and also the mechanism of its binding by an antibody, called amboceptor, with two receptors, one of which bound the antigen, and the other of which bound complement (28).

These three great discoveries relating to host defense mechanisms—phagocytic cells, antibodies, and complement—provided the foundation for building the field of host resistance or immunology. All three were reported within the relatively short time span of a decade, 1884 to 1895. Their importance was quite properly reflected by the fact that several of the early Nobel Prizes were awarded to the pioneers in this area: the first such award to Behring in 1901, to Koch in 1905, to both Metchnikoff and Ehrlich in 1908, and to Bordet in 1919. The only name missing from this list is, of course, that of Pasteur, who unfortunately died before Nobel Prizes were awarded.

This is not the time or place to recount details of the innumerable advances, large and small, that have added to this foundation to produce the skyscraper edifice of today, but a few general summary statements are perhaps in order. Knowledge on the role of phagocytic cells and features of their interactions with parasites has been extended to the subcellular and even the molecular level, which would amaze and delight Metchnikoff were he able to survey the modern scene. The present knowledge on the molecular structure of antibodies, on their diversity and selective mechanism of clonal expansion, on their specificities and activities, would please and delight Paul Ehrlich, especially since his theories have proved to be correct in nearly every regard! Pasteur and Behring would be gratified indeed if they could see today's effective, safe immunization procedures for a wide range of microbial infectious diseases. Bordet would be awestruck with the explosion of information on the complex complement system, the isolation of its components and establishment of their interactions with one another as well as their actions on other host-defense systems, all of which occurred as a result of his simple test tube discovery! Finally, another more recent development, which has changed the face of the host resistance field, deserves special mention; namely, the discoveries, beginning about 1950, that lymphocytes were not inert, uniform cells in dormant or terminal states, but rather constituted a large family of cells, each with its own life history, distribution and potential, many of which play a central role in the operation of the classical immune systems—phagocytic cells, antibodies, and complement.

ACKNOWLEDGMENT

The author would like to acknowledge his extensive use of "The History of Bacteriology", The Heath Clark Lectures delivered at The London School of Hygiene and Tropical Medicine in 1936 (5) as a source of historical perspective and of references on the early history of bacteriology and immunology. Professor Bulloch worked in these fields during their formative years, and he knew personally many of the pioneers who made important contributions. His views were probably not biased as a result of the French-German polemic that ranged during the years following the war of 1870, thus making him in my opinion, a particularly valuable reporter on the people and events discussed in this chapter.

REFERENCES

1. Stettler, A. (1972): History of concepts of infection and defense. *Gesnerus*, 29:255.
2. Silverstein, A. M., and Bialasiewicz, A. A. (1980): A history of theories of acquired immunity. *Cell. Immunol.*, 51:151.
3. Duclaux, E. (1920): *Pasteur, The History of a Mind*, translated by E. F. Smith and F. Hedges. W. B. Sanders Co., Philadelphia and London.
4. Dubos, R. J. (1950): *Louis Pasteur, Free Lance of Science*, Little Brown and Co., Boston.
5. Bulloch, W. (1938): *The History of Bacteriology*. Oxford University Press, London, New York, Toronto.
6. Metchnikoff, O. (1921): *Life of Elie Metchnikoff*. Houghton Mifflin Co., Boston and New York.
7. Löffler, F. (1884): Untersuchungen über die Bedeutung der Microorganismen für die Entstehung der Diphtherie beim Menschen, bei der Taube und beim Kalbe, Mitth. an das kaiserle. *Gesundheitsamt*, 2:421.

8. Kitasato, S. (1889): Über den Tetanusbacillus, *Z. Hyg.*, 7:225.
9. Fraenkel, C. (1890): Untersuchungen über Bacteriengifte. Immunisirungsversuche bei Diphtherie, *Berl. Wochenschr.*, 27:1133.
10. Behring, E., and Kitasato, S. (1890): Über das Zustandekommen der Diphtherie-Immunität und Tetanus-Immunität bei Thieren, *Dsch. Med. Wochenschr.*, 26:1113.
11. Behring, E. (1890): Über das Zustandekommen der Diphtherie-Immunität bei Thieren. *Dtsch. Med. Wochenschr.*, 26:1145.
12. Ehrlich, P. (1891): Experimentelle Untersuchungen über Immunität, I. Über Ricin, II. Über Abrin, *Dtsch. Med. Wochenschr.*, 27:976, 1218.
13. Durham, H. E. (1896): On a special action of the serum of highly immunized animals and its use for diagnostic and other purposes. *Proc. R. Soc. Lond.*, 59:224.
14. Gruber, M., and Durham, H. E. (1896): Eine neue Methode zur raschen Erkennung des Choleravibrio und des Typhusbacillus, *Münch. Med. Wochenschr.*, 43:285.
15. Widal, F. (1896): Sérodiagnostic de la fièvre typhoïde. *Bull. Mém. Soc. Méd. d'Hôp. Paris*, 3rd series, 13:561.
16. Kraus, R. (1897): Über specifische Reaktionen in keimfreien Filtraten aus Cholera-Typhus-Pestbouillonculturen erzeugt durch homologes Serum. *Wien. Klin. Wochenschr.*, 10:736.
17. Landsteiner, K. (1945): *The Specificity of Serological Reactions*, revised edition. Harvard University Press, Cambridge, Massachusetts.
18. Silverstein, A. M. (1979): History of Immunology. Cellular versus Humoral Immunity: Determinants and Consequences of an Epic 19th Century Battle, *Cell. Immunol.*, 48:208.
19. Nuttall, G. (1888): Experimente über die bacterienfeindlichen Einflüsse des thierischen Körpers, *Z. Hyg.*, 4:353.
20. Nissen, F. (1889): Zur Kenntniss der bacterienvernichtenden Eigenschaft des Blutes, *Z. Hyg.*, 6:487.
21. Buchner, H. (1889): Über die bacterientödtende Wirkung des zellfreien Blutserums, *Zentralbl. Bakteriol. [Orig]*, 5:817.
22. Behring, E., and Nissen, F. (1890): Über bacterienfeindliche Eigenschaften verschiedener Blutserumarten; ein Beitrag zur Immunitätsfrage, *Z. Hyg.*, 8:412.
23. Pfeiffer, R. (1894): Weitere Untersuchungen über das Wesen der Choleraimmunität und über specifisch bactericide Processe. *Z. Hyg. Infections*, 18:1.
24. Fraenkel, C., and Sobernheim, G. (1894): Versuche über das Zustandekommen der künstlichen Immunität. *Hyg. Rundsch. (Berlin)*, 4:97; 145.
25. Bordet, J. (1895): Les leucocytes et les propriétés actives du sérum chez les vaccinés, *Ann. Inst. Pasteur (Paris)*, 9:462.
26. Bordet, J. (1898): Sur l'agglutination et la dissolution des globules rouges par le sérum d'animaux injectés de sang défibriné, *Ann. Inst. Pasteur (Paris)*, 7:688.
27. Ehrlich, P., and Morgenroth, J. (1899): Über Haemolysine. *Berl. Klin. Wochenschr.*, 36:481.
28. Ehrlich, P., and Morgenroth, J. (1899): Zur Theorie der Lysinwirkung. *Berl. Klin. Wochenschr.*, 36:6.

Advances in Host Defense Mechanisms, Vol. 1,
edited by John I. Gallin and Anthony S. Fauci,
Raven Press, New York © 1982.

Monocyte and Macrophage Development

David W. Golde and William G. Hocking

*Division of Hematology-Oncology, Department of Medicine, UCLA School of Medicine,
Los Angeles, California 90024*

Cells of the monocyte-macrophage series constitute the mononuclear phagocyte system. These cells are ubiquitous in mammalian tissues, and they function critically in the ecology of the body. Phylogenetically the mononuclear phagocyte is one of the most primitive cell types. Cells homologous to the mononuclear phagocyte are found in early life forms, and single-cell protozoa such as the amoeba have considerable similarity to the mammalian macrophage. Ontogenically the macrophage has its origin in the yolk sac (70), but the cells of the mononuclear phagocyte system in the adult derive from a common ancestor in the bone marrow (14).

The mononuclear phagocytes function in five main areas.

(a) They participate in host defense against microorganisms and are particularly effective in containing obligate intracellular microorganisms.

(b) They are the principal cellular element involved in removal of damaged, senescent, or dying cells, and they metabolize organic debris and sequester non-metabolizable inorganic materials.

(c) The mononuclear phagocytes participate in bidirectional cellular interactions with lymphocytes, which are important in humoral and cellular immune function.

(d) The mononuclear phagocytes also function in producing bioactive materials important in regulating other cellular functions. Such factors include colony-stimulating activity, plasminogen activator, complement components, pyrogen, lymphocyte-activating factor, and prostaglandins (13,72).

(e) The macrophage may be important in the control of neoplasia (31).

Cells of the mononuclear phagocyte series are concentrated in organs of the reticuloendothelial system. This system is usually represented by the spleen, liver, and bone marrow. Although macrophages, fibroblasts, and endothelial cells are anatomically associated in reticuloendothelial tissues, these cells are not developmentally closely related. Mononuclear phagocytes derive from hematopoietic cell precursors in the bone marrow, whereas the endothelial cells and fibroblasts are unrelated to hematopoietic stem cells and are derived from the endoderm and mesenchyme, respectively (45). The prefix reticulo is frequently used imprecisely with respect to macrophages. Reticulin is a silver-staining precollagen produced by fibroblasts. Reticulum or reticular cells are probably a subclass of fibroblasts, although the nomenclature is used by various investigators to connote different cells. We suggest avoiding confusing nomenclature by referring to cells of the mononuclear phagocyte system as monocytes and macrophages, or by their special names, depending on the tissue of residence (for example, the Kupffer cell of the liver, the Langerhans cell of skin, and the alveolar macrophage). The term fibroblast should refer to those cells producing collagen and its precursors.

STEM CELLS AND THE REGULATION OF MONOCYTOPOIESIS

All of the circulating cellular elements of blood are ultimately derived from a pluripotent stem cell in the bone marrow. A stem cell may be defined as a cell with extensive capacity for self-renewal (production of identical daughter cells) and the ability to give rise to more differentiated cells of several lineages (Fig. 1). A myeloid stem cell has been identified which no longer has the capacity to differentiate along the lymphoid pathway, but gives rise to precursor cells for erythrocytes, megakaryocytes, monocytes, and granulocytes (1). The stem cells cannot be identified morphologically, and there is no definitive assay for pluripotent stem cells in man, although multipotent hematopoietic precursors can now be cultivated *in*

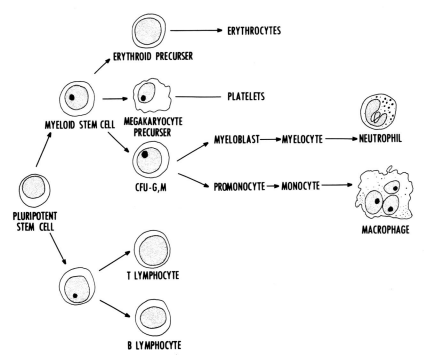

FIG. 1. Schematic representation of hematopoiesis and lymphopoiesis. Monocytes and macrophages share a common pluripotent myeloid stem cell with other cells of bone marrow origin. The committed precursor of granulocytes is the same as the monocyte-macrophage precursor.

vitro (29). The myeloid stem cell gives rise to "committed" precursor cells that have extensive capacity for replication; however, these committed cells are restricted to maturation along one or at most two cell lineages. Committed precursors have been defined for each bone marrow cell lineage, and these cells can be assayed *in vitro* by their ability to give rise to colonies of differentiated descendants in soft-gel culture in the presence of appropriate humoral stimulation (42,68).

There is considerable evidence to indicate that monocytes and granulocytes derive from a common progenitor cell (68). This common precursor is referred to as the colony-forming unit-granulocyte, monocyte (CFU-G,M) because of its ability to give rise to colonies of mononuclear phagocytes and granulocytes in bone marrow cultures. It has been shown by transfer of single cells that such precursor cells are capable of maturation along both pathways (67). Thus, mixed colonies containing both monocytes and neutrophils are frequently identified in these semisolid gel cultures. It is uncertain at what stage a precursor cell becomes committed to either monocytic or granulocytic differentiation. It was believed that the decision was made at the CFU-G,M level; however, recent experience with human leukemia myeloid cell lines has brought this concept into question. Two human myeloid leukemic cell lines referred to as HL-60 and KG-1 have been developed (23,56), and these are both able to differentiate along the monocyte-macrophage pathway in the presence of certain phorbol esters (57,84). The HL-60 cells are usually at the progranulocyte level, whereas most of the KG-1 cells are at the myeloblast stage of development. Thus it appears that early morphologically identifiable myeloid elements are capable of differentiation along the mononuclear phagocyte pathway.

The growth of granulocyte and monocyte colonies in semisolid gel culture requires the presence of a hormone referred to as colony-stimulating factor (CSF) (6,42,68). Colony-stimulating factor has been identified in many murine tissues; however, the prominent sources of human CSF are cells of the mononuclear phagocyte series and activated T lymphocytes (12,13,41,43). The CSFs appear to represent a family of glycoprotein hormones containing sialic acid and generally ranging in molecular weight between 20,000 and 50,000 (60). It now seems clear that the macrophage-stimulating factor first described by Stanley and co-workers is identical to CSF (91). A CSF has been isolated and purified from murine L cells which stimulates only the growth of mononuclear phagocytes *in vitro* (92). This material has been purified some 100,000-fold. It is active on mouse bone marrow cells at concentrations of 10^{-11} M. A radioimmunoassay has been developed for this CSF as well as a radioreceptor assay (48). A CSF has also been purified from mouse-lung-conditioned medium (11), although no human CSF has been purified to homogeneity. Human CSF may be obtained from placenta (77), from lung-conditioned medium (33), and from various leukocyte preparations. We have partially purified a CSF from a human T-lymphocyte cell line (46,61). This CSF has a molecular weight of 34,000 and stimulates the production of both granulocytes and monocytes *in vitro*.

It has been convincingly demonstrated that human blood monocytes and tissue macrophages produce CSF (6,12,41,43). The release of CSF by mononuclear phagocytes *in vitro* is augmented by a number of materials that have in common the property of activating macrophages. These include endotoxin, bacillus Calmette-Guerin, poly-IC, glucan, etc. (10,15,27,85). Neoplastic monocytes in monocytic leukemia retain the ability to elaborate CSF (47), and a human monocytic cell line has been developed which produces this regulator (26). The concept has evolved that circulating and resident mononuclear phagocytes may respond to appropriate stimuli by increasing production of CSF and thereby increasing proliferation of monocyte precursors. The T lymphocytes are also important producers of CSF when the lymphocytes are activated by either lectins or antigens. Thus, immunologic reactions involving T-cell activation can lead to increased CSF production and increased numbers of mononuclear phagocytes produced by the bone marrow (13).

In most regulated systems there is a balance between positive feedback and inhibition. Thus, it has been postulated that monocyte production is regulated by the positive feedback of CSF and inhibitory factors also elaborated by the mature mononuclear phagocytes. Kurland and colleagues have provided evidence indicating that prostaglandins constitute part of the negative feedback loop (58). Monocytes and macrophages produce prostaglandins of the E series (PGE), and these prostaglandins have a direct inhibitory effect on mononuclear phagocyte production. Prostaglandins apparently have little effect on granulocyte production *in vitro* (80). Exposure of macrophages to high concentrations of CSF leads to an increase in the synthesis of PGE. Thus, it is believed that prostaglandins may act to limit excessive monocyte production. Granulocytes also produce an inhibitor that limits proliferation of CFU-G,M. This inhibitor produced by neutrophils has been identified as lactoferrin, which suppresses CSF production by mononuclear phagocytes (8,80). The precise physiologic relevance of these inhibitor molecules in the intact organism has not been clearly delineated. It is relatively well established that monocyte production is stimulated by CSF, and there are several negative-feedback-regulator candidates, the most important of which appear to be PGE and lactoferrin.

MONOCYTE KINETICS

The monocyte is the circulating element of the mononuclear phagocyte series. Ultimately, the monocyte develops into a macrophage. There are a minimum of three and probably more generations between the earliest morphologically identifiable precursor and the mature circulating monocyte. The generation time for promonocytes in the mouse has been estimated to be about 16 to 19 hr. The promonocyte cell cycle time in man is approximately 2 days. The ^{3}H-thymidine-labeling index for promonocytes is about 80% (97), indicating that, at any given time, the majority of these cells are in the DNA synthetic phase of the cycle. Usually, the S phase comprises about 60% to 70% of the total cell cycle time. The total number of monocytes in the bone marrow in man has been estimated to be about 7.3×10^9 cells. Monocytes leave the bone marrow within 24 hr of completing their last division (97,103). There is no marrow reserve pool of monocytes comparable to the large bone marrow granulocyte reserve compartment.

The half-time of disappearance of labeled monocytes from the circulation appears to be about 71 hr (97). These data were obtained using ^{3}H-thymidine as a marker of newly formed monocytes. Other investigators have found a considerably shorter half-life (8.4 hr) when DF^{32}P was used as a label (69). It may be that the cells were damaged by manipulation during the labeling process. Studies in the mouse indicate that there is no substantial marginated pool of monocytes (96). Thus, unlike the blood granulocyte pool, which consists of approximately 50% marginated cells, the blood monocyte pool is composed almost entirely of circulating elements. The circulating monocytes have some capacity for proliferation, but the ^{3}H-thymidine-labeling index usually is less than 1%. The average number of blood monocytes in adult man is estimated at 1.7×10^9 cells. The blood monocytes leave the peripheral blood in a random fashion at a rate of approximately 1.6×10^7 cells/hr. Once the monocytes enter the tissues they are not believed capable of reentering the circulation.

MATURATION OF MONONUCLEAR PHAGOCYTES

The earliest morphologically identifiable mononuclear phagocyte progenitor in the bone marrow is the promonocyte. The promonocyte is a cell of approximately 10 to 18 μm in diameter. It has a well-developed Golgi complex and contains peroxidase-positive granules. The promonocyte has poorly developed phagocytic capacity and has few receptors for the Fc portion of IgG (16). The mature monocyte has a diameter of approximately 12 to 20 μm and usually has an oval or horseshoe-shaped nucleus. Nucleoli are not observed, and the chromatin is usually loose and not highly condensed. The abundant cytoplasm is grayish or blue in color, and there are occasional vacuoles and peroxidase-containing granules (76) (Fig. 2). A population of peroxidase-negative granules has also been identified in the monocyte (74,75). When the monocyte leaves the circulation it enters the tissues where, if it remains viable, it will mature into a macrophage. The macrophage is a large cell which, in the giant cell form, can reach a size of greater than 100 μm in diameter. The macrophage has one or several nuclei, usually with peripherally condensed chromatin, with expansive and heavily vacuolated cytoplasm. Mature macrophages normally lose cytochemical peroxidase activity. The mature macrophage is an efficient phagocyte and a highly motile cell. It is capable of ingesting and killing large numbers of microorganisms, and it has the capacity to sequester inorganic and nondigestible material. It is difficult to examine the maturational sequence of the mononuclear phagocyte in fresh tissue. We have used an *in vitro* culture method to study the differentiation of macrophages from normal human bone marrow (3). Promonocytes are the first recognizable cell in the monocytic series, and they are the precursor of the circulating monocyte. Promonocytes were numerous during the first several days of culture, and peroxidase reaction product could be found in the rough endoplasmic reticulum, the Golgi area, and in the cytoplasmic granules. As

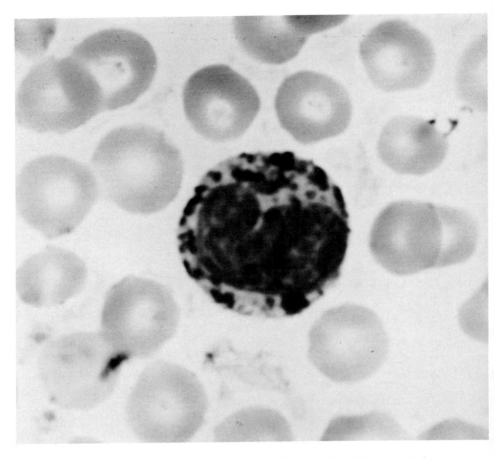

FIG. 2. Peripheral blood monocyte stained for peroxidase (dark granules).

the cells developed into macrophages, peroxidase synthesis stopped, although some peroxidase-containing granules persisted. The mature macrophages later in culture (14 days) contained granules without peroxidase activity. Macrophages are in close association with one another in these cultures, and their surface membranes interdigitate in a manner characteristic of epithelioid cells. Specialized zones of adherence can be observed at various contact points between these macrophages which have the appearance of septate junctions (Fig. 3). Multinucleated giant cells form *in vitro* by the processes of cell fusion and nuclear endoreduplication.

When viewed in the scanning electron microscope the characteristic ruffled membrane of macrophages can be observed (Fig. 4). The macrophage adheres to the substratum by a large process referred to as a lamellipodium, and the cells can become extensively adherent and spread out on the culture surface (Fig. 5). Macrophages are also capable of sending pseudopodia in several directions, and their

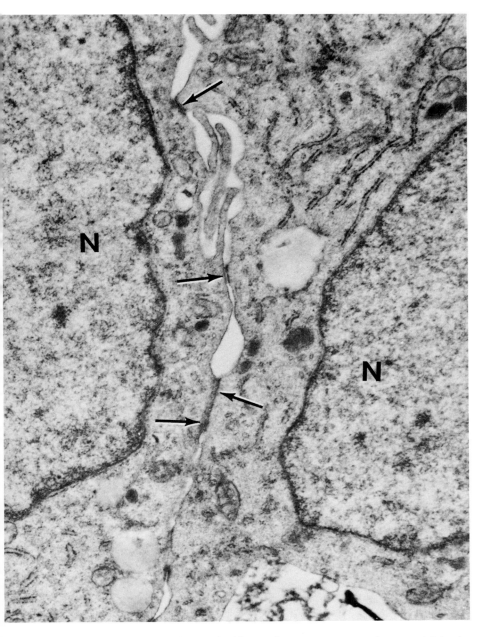

FIG. 3. Transmission electron micrograph of human bone-marrow macrophages maintained in liquid culture. Close intercellular contacts *(arrows)* occur in these cultures (× 17,000).

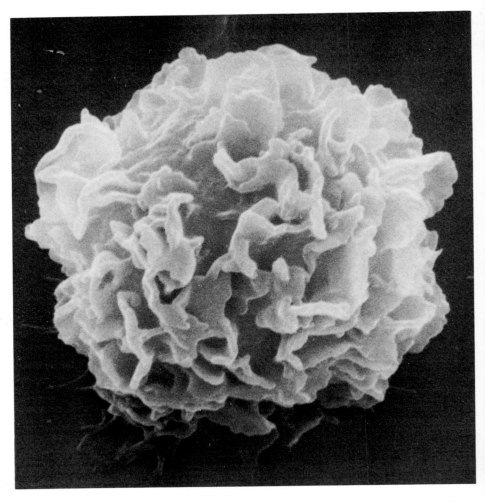

FIG. 4. Scanning electron micrograph of a human alveolar macrophage showing extensive ruffling of the cell membrane (× 12,000).

motility largely depends on extension of pseudopodia followed by a flowing of the cell membrane and cytoplasm over the attached area.

ORIGIN AND KINETICS OF TISSUE MACROPHAGES

Tissue macrophages exist in many forms, including the alveolar macrophage of the lung, the hepatic Kupffer cell, the giant cell of granulomata, the dermal Langerhans cell, peritoneal and pleural macrophages, and the osteoclast. Studies in animals have shown that the alveolar macrophages and hepatic Kupffer cells have their origin in a bone marrow progenitor (9,37,54,95,99,101). These studies have

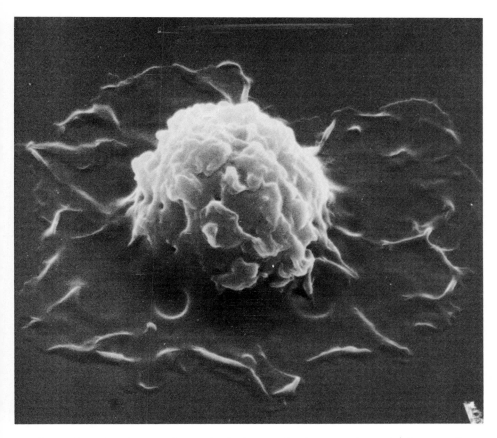

FIG. 5. Scanning electron micrograph of a human alveolar macrophage showing extensive spreading and attachment by a lamellipodium (× 4,600).

generally used a model whereby the animal receives lethal whole-body irradiation and then infusion of donor bone marrow cells. The tissue macrophages are identified by enzymatic, antigenic, and karyotypic markers. Recent studies in mice also suggest that under unperturbed conditions the alveolar macrophages have their origin in circulating monocytes which derive from the bone marrow compartment (4). Other studies in parabiotic animals, however, do not support these findings, and suggest that the alveolar macrophage compartment is not sustained by the influx of monocytes but rather by endogenous replication (22,98). A number of studies in rodents have shown that the Kupffer cell and alveolar macrophage have proliferative capability (54,59,60).

We have used the circumstance of allogeneic bone marrow transplantation between HLA-matched siblings of opposite sex to study the origin of alveolar macrophages in man (38,94). In female patients receiving transplants from male donors we found that the alveolar macrophages were of donor origin as determined by the presence of the fluorescent Y chromosome. Alternatively, in male recipients of transplants from female donors the Y chromosome disappeared from the alveolar macrophages. An estimate of the Y-body disappearance time suggested that complete replacement of the alveolar macrophage compartment occurred by 100 days after transplantation. Replacement of the alveolar macrophages with cells of donor type was noted to occur in patients given lethal whole-body irradiation as well as those receiving only cyclophosphamide conditioning. Similar studies performed in patients who died after receiving grafts from donors of opposite sex indicated that hepatic macrophages (Kupffer cells) are also replaced by cells of donor origin (36).

We had previously demonstrated that the alveolar macrophage has proliferative capacity (40). In these studies, we exposed lavaged macrophages from normal donors to ^{3}H-thymidine, and we found that the ^{3}H-thymidine-labeling index varied between 0.35% and 1.25%. The uptake of thymidine was blocked by hydroxyurea and cytosine arabinoside, indicating that the thymidine incorporation was for scheduled DNA synthesis and not DNA repair. The low ^{3}H-thymidine-labeling index suggests that only a small percentage of the alveolar macrophage population is proliferating at any given time. On the other hand, this proliferative rate may be sufficient to maintain the total alveolar macrophage population if, as believed, these are long-lived cells. The life-span of the alveolar macrophage in man, however, is unknown.

Although there have been no good studies of the kinetics of human alveolar macrophages in the steady state, it seems likely that, although they originate in the bone marrow and may be replaced by circulating monocytes entering the lung tissue, the alveolar macrophage population can probably be maintained by local proliferation. Thus, in situations of chronic bone marrow aplasia, it is likely that the tissue macrophage populations remain intact even though the bone marrow is nonfunctional. This hypothesis was tested in a limited manner by studying patients with acute leukemia who were undergoing induction chemotherapy and who had no circulating monocytes for a period of several months (44). These leukemic patients had normal numbers of alveolar macrophages obtained by bronchopulmonary lavage. These cells retained their limited proliferative capacity as evidenced by scheduled uptake of ^{3}H-thymidine. Most evidence suggests that, although the resident macrophage of the lung may participate in defense against pulmonary infections, an influx of mononuclear phagocytes from the peripheral blood is the main source of macrophage host defense cells present in the lung during granulomatous inflammation (90). The proliferative capacity of rodent alveolar macrophages has been widely demonstrated (28,59,88).

We obtained evidence that macrophages in patients with chronic myelogenous leukemia derive from the neoplastic clone in experiments demonstrating that the marrow-derived macrophages contain the Philadelphia chromosome marker (39). Others have adduced similar evidence using studies of female patients heterozygous for glucose-6-phosphate dehydrogenase (30). In these latter studies, monocyte-derived macrophages were shown to possess only one enzyme type, indicating that they were clonally derived from the neoplastic progenitor. These observations suggest that tissue macrophages in chronic myelogenous leukemia are involved in the neoplastic process.

There is also evidence to indicate that the dermal Langerhans cell is of bone marrow origin (35,52). Recent findings concerning the osteoclast have had important clinical implications. In murine osteopetrosis there is a deficiency of osteoclast activity. This defect can be corrected by transplantation of normal bone marrow or spleen cells (100). These observations suggested that a progenitor cell in the donor bone marrow and spleen was capable of differentiating to an osteoclast. Further direct evidence for this hypothesis was obtained using the beige mouse model in which giant lysosomes were found in the osteoclasts that could be transplanted into osteopetrotic mice (2). The important implication of these findings for man has been the successful treatment of human osteopetrosis by bone marrow transplantation (17). In these human studies, the osteoclast in the recipient was shown to be of donor origin. Thus, it appears that osteoclasts are a specialized form of tissue macrophage concerned with bone resorption.

THE PULMONARY ALVEOLAR MACROPHAGE

The pulmonary alveolar macrophage (PAM) is the principal mononuclear phagocyte of the lung (50). With the development of bronchopulmonary lavage techniques, this cell has become the most accessible human tissue macrophage.

The technique of bronchopulmonary lavage was first developed using a rabbit model (71). This method allows harvesting of viable bronchoalveolar cells. The technique was later modified and applied to human studies (32). Development of the flexible fiberoptic bronchoscope, however, has facilitated the widespread application of bronchopulmonary lavage in man (50), allowing an easily available source of PAM for study.

The PAM is heterogeneous in size, varying from 15 to 50 μm in diameter. The cytoplasm contains numerous granules and vacuoles, and the nuclear to cytoplasmic ratio averages 1:3. The PAM stains strongly for α-naphthyl butyrate esterase and with periodic acid-Schiff reagent, less intensely with oil red 0, and does not stain for peroxidase.

Transmission electron microscopy demonstrates an eccentric nucleus and prominent nucleolus (Fig. 6). Occasional PAMs are multinucleate. The cytoplasm contains a prominent Golgi apparatus, mitochondria, rough endoplasmic reticulum, and free ribosomes (19,49,64,81). The most distinctive cytoplasmic feature is the presence of many membrane-bound cytoplasmic granules, the primary lysosomes (102). These inclusions contain cathepsins, lysozyme, β-glucuronidase, β-galactosidase, aryl sulfatase, acid ribonuclease, and phospholipases (20,34,73,81,89, 93,104). Although peroxidase is not demonstrated by cytochemical techniques, some peroxidatic activity is present in the PAM (25,79). Secondary lysosomes are more heterogeneous and contain cellular debris and substances ingested from the extracellular environment. These inclusions are formed by fusion of a primary lysozyme with a digestive vacuole (73). Alveolar macrophages obtained from smok-

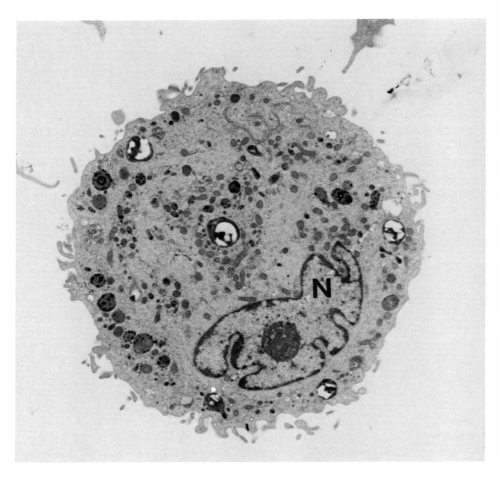

FIG. 6. Transmission electron micrograph of a human alveolar macrophage obtained by bronchopulmonary lavage from a nonsmoker (× 12,600).

ers contain unique "smoker's inclusions" (7) (Fig. 7). These inclusions are of heterogeneous composition but they contain needlelike structures composed of aluminum silicate crystals present in inhaled smoke. The PAM surface has been studied by scanning electron microscopy (82). The cell surface membrane is normally highly ruffled, and the PAM attaches to glass by lamellipodia and filopodia.

Metabolic features of the PAM are distinctive. The basal respiratory rate is greater than that of other phagocytes, but during phagocytosis only a modest respiratory "burst" occurs, in contrast to the large burst observed in polymorphonuclear leukocytes and peritoneal macrophages (78). Although other phagocytic cells primarily depend on energy derived from glycolysis during phagocytosis, the PAM requires both glycolysis and oxidative metabolism for this process (18,19,66,78). Freshly

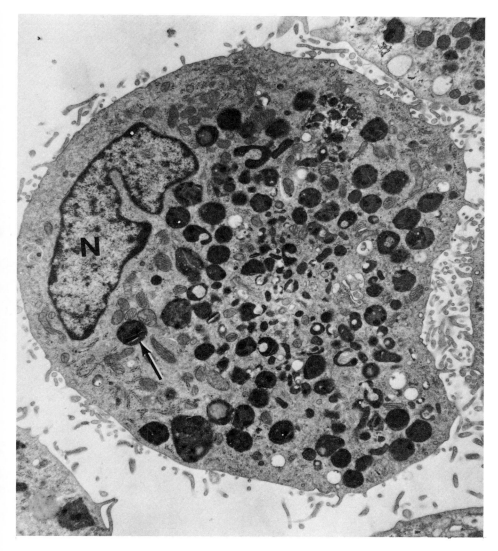

FIG. 7. Transmission electron micrograph of an alveolar macrophage obtained by broncho-pulmonary lavage from a heavy cigarette smoker. "Smoker's inclusions" are numerous, and needlelike crystals are visible in some *(arrow)* ($\times$ 8,500).

harvested PAMs contain high levels of cytochrome oxidase and low levels of pyruvate kinase and phosphofructokinase, whereas the pattern is reversed in peritoneal macrophages. When PAMs are incubated in an anaerobic environment the enzymatic pattern becomes similar to that of the peritoneal macrophage (87).

The PAM is critical to the defense of the lung against inhaled microorganisms, particularly those capable of intracellular replication. The PAM possesses surface membrane receptors for the Fc fragment of IgG and C'3, which are important in particle recognition, attachment, and ingestion (24,65,83,86). After exposure of these cells to specific or nonspecific immune stimulants, the number and affinity of these receptors increases, accompanied by increased numbers of mitochondria and lysosomes, increased lysosomal enzyme activities, and increased metabolic and phagocytic activities. These changes characterize the state of macrophage activation epitomized by enhanced ability to kill infectious agents (62,63).

The antimicrobial killing mechanisms used by the PAM probably include: (a) peroxidation of microbes in the presence of halide, hydrogen peroxide, and peroxidase (25,79); (b) lysosomal enzyme release (21,93); (c) catalase (55,93); (d) superoxide anion (5); (e) lysosomal cationic proteins. The PAM is the critical effector in pulmonary cell-mediated immune reactions. Both activation of the resident population and recruitment of circulating monocytes into the alveoli are probably involved in the response to lung infections. The PAM produces chemotactic factors that attract inflammatory cells to the lung (51,53). In addition, the production of CSF may increase the production of polymorphonuclear and mononuclear phagocytes in the bone marrow (43).

CONCLUSION

Thus, cells within the monocyte macrophage series play a pivotal role in the complex mechanisms of host defenses. They originate ontologically in the yolk sac, and in the adult, they derive from a common stem cell in the bone marrow. The cells undergo a series of developmental steps and seed multiple organ systems, displaying a broad range of functional capabilities from defense against microbial invaders, to removal of various forms of debris, to participating in the cellular interactions of immunoregulation, to secreting a variety of bioactive materials, and to playing a potentially important role in control of neoplastically transformed cells. Further study of this ontologically ancient cell will surely provide greater insight into the complex mechanisms of host defense.

ACKNOWLEDGMENT

Supported by United States Public Health Services grants CA 15688 CA 30388 and RR 00865.

REFERENCES

1. Abramson, S., Miller, R. G., and Phillips, R. A. (1977): The identification in adult bone marrow of pluripotent and restricted stem cells of the myeloid and lymphoid systems. *J. Exp. Med.*, 145:1567–1579.
2. Ash, P., Loutit, J. F., and Townsend, K. M. S. (1980): Osteoclasts derived from haematopoietic stem cells. *Nature (London)*, 283:669–670.
3. Bainton, D. F., and Golde, D. W. (1978): Differentiation of macrophages from normal human bone marrow in liquid culture. *J. Clin. Invest.*, 61:1555–1569.

4. Blussé van Oud Alblas, A., and Van Furth, R. (1979): Origin, kinetics, and characteristics of pulmonary macrophages in the normal steady state. *J. Exp. Med.*, 149:1504–1518.
5. Boxer, L. A., Ismail, G., Allen, J. M., and Baehner, R. L. (1979): Oxidative metabolic responses of rabbit pulmonary alveolar macrophages. *Blood*, 53:486–491.
6. Brennan, J. K., Lichtman, M. A., DiPersio, J. F., and Abboud, C. N. (1980): Chemical mediators of granulopoiesis: a review. *Exp. Hematol.*, 8:441–464.
7. Brody, A. R., and Craighead, J. E. (1975): Cytoplasmic inclusions in pulmonary macrophages of cigarette smokers. *Lab. Invest.*, 32:125–132.
8. Broxmeyer, H. E., Smithyman, A., Eger, R. R., Meyers, P. A., and de Sousa, M. (1978): Identification of lactoferrin as the granulocyte-derived inhibitor of colony-stimulating activity production. *J. Exp. Med.*, 148:1052–1067.
9. Brunstetter, M. A., Hardie, J. A., Schiff, R., Lewis, J., and Cross, C. (1971): The origin of pulmonary alveolar macrophages: studies of stem cells using the Es-2 marker of mice. *Arch. Intern. Med.*, 127:1064–1068.
10. Burgaleta, C., and Golde, D. W. (1977): Effect of glucan on granulopoiesis and macrophage genesis in mice. *Cancer Res.*, 37:1739–1742.
11. Burgess, A. W., Camakaris, J., and Metcalf, D. (1977): Purification and properties of colony-stimulating factor from mouse lung-conditioned medium. *J. Biol. Chem.*, 252:1998–2003.
12. Chervenick, P. A., and LoBuglio, A. F. (1972): Human blood monocytes: stimulators of granulocyte and mononuclear colony formation in vitro. *Science*, 178:164–166.
13. Cline, M. J., and Golde, D. W. (1979): Cellular interactions in haematopoiesis. *Nature (London)*, 277:177–181.
14. Cline, M. J., Lehrer, R. I., Territo, M. C., and Golde, D. W. (1978): Monocytes and macrophages: functions and diseases. *Ann. Intern. Med.*, 88:78–88.
15. Cline, M. J., Rothman, B., and Golde, D. W. (1974): Effect of endotoxin on the production of colony-stimulating factor by human monocytes and macrophages. *J. Cell. Physiol.*, 84:193–196.
16. Cline, M. J., and Sumner, M. A. (1972): Bone marrow macrophage precursors. I. Some functional characteristics of the early cells of the mouse macrophage series. *Blood*, 40:62–69.
17. Coccia, P. F., Krivit, W., Cervenka, J., Clawson, C., Kersey, J. H., Kim, T. H., Nesbit, M. E., Ramsay, N. K. C., Warkentin, P. I., Teitelbaum, S. L., Kahn, A. J., and Brown, D. M. (1980): Successful bone-marrow transplantation for infantile malignant osteopetrosis. *N. Engl. J. Med.*, 302:701–708.
18. Cohen, H. J., and Chovaniec, M. E. (1978): Superoxide production by digitonin-stimulated guinea pig granulocytes: the effects of N-ethyl maleimide, divalent cations, and glycolytic and mitochondrial inhibitors on the activation of the superoxide generating system. *J. Clin. Invest.*, 61:1088–1096.
19. Cohen, A. B., and Cline, M. J. (1971): The human alveolar macrophage: isolation, cultivation in vitro, and studies of morphologic and functional characteristics. *J. Clin. Invest.*, 50:1390–1398.
20. Cohn, Z. A., and Wiener, E. (1963): The particulate hydrolases of macrophages. I. Comparative enzymology, isolation, and properties. *J. Exp. Med.*, 118:991–1008.
21. Cohn, Z. A., and Wiener, E. (1963): The particulate hydrolases of macrophages. II. Biochemical and morphological response to particle ingestion. *J. Exp. Med.*, 118:1009–1020.
22. Collins, F. M., and Auclair, L. K. (1980): Mononuclear phagocytes within the lungs of unstimulated parabiotic rats. *J. Reticuloendothel. Soc.*, 27:429–441.
23. Collins, S. J., Gallo, R. C., and Gallagher, R. E. (1977): Continuous growth and differentiation of human myeloid leukaemic cells in suspension culture. *Nature (London)*, 270:347–349.
24. Daughaday, C. C., and Douglas, S. D. (1976): Membrane receptors on rabbit and human pulmonary alveolar macrophages. *J. Reticuloendothel. Soc.*, 19:37–45.
25. Davis, G. S., Mortara, M., Pfeiffer, L. M., and Green, G. M. (1977): Bactericidal and biochemical peroxidase activity in human alveolar macrophages. (Abstr.) *Am. Rev. Resp. Dis.*, 115:210a.
26. DiPersio, J. F., Brennan, J. K., and Lichtman, M. A. (1978): Granulocyte growth modulators elaborated by human cell lines. In: *Hematopoietic Cell Differentiation. ICN-UCLA Symposia on Molecular and Cellular Biology, Volume X*, edited by D. W. Golde, M. J. Cline, M. J. Metcalf, and C. F. Fox, pp. 433–444. Academic Press, New York.
27. Eaves, A. C., and Bruce, W. R. (1974): In vitro production of colony-stimulating activity. I. Exposure of mouse peritoneal cells to endotoxin. *Cell Tissue Kinet.*, 7:19–30.
28. Evans, M. J., Cabral, L. J., Stephens, R. J., and Freeman, G. (1973): Cell division of alveolar macrophages in rat lung following exposure to NO_2. *Am. J. Pathol.*, 70:199–206.

29. Fauser, A. A., and Messner, H. A. (1979): Identification of megakaryocytes, macrophages, and eosinophils in colonies of human bone marrow containing neutrophilic granulocytes and erythroblasts. *Blood*, 53:1023–1027.
30. Fialkow, P. J., Jacobson, R. J., and Papayannopoulou, T. (1977): Chronic myelocytic leukemia: Clonal origin in a stem cell common to the granulocyte, erythrocyte, platelet and monocyte/macrophage. *Am. J. Med.*, 63:125–130.
31. Fink, M. A., Editor (1976): *The Macrophage in Neoplasia*. Academic Press, New York.
32. Finley, T. N., Swenson, E. W., Curran, W. S., Huber, G. L., and Ladman, A. J. (1967): Bronchopulmonary lavage in normal subjects and patients with obstructive lung disease. *Ann. Intern. Med.*, 66:651–658.
33. Fojo, S. S., Wu, M.-C., Gross, M. A., Purcell, Y., and Yunis, A. A. (1978): Purification and characterization of a colony stimulating factor from human lung. *Biochemistry*, 17:3109–3116.
34. Franson, R. C., and Waite, M. (1973): Lysosomal phospholipases A_1 and A_2 of normal and bacillus Calmette Guérin-induced alveolar macrophages. *J. Cell Biol.*, 56:621–627.
35. Frelinger, J. G., Hood, L., Hill, S., and Frelinger, J. A. (1979): Mouse epidermal Ia molecules have a bone marrow origin. *Nature (London)*, 282:321–323.
36. Gale, R. P., Sparkes, R. S., and Golde, D. W. (1978): Bone marrow origin of hepatic macrophages (Kupffer cells) in humans. *Science*, 201:937–938.
37. Godleski, J. J., and Brain, J. D. (1972): The origin of alveolar macrophages in mouse radiation chimeras. *J. Exp. Med.*, 136:630–643.
38. Golde, D. W. (1977): Kinetics and function of the human alveolar macrophage. *J. Reticuloendothel. Soc.*, 22:223–230.
39. Golde, D. W., Burgaleta, C., Sparkes, R. S., and Cline, M. J. (1977): The Philadelphia chromosome in human macrophages. *Blood*, 49:367–370.
40. Golde, D. W., Byers, L. A., and Finley, T. N. (1974): Proliferative capacity of human alveolar macrophage. *Nature (London)*, 247:373–375.
41. Golde, D. W., and Cline, M. J. (1972): Identification of the colony-stimulating cell in human peripheral blood. *J. Clin. Invest.*, 51:2981–2983.
42. Golde, D. W., and Cline, M. J. (1974): Regulation of granulopoiesis. *N. Engl. J. Med.*, 291:1388–1395.
43. Golde, D. W., Finley, T. N., and Cline, M. J. (1972): Production of colony-stimulating factor by human macrophages. *Lancet*, ii:1397–1399.
44. Golde, D. W., Finley, T. N., and Cline, M. J. (1974): The pulmonary macrophage in acute leukemia. *N. Engl. J. Med.*, 290:875–878.
45. Golde, D. W., Hocking, W. G., Quan, S. G., Sparkes, R. S., and Gale, R. P. (1980): Origin of human bone marrow fibroblasts. *Br. J. Haematol.*, 44:183–187.
46. Golde, D. W., Quan, S. G., and Cline, M. J. (1978): Human T lymphocyte cell line producing colony-stimulating activity. *Blood*, 52:1068–1072.
47. Golde, D. W., Rothman, B., and Cline, M. J. (1974): Production of colony-stimulating factor by malignant leukocytes. *Blood*, 43:749–756.
48. Guilbert, L. J., and Stanley, E. R. (1980): Specific interaction of murine colony-stimulating factor with mononuclear phagocytic cells. *J. Cell Biol.*, 85:153–159.
49. Harris, J. O., Swenson, E. W., and Johnson, J. E., III. (1970): Human alveolar macrophages: comparison of phagocytic ability, glucose utilization, and ultrastructure in smokers and nonsmokers. *J. Clin. Invest.*, 49:2086–2096.
50. Hocking, W. G., and Golde, D. W. (1979): The pulmonary-alveolar macrophage. *N. Engl. J. Med.*, 301:580–587; 639–645.
51. Hunninghake, G. W., Gallin, J. I., and Fauci, A. S. (1978): Immunologic reactivity of the lung: the in vivo and in vitro generation of a neutrophil chemotactic factor by alveolar macrophages. *Am. Rev. Resp. Dis.*, 117:15–23.
52. Katz, S. I., Tamaki, K., and Sachs, D. H. (1979): Epidermal Langerhans cells are derived from cells originating in bone marrow. *Nature (London)*, 282:324–326.
53. Kazmierowski, J. A., Gallin, J. I., and Reynolds, H. Y. (1977): Mechanism for the inflammatory response in primate lungs: demonstration and partial characterization of an alveolar macrophage-derived chemotactic factor with preferential activity for polymorphonuclear leukocytes. *J. Clin. Invest.*, 59:273–281.
54. Kelly, L. S., and Dobson, E. L. (1971): Evidence concerning the origin of liver macrophages. *Br. J. Exp. Pathol.*, 52:88–99.

55. Klebanoff, S. J. (1969): Antimicrobial activity of catalase at acid pH. *Proc. Soc. Exp. Biol. Med.*, 132:571–574.
56. Koeffler, H. P., and Golde, D. W. (1978): Acute myelogenous leukemia: a human cell line responsive to colony-stimulating activity. *Science*, 200:1153–1154.
57. Koeffler, H. P., and Golde, D. W. (1980): Human myeloid leukemia cell lines: a review. *Blood*, 56:344–350.
58. Kurland, J. I., Bockman, R. S., Broxmeyer, H. E., and Moore, M. A. S. (1978): Limitation of excessive myelopoiesis by the intrinsic modulation of macrophage-derived prostaglandin E. *Science*, 199:552–555.
59. Lin, H.-S., Kuhn, C., and Kuo, T.-T. (1975): Clonal growth of hamster free alveolar cells in soft agar. *J. Exp. Med.*, 142:877–886.
60. Lusis, A. J. (1980): Hematopoietic growth factors. In: Growth factors, moderated by D. W. Golde. *Ann. Intern. Med.*, 92:656–658.
61. Lusis, A. J., Quon, D. H., and Golde, D. W. (1981): Purification and characterization of a human T-lymphocyte-derived granulocyte-macrophage colony-stimulating factor. *Blood*, 57:13–21.
62. Mackaness, G. B. (1964): The immunological basis of acquired cellular resistance. *J. Exp. Med.*, 120:105–120.
63. Mackaness, G. B. (1970): The mechanism of macrophage activation. In: *Infectious Agents and Host Reactions*, edited by S. Mudd, pp. 61–75. W. B. Saunders Co., Philadelphia.
64. Mann, P. E. G., Cohen, A. B., Finley, T. N., and Ladman, A. J. (1971): Alveolar macrophages. Structural and functional differences between nonsmokers and smokers of marijuana and tobacco. *Lab. Invest.*, 25:111–120.
65. Mantovani, B., Rabinovitch, M., and Nussenzweig, V. (1972): Phagocytosis of immune complexes by macrophages. Different roles of the macrophage receptor sites for complement (C3) and for immunoglobulin (IgG). *J. Exp. Med.*, 135:780–792.
66. Mason, R. J., Stossel, T. P., and Vaughan, M. (1973): Quantitative studies of phagocytosis by alveolar macrophages. *Biochim. Biophys. Acta*, 304:864–870.
67. Metcalf, D. (1971): Transformation of granulocytes to macrophages in bone marrow colonies in vitro. *J. Cell. Physiol.*, 77:277–280.
68. Metcalf, D. (1977): *Hematopoietic Colonies. In Vitro Cloning of Normal and Leukemic Cells.* Springer-Verlag, Berlin.
69. Meuret, G. (1972): Monozytopoese und Kinetik der Blutmonozyten beim Menschen. *Blut*, 24:337–345.
70. Moore, M. A. S., and Metcalf, D. (1970): Ontogeny of the haemopoietic system: yolk sac origin of in vivo and in vitro colony forming cells in the developing mouse embryo. *Br. J. Haematol.*, 18:279–296.
71. Myrvik, Q. N., Leake, E. S., and Fariss, B. (1961): Studies on pulmonary alveolar macrophages from the normal rabbit: a technique to procure them in a high state of purity. *J. Immunol.*, 86:128–132.
72. Nathan, C. F., Murray, H. W., and Cohn, Z. A. (1980): The macrophage as an effector cell. *N. Engl. J. Med.*, 303:622–626.
73. Nichols, B. A. (1976): Normal rabbit alveolar macrophages. II. Their primary and secondary lysosomes as revealed by electron microscopy and cytochemistry. *J. Exp. Med.*, 144:920–932.
74. Nichols, B. A., and Bainton, D. F. : Differentiation of human monocytes in bone marrow and blood. Sequential formation of two granule populations. *Lab. Invest.*, 29:27–40.
75. Nichols, B. A., and Bainton, D. F. (1975): Ultrastructure and cytochemistry of mononuclear phagocytes. In: *Mononuclear Phagocytes in Immunity, Infection and Pathology,* edited by R. van Furth, pp. 17–55. Blackwell Scientific Publications Ltd., Oxford.
76. Nichols, B. A., Bainton, D. F., and Farquhar, M. G. (1971): Differentiation of monocytes. Origin, nature, and fate of their azurophil granules. *J. Cell Biol.*, 50:498–515.
77. Nicola, N. A., Metcalf, D., Johnson, G. R., and Burgess, A. W. (1978): Preparation of colony stimulating factors from human placenta conditioned medium. *Leukemia Res.*, 2:313–322.
78. Oren, R., Farnham, A. E., Saito, K., Milofsky, E., and Karnovsky, M. L. (1963): Metabolic patterns in three types of phagocytizing cells. *J. Cell Biol.*, 17:487–501.
79. Paul, B. B., Strauss, R. R., Selvaraj, R. J., and Sbarra, A. J. (1973): Peroxidase mediated antimicrobial activities of alveolar macrophage granules. *Science*, 181:849–850.

80. Pelus, L. M., Broxmeyer, H. E., Kurland, J. I., and Moore, M. A. S. (1979): Regulation of macrophage and granulocyte proliferation. Specificities of prostaglandin E and lactoferrin. *J. Exp. Med.*, 150:277–292.
81. Pratt, S. A., Smith, M. H., Ladman, A. J., and Finley, T. N. (1971): The ultrastructure of alveolar macrophages from human cigarette smokers and nonsmokers. *Lab. Invest.*, 24:331–338.
82. Quan, S. G., and Golde, D. W. (1977): Surface morphology of the human alveolar macrophage. *Exp. Cell Res.*, 109:71–77.
83. Reynolds, H. Y., Atkinson, J. P., Newball, H. H., and Frank, M. M. (1975): Receptors for immunoglobulin and complement on human alveolar macrophages. *J. Immunol.*, 114:1813–1819.
84. Rovera, G., O'Brien, T. G., and Diamond, L. (1979): Induction of differentiation in human promyelocytic leukemia cells by tumor promoters. *Science*, 204:868–870.
85. Ruscetti, F. W., and Chervenick, P. A. (1974): Release of colony-stimulating factor from monocytes by endotoxin and polyinosinic-polycytidylic acid. *J. Lab. Clin. Med.*, 83:64–72.
86. Shurin, S. B., and Stossel, T. P. (1978): Complement (C3)-activated phagocytosis by lung macrophages. *J. Immunol.*, 120:1305–1312.
87. Simon, L. M., Robin, E. D., Phillips, J. R., Acevedo, J., Axline, S. G., and Theodore, J. (1977): Enzymatic basis for bioenergetic differences of alveolar versus peritoneal macrophages and enzyme regulation by molecular O_2. *J. Clin. Invest.*, 59:443–448.
88. Soderland, S. C., and Naum, Y. (1973): Growth of pulmonary alveolar macrophages in vitro. *Nature (London)*, 245:150–152.
89. Sorber, W. A., Leake, E. S., and Myrvik, Q. N. (1974): Isolation and characterization of hydrolase-containing granules from rabbit lung macrophages. *J. Reticuloendothel. Soc.*, 16:184–192.
90. Spector, W. G., and Lykke, A. W. J. (1966): The cellular evolution of inflammatory granulomata. *J. Pathol. (London)*, 92:163–177.
91. Stanley, E. R., Cifone, M., Heard, P. M., and Defendi, V. (1976): Factors regulating macrophage production and growth: identity of colony-stimulating factor and macrophage growth factor. *J. Exp. Med.*, 143:631–647.
92. Stanley, E. R., and Heard, P. M. (1977): Factors regulating macrophage production and growth. Purification and some properties of the colony stimulating factor from medium conditioned by mouse L cells. *J. Biol. Chem.*, 252:4305–4312.
93. Stossel, T. P., Mason, R. J., Pollard, T. D., and Vaughan, M. (1972): Isolation and properties of phagocytic vesicles. II. Alveolar macrophages. *J. Clin. Invest.*, 51:604–614.
94. Thomas, E. D., Ramberg, R. E., Sale, G. E., Sparkes, R. S., and Golde, D. W. (1976): Direct evidence for a bone marrow origin of the alveolar macrophage in man. *Science*, 192:1016–1018.
95. Van Furth, R. (1970): Origin and kinetics of monocytes and macrophages. *Semin. Hematol.*, 7:125–141.
96. Van Furth, R., and Cohn, Z. A. (1968): The origin and kinetics of mononuclear phagocytes. *J. Exp. Med.*, 128:415–435.
97. Van Furth, R., Raeburn, J. A., van Zwet, T. L. (1979): Characteristics of human mononuclear phagocytes. *Blood*, 54:485–500.
98. Volkman, A. (1976): Disparity in origin of mononuclear phagocyte populations. *J. Reticuloendothel. Soc.*, 19:249–268.
99. Volkman, A., and Gowans, J. L. (1965): The origin of macrophages from bone marrow in the rat. *Br. J. Exp. Pathol.*, 46:62–70.
100. Walker, D. G. (1975): Control of bone resorption by hematopoietic tissue. The induction and reversal of congenital osteopetrosis in mice through use of bone marrow and splenic transplants. *J. Exp. Med.*, 142:651–663.
101. Weiden, P. L., Storb, R., and Tsoi, M.-S. (1975): Marrow origin of canine alveolar macrophages. *J. Reticuloendothel. Soc.*, 17:342–345.
102. Weissmann, G. (1967): The role of lysosomes in inflammation and disease. *Annu. Rev. Med.*, 18:97–112.
103. Whitelaw, D. M., and Batho, H. F. (1975). Kinetics of monocytes. In: *Mononuclear Phagocytes in Immunity, Infection, and Pathology*, edited by R. van Furth, pp. 175–188. Blackwell Scientific Publications Ltd., Oxford.
104. Yarborough, D. J., Meyer, O. T., Dannenberg, A. M., Jr., and Pearson, B. (1967): Histochemistry of macrophage hydrolases. III. Studies on β-galactosidase, β-glucuronidase and aminopeptidase with indolyl and naphthyl substrates. *J. Reticuloendothel. Soc.*, 4:390–408.

Advances in Host Defense Mechanisms, Vol. 1,
edited by John I. Gallin and Anthony S. Fauci,
Raven Press, New York © 1982.

Mononuclear Cell Phagocytic Mechanisms and Host Defense

Frank M. Griffin, Jr.

Division of Infectious Diseases, Department of Medicine, University of Alabama in Birmingham, Birmingham, Alabama 35294

The mononuclear phagocyte system, which consists of circulating monocytes and tissue macrophages, is one of two major phagocytic cell systems, the other being polymorphonuclear neutrophils. The development, maturation, kinetics, and distribution of cells of the mononuclear phagocyte system are discussed by Dr. Golde and Dr. Hocking in the preceding chapter. From their account of the development of some of the specialized functions and organelles of monocytes and macrophages, it is apparent that, during their maturation, these cells acquire the tools that equip them to phagocytize both foreign invaders such as pathogenic microorganisms and endogenous invaders such as neoplastic cells.

Much of the experimental work on phagocytic mechanisms has been performed with macrophages, the tissue form of the mononuclear phagocyte. However, less extensive studies of phagocytosis by neutrophils and other phagocytic cells suggest that there are far more similarities than differences between the mechanisms by which different cell types perform this function. Thus, although the cell of emphasis in this article will be the macrophage, studies that have taught us important lessons about phagocytic mechanisms will be discussed, regardless of the cell type with which experiments were performed.

In the subsequent discussion, we will see that phagocytosis is an intriguing process that involves not only the phagocytic cell itself but also immunoglobulin, the complement system, lymphocytes, and certain lymphocyte products. Moreover, an understanding of the mechanisms of phagocytosis requires at least a working knowledge of cell-surface organization, receptor-ligand interactions, cell surface to cell interior communication, and the intracellular contractile apparatus.

Several studies performed during the past few years have changed the way we view both the process of phagocytosis itself and the roles of opsonins and receptors in phagocytosis. This chapter will emphasize these studies and will discuss the possible relevance of the newer findings to host defense against pathogenic microorganisms.

THE THREE STEPS OF PHAGOCYTOSIS

The process of phagocytosis is most conveniently divided into three distinct steps: particle attachment, generation and transmission of the phagocytic signal, and particle ingestion.

The first step, particle attachment, involves the apposition of the phagocytic cell's plasma membrane to the particle surface. It can occur even in the absence of cellular metabolism and is almost solely dependent on the surface properties of the particle and the surface properties of the cell.

The second step, signal generation and transmission, is the least understood. Before it can be ingested, a particle must bind to the surface of the phagocytic cell; thus, it seems clear that the attachment step results in physical and/or chemical changes in the cell that trigger ingestion of the particle. To date we have no clear idea of what these changes are or how they are translated into the motive force necessary for particle engulfment.

The third step, particle ingestion, involves the extension of cellular pseudopods around the particle and fusion of the leading edges of pseudopod plasma membrane to enclose the particle in a phagocytic vacuole. This process uses energy, is regulated by both the cell surface and the particle surface, and is carried out by the intracellular contractile machinery.

PARTICLE RECOGNITION AND ATTACHMENT

A phagocytic cell constantly comes into contact with numerous particulate materials; yet it attaches and ingests only selected particles. The cell must therefore be able to identify its intended meal. It can do so because its plasma membrane bears structures that recognize specific molecules on the surfaces of certain particles.

Particle recognition and attachment have been most extensively studied using particles that require immunologic coating, or opsonization, in order to be bound by phagocytic cells. It was known in the late 19th century that serum factors enhanced the rate of uptake of certain bacteria by neutrophils, but it was not clear whether these factors exerted their effects on the bacteria or on the cells. In 1903 Wright and Douglas (170) were the first to show that these factors had no effect on the cells but instead altered the bacteria such that they were more appetizing to the cells. The rapid expansion in our understanding of immunoglobulin and complement chemistry in the middle of the 20th century made it apparent that the opsonic serum factors were IgG and C3b, defined the roles of these molecules in the attachment step of phagocytosis, and led to the concept that plasma membrane receptors, which specifically recognize portions of these molecules, are the means by which phagocytic cells recognize and attach to their surfaces particles coated with these ligands.

When certain otherwise nonattachable particles are coated with IgG molecules directed against their surfaces, they can be recognized and attached by phagocytic cells (6,13,23,72–75,90,99,112,117,154). Attachment is mediated by the Fc portion of the IgG molecule, since particles coated with F(ab′)$_2$ fragments of IgG are not attached, and Fc fragments, but not Fab fragments, of IgG can compete for binding sites on the cell surface and block the attachment of IgG-coated particles (9,23,62).

The specificity with which the Fc portion of IgG interacts with the phagocytic cell surface supports the concept that these cells bear molecules on their plasma membranes that are Fc receptors. So also does the finding that the ability of the cells to bind IgG molecules exhibits saturation kinetics (2,6,62,157,171). Moreover, several investigators have recently isolated molecules from the plasma membranes of phagocytic cells that bind specifically to the Fc portion of IgG (5,38,86,92,93,98). The molecular weights of the molecules identified have ranged from 35,000 to more than 120,000 daltons, suggesting either that some of the molecules are non-specific binders of certain proteins, that the molecules are the same but either aggregate or become partially degraded under the experimental conditions used to isolate them, or that there are several classes of Fc receptors. There is, in fact, good evidence that mouse macrophages have two classes of Fc receptors: one that recognizes mouse IgG2a, is trypsin-sensitive, and mediates particle binding but may be incapable of promoting particle ingestion, and another that recognizes mouse IgG1 and IgG2b, is trypsin-resistant, and promotes particle ingestion as well as attachment (52,63,69,102,138,155–157,159,160).

A molecule generated by the activation of complement also serves to bind particles to phagocytic cells. Complement activation may occur by either the classical or the alternative pathway (44). The classical pathway is initiated by the binding of Cl to antigen-antibody complexes, such as those formed by the interaction of either IgG or IgM with appropriate antigens on the surface of a particle. The alternative pathway can be initiated by the interaction of certain complement components with lipo-polysaccharides or polysaccharides, such as those contained in the cell walls and capsules of bacteria and other microorganisms. Both pathways converge at C3, resulting in the cleavage of C3 into two fragments, C3a and C3b. The major fragment, C3b, binds to the surface of the particle via a labile binding site. The particle can then be bound to the surface of the phagocytic cell via a different molecular site, the stable binding site.

The concept that binding of C3b-coated particles to the phagocytic cell surface is mediated by specific C3b receptors is supported by several findings. First, binding of complement-coated particles to the cell surface is strictly dependent on the presence of C3b on the particle surface; when these particles are coated with other complement components, including other fragments of C3, they are not bound (14,21,48,54,60,71,74,88,126). Second, binding of C3b-coated particles can be blocked by either fluid phase C3 or C3b but not by other complement components, other C3 fragments, or other serum proteins (126). Third, the ability of phagocytic cells to bind C3b-coated particles can be abolished by treating the cells with trypsin (14,54,71,88), suggesting that the recognition site for the C3b molecule is an externally disposed, trypsin-sensitive plasma membrane protein. Finally, Fearon (40) has recently isolated from the plasma membranes of human erythrocytes a 205,000-dalton protein that specifically binds C3b. By treating monocytes and neutrophils with antibody to this protein, he was able to block completely the binding of C3b-coated particles to their surfaces. The protein therefore appears to be the receptor for C3b on both phagocytic and nonphagocytic cells.

As with Fc receptors, phagocytic cells have two classes of C3 receptors, one that recognizes C3b, the other that recognizes C3bi, the form of C3b that has been nicked by C3b inactivator (21,126). It is not known at present whether or not these receptors differ in their phagocytosis-promoting potential.

Based on the findings cited above, it seems very likely that specific receptors mediate the attachment of immunologically coated particles to the plasma membranes of phagocytic cells and are therefore responsible for the first step of immunologically mediated phagocytosis.

Many particles, e.g., most nonencapsulated bacteria, do not require opsonization but can be bound and ingested in their native states (10,25–27,41,42,52,59,60,64, 68,76,94,103,104,116,118,127,129,158). Early investigators hypothesized that either the net surface charge or the hydrophobicity of a particle determined whether or not it could be recognized by phagocytic cells (41,104,116). However, experimental evidence in support of that concept has been difficult to obtain. Phagocytic cells attach and ingest particles that differ considerably in these surface properties, and modification of either the net surface charge or the hydrophobicity of a particle does not predictably influence its ingestibility (85,119). It remains possible that these nonspecific surface properties account for the recognition of some particles (e.g., polystyrene latex beads) by phagocytic cells; however, it seems likely that more specific mechanisms are involved in the recognition of most physiologically relevant particles.

The principles derived from the study of immunologically mediated particle attachment led some investigators to propose that nonimmunologically mediated particle binding was also dependent on the interaction of specific molecules of the particle surface with receptors for these molecules on the phagocytic cell's plasma membrane. Results of several recent studies support that view. The complement receptor itself can serve as the receptor for some bacteria directly (42). Terminal mannose residues on the plasma membranes of mouse peritoneal macrophages are required in order for the cells to bind certain strains of *Escherichia coli* and *Salmonella typhi* (10); a glucose-binding receptor on the surface of *Dictyostelium discoideum* is responsible for binding *E. coli* that bear terminal glucose residues (127,158); and the wheat germ agglutinin receptor of *Dictyostelium* is also the receptor for certain yeasts (68,129). In these instances, particle recognition is accomplished by the interaction of lectinlike molecules on the surface of either the particle or the cell with specific sugars on the surface of the other. Czop and her colleagues (25–27) have found that chemical modification of the surfaces of certain particles that are not recognized in their native states, exposes a site on the particle surface that can be recognized by human monocytes. Both these modified particles and several particles that are attached and ingested in their native states (e.g., zymosan) are recognized and bound by monocytes via a "recognition unit" on the monocytes' plasma membrane; the unit is exquisitely trypsin susceptible and clearly distinct from the cells' Fc and C3b receptors.

These results support the concept that the ability of phagocytic cells to recognize and attach a particle is mediated by the interaction of specific plasma membrane receptors with specific molecular sites on the particle's surface. When these molecules are serum components such as IgG and C3b, they are extrinsic ligands; when natural components of the particle itself, they are intrinsic ligands. Further investigation seems likely to result in the identification, and eventually the isolation, of more and more intrinsic ligands and of molecules on phagocytic cells that serve as their receptors.

GENERATION AND TRANSMISSION OF THE PHAGOCYTIC SIGNAL

Attachment of a particle bearing either extrinsic or intrinsic ligands on its surface to appropriate receptors on the cell is a prerequisite for ingestion of the particle. Engagement of these receptors leads to a cellular response, namely pseudopod extension around the bound particle. Since the stimulus, particle attachment, is a cell surface event, and since the response, particle ingestion, is an intracellular event, it follows that there must be a means of communication between the cell surface and its intracellular compartment, i.e., a signal. At present, the existence of a phagocytic signal is largely theoretical and the evidence for its existence chiefly inferential. However, several candidates have been advanced as at least components of the signal.

Cyclic nucleotides are messengers in many receptor-response reactions in a variety of cells (15,22,65,82,130,168). Muschel et al. (105,106) derived from a macrophage-like murine cell line mutants that retained the ability to bind and ingest latex beads and to bind IgG-coated sheep erythrocytes but that had lost the ability to ingest these erythrocytes. When incubated for 18 hr with either 8 Br-cAMP, cholera toxin, or isoproterenol, or when treated overnight with a phosphodiesterase inhibitor, maneuvers that increased intracellular cAMP levels, these cells regained the ability to phagocytize IgG-coated erythrocytes. These investigators were able to demonstrate a similar requirement for cAMP in Fc receptor-mediated phagocytosis by nonmutant, parental cells whose Fc receptor function had been impaired by pretreating the cells with insulin (106). These results certainly support a role for a cAMP-mediated function in phagocytosis. However, because the cells had to be exposed to elevated levels of cAMP for several hours before augmented Fc receptor function could be detected, it seems unlikely that a reaction involving this nucleotide is itself the phagocytic signal. Furthermore, alteration of extracellular cAMP concentration does not consistently affect phagocytosis (15,24,97,149,163), and intracellular levels of cAMP do not change consistently during phagocytosis (12,94,110,144).

Pearlman and colleagues (111) found that an esterase activity was required in order for guinea pig neutrophils to ingest complement-coated erythrocytes; and Musson and Becker (107) have used esterase inhibitors to generate evidence that at least two esterase activities, one of which is activated by receptor-ligand binding, are required for complement receptor-mediated phagocytosis by human neutrophils.

We have recently found that the protease inhibitor tosyl-L-lysine chloromethyl ketone (TLCK), at concentrations that do not impair several other macrophage functions, strikingly inhibits Fc receptor-mediated phagocytosis by mouse peritoneal macrophages (Shaw and Griffin, Jr., *in preparation*). And evidence has recently been presented that a methylation reaction is required for all types of cell movement (113,114), including phagocytosis by some but not all phagocytic cells (89,150). These results provide strong evidence that certain chemical changes, induced by the attachment of a particle to the surface of the phagocytic cell, are necessary in order for ingestion to proceed. Our information is currently insufficient, however, to identify the biochemical pathways which constitute the phagocytic signalling mechanism.

Despite our ignorance of the chemical nature of the phagocytic signal, we do know some of its features. Not all of the particles that are attached to the phagocytic cell's surface are ingested (14,28,39,47,52–60,77,95,96,100,101,105,106,108,118, 119,135,136). And those particles bound by means that do not generate the signal are not ingested when the cell is fed particles that bind to its plasma membrane, generate a phagocytic signal, and are themselves ingested (54,57,59), indicating that either the signal itself or its effects on the cell are quite localized. Macrophages and neutrophils treated with 2-deoxyglucose lose their ability to phagocytize particles via their Fc and C3 receptors but retain the ability to bind particles by these receptors and to bind and ingest particles via other receptors (16,100,101). These results suggest that 2-deoxyglucose treatment selectively dissociates certain cell surface events, engagement of the macrophage's Fc and C3b receptors, from the intracellular machinery of phagocytosis; that is, that it blocks either the generation or the transmission of the phagocytic signal. These results and those of Muschel et al. (105,106), cited above, suggest also that the signal for immunologically mediated phagocytosis may be different from that for nonimmunologically mediated phagocytosis.

PARTICLE INGESTION

Once the phagocytic signal has been generated and transmitted, the cell responds by extending pseudopods around the bound particle and eventually enclosing it within a phagocytic vacuole. The ingestion process depends on surface properties of both the cell and the particle and on certain intracellular events.

Surface Requirements for Particle Ingestion

Repeated Receptor-Ligand Binding is Required During the
Ingestion Phase of Phagocytosis

When the plasma membrane of a neuron receives a stimulus of sufficient magnitude, it responds by propagating an action potential that is cell-wide and quantitatively invariant (128). There is no graded response to subthreshold increments of the stimulus, but rather an "all or none" response, determined by whether or not the threshold stimulus is achieved. Our finding of the macrophage's ability to distinguish between two types of particles bound to its plasma membrane and ingest one while not ingesting the other indicates that the response to a phagocytic stimulus, or signal, is not a cell-wide response (54,57,59). Phagocytic cells are able to ingest particles that vary considerably in size and shape. There appears to be no particle too small to signal its own ingestion, suggesting that there is no absolute threshold that a phagocytic signal must achieve in order to initiate ingestion. And, both during its formation and after its completion, the size and shape of a phagosome conform precisely to the size and shape of the particle ingested (57), suggesting that the particle itself finely regulates its own engulfment.

These findings raise several important questions about the regulation of ingestion. (a) Are there phagocytic signals of varying magnitudes? (b) How does the cell determine precisely the quantity of its response to a phagocytic signal of a given magnitude? (c) How does the cell's plasma membrane fit so tightly with the surface of the particle?

These questions have been answered at least in part by studies of the interaction of mouse peritoneal macrophages with particles coated with ligands on only a portion of their surfaces. The initial attachment of a ligand-coated particle to the phagocytic cell's surface occurs via the interaction of ligands located on only a small arc of the particle's surface with specific receptors on only a small portion of the cell's plasma membrane. Whereas only a minority of the total number of ligands on the particle are bound by receptors during this initial particle-cell encounter, it is these few ligand-receptor interactions that generate at least the initial phagocytic signal and initiate particle ingestion. It was possible that these initial ligand-receptor bonds triggered intracellular events that destined the attached particle for ingestion, and that ligands located over the remainder of the particle surface and receptors lying outside this zone of initial attachment were superfluous to the ingestion process. If this were the case, then a particle with ligands located on only one hemisphere of its circumference should be ingestible, and phagocytic cells whose receptors lying outside the initial attachment zone were removed should be able to ingest a particle previously attached via appropriate receptors. However, we found that particles coated with either IgG or C3b ligands on only one arc of their circumference were not ingested, and particles diffusely coated with IgG and bound by macrophages' Fc receptors could not be ingested by macrophages whose remaining Fc receptors had been functionally removed from their plasma membranes (56,57).

These results indicate that not only are ligands and receptors the determinants of particle attachment and signal generation, but that they also play a key role in the ingestion process. However, the results do not define precisely the role of ligand-receptor interactions outside the zone of initial particle attachment. It was possible that the initial ligand-receptor interactions activated intracellular machinery that committed the cell to pseudopod extension of a degree sufficient for the ingestion of the attached particle, and that ligands located over the remainder of the particle acted only as "passive" binding sites for plasma membrane receptors on advancing pseudopods. Alternatively, repetitive receptor-ligand interactions may have been required in order to generate repeated phagocytic signals necessary for the continued extension of plasma membrane pseudopods and, therefore, for completion of the ingestion process.

We recently sought to distinguish between these possibilities (137). The Fc receptors of resident mouse peritoneal macrophages mediate both the attachment and the ingestion of IgG-coated particles; engagement of these receptors, therefore, generates a phagocytic signal. The C3b receptors of these cells, on the other hand, mediate efficient attachment of C3b-coated particles but do not promote their ingestion; these receptors are nonsignal-generating. We bound sheep erythrocytes coated with both IgG and C3b to macrophages at 4°C; attachment occurred both via the cells' Fc receptors and via their C3b receptors, but ingestion could not proceed at this temperature. The Fc receptors lying outside the zone of particle attachment were specifically blocked by treating the preparations with antimacrophage serum at 4°C, treatment that does not disrupt previously established IgG-Fc receptor bonds and does not affect the ability of macrophages' C3b receptors to bind C3b ligands (14,54,56,57,59,70). Cultures were then placed at 37°C, conditions that are permissive both for phagocytic signal transmission by IgG-Fc receptor bonds previously formed at 4°C (57) and for particle ingestion (56,57).

The protocol used was intended to provide an initial phagocytic signal in the form of engagement of the macrophages' Fc receptors by particle-bound IgG. However, completion of particle ingestion, if it occurred, would have to proceed via macrophage C3b receptor binding to particle-bound C3b, interactions that are incapable of generating a phagocytic signal but that are quite efficient at promoting particle binding and which should be excellent "passive" guides for directing pseudopod flow around the particle if the initial IgG-Fc receptor interactions generated a sufficient phagocytic signal. These erythrocytes were not ingested (137), strongly suggesting that sequential binding of receptors to ligands over the entire particle surface is required not only to direct pseudopod flow but also to generate repeated phagocytic signals throughout the phagocytic process. This mechanism is not surprising, for it is the most efficient means by which phagocytosis could occur, and it provides the phagocytic cell with the maximum capability to regulate the process.

Based on these results, we envision that phagocytosis occurs in the following manner: The engagement of receptors by particle-bound ligands at the site of initial attachment of the particle to the cell generates a signal that is transmitted intracellularly, resulting in the local formation of a small pseudopod. Receptors on advancing pseudopods bind to ligands located farther along the particle surface, generating additional phagocytic signals that result in further pseudopod extension. The cycle of ligand-receptor binding → intracellular signal transmission → local pseudopod extension must be repeated many times until the leading edges of plasma membrane meet and fuse to enclose the particle within a phagocytic vacuole.

Receptor Mobility During Phagocytosis

Biochemical and morphologic evidence suggests that reorganization of plasma membrane receptors and other plasma membrane components occurs when the receptors are engaged by ligands. Amino acid transport sites (153) and other proteins (166,167) on the plasma membranes of neutrophils were preserved when each neutrophil consumed a meal of latex particles sufficient to result in interiorization of 35% of its plasma membrane, suggesting that during ingestion these sites move to regions of the plasma membrane not incorporated into the phagocytic vacuole. Freeze-fracture studies have demonstrated that molecules redistribute within the plasma membrane after macrophages have bound particles coated with immunologic ligands (37). And, both Fc and C3b receptors of macrophages, although inherently randomly distributed, will, under certain conditions, migrate to one pole of the cell when engaged by their ligands (124,161).

Studies by Michl and co-workers (102) suggest that the ability of a receptor to migrate within the plane of the macrophage plasma membrane is a determinant of whether or not that receptor can promote particle ingestion. The Fc receptor of both resident and thioglycollate-elicited mouse peritoneal macrophages mediates both attachment and ingestion of IgG-coated particles. The C3b receptor of resident macrophages, as indicated above, mediates only attachment of C3b-coated particles, whereas the C3b receptor of thioglycollate-elicited macrophages promotes ingestion as well. Michl and colleagues (102) found that when macrophages were plated on glass coverslips coated with antigen-antibody complexes, the Fc receptors of both resident and thioglycollate-elicited macrophages migrated to the glass-adherent surface of the cell. When macrophages were plated on coverslips coated with antigen-antibody-complement complexes, the C3b receptors of thioglycollate-elicited macrophages also redistributed, whereas the C3b receptors of resident macrophages did not. We have found that the C3b receptors of resident macrophages treated with a lymphokine preparation that imparts to these cells the ability to ingest C3b-coated particles (see below) likewise migrate to the glass-adherent surface of macrophages plated on antigen-antibody-complement complexes (58). The ability of Fc and C3b receptors to redistribute on the macrophage surface correlates exactly with their ability to promote ingestion, suggesting that movement of receptors within the cell's plasma membrane, induced by engagement of the appropriate ligand, may be an essential step in the ingestion process.

Intracellular Events During Phagocytosis

Metabolism of Phagocytizing Cells

Particle ingestion is an energy-requiring process, for it cannot proceed either at low temperatures or in the presence of inhibitors of anaerobic glycolysis such as sodium fluoride and iodoacetate (79–81,119,131,132). Except in the alveolar macrophage (80,109), low oxygen tension and inhibitors of oxidative metabolism, such as potassium cyanide, do not affect the ability of the cells to phagocytize (79–81,123). Thus, the energy for phagocytosis by most cells is generated by anaerobic glycolysis, and for many years it has been assumed that adenosine triphosphate (ATP) is the energy source (79–81,131,132).

However, there is no change in total intracellular ATP levels in neutrophils or in macrophages during phagocytosis, and, in experiments by Michl and co-workers (101), depletion of intracellular ATP levels by 83% failed to alter the ability of mouse peritoneal macrophages to phagocytize any particle tested. These findings led Loike and colleagues (91) to examine carefully ATP turnover in mouse peritoneal macrophages. These investigators found that, although the total quantity of intracellular ATP did not change, the rate of ATP turnover increased dramatically during phagocytosis. This finding led them to search for additional reservoirs of high-energy phosphate bonds that might rapidly replenish ATP during its consumption. They found that, like muscle cells, macrophages contain large quantities of creatine phosphate, the levels of which fall dramatically during phagocytosis. These results strongly suggest that ATP is, in fact, the energy source for phagocytosis by macrophages and that intracellular levels of ATP are preserved during phagocytosis by the phosphorylation of adenosine diphosphate (ADP) by creatine phosphate and perhaps by other reservoirs of high-energy phosphate bonds as well.

Whereas anaerobic glycolysis provides all, or nearly all, of the energy for phagocytosis in most phagocytic cells, it is not the only metabolic pathway the activity of which increases during phagocytosis. Oxygen consumption and metabolism are enhanced, and the activity of the hexose monophosphate shunt is greatly stimulated as well (28,79–81,131). These pathways are not required for ingestion, but they are required for intracellular microbial killing and are discussed in detail elsewhere in this volume.

The Machinery of Phagocytosis

As previously noted, ingestion requires that the cell extend pseudopods around the attached particle until the leading edges of pseudopod plasma membrane meet and fuse to enclose the particle in a phagocytic vacuole. It is this function for which metabolic energy is required.

The first indication of how pseudopod extension occurs was obtained from morphologic data and shortly thereafter from indirect biochemical studies and from one clinical study. Electron microscopic studies revealed that actin filaments were present in huge aggregates in pseudopods enveloping particles but formed only a thin subplasmalemmal rim in the regions of the cells not involved in particle ingestion (57,122). Actin and myosin were identified in the cytoplasm of phagocytic cells (3,4,17,115,143) and were found in greatest concentration at sites participating in particle ingestion (143); and cytochalasin B, a compound that impairs actin gelation (67,141,142) and microfilament function (8), was found to inhibit phagocytosis (8,139,173). The critical importance of actin in phagocytosis in vivo was demonstrated by studies of a patient with recurrent, severe, systemic bacterial infections. His neutrophils were unable to move randomly, to respond to chemotactic stimuli, or to phagocytize. They contained normal quantities of actin, but, unlike actin from neutrophils of normal controls, it failed to polymerize in the presence of 0.6 M KCl (17).

These findings led Stossel and colleagues (17,18,66,67,145,147,148,172) to explore the possibility that actin filaments provide the motive force of phagocytosis. Over the past several years, these investigators have isolated from macrophages several proteins that, when incubated in appropriate combination *in vitro*, undergo sol-gel transformations that very likely account for the mechanism by which cellular functions that require movement of all or parts of a phagocytic cell (random motility, movement in response to chemotactic agents, and phagocytosis) occur. These investigators first isolated actin, myosin, and an actin-binding protein (ABP) from the cytosol of alveolar macrophages. When incubated *in vitro*, ABP caused actin to gel; the addition of myosin caused the gel to contract (148). Since during phagocytosis most of the ABP shifts from the plasma membrane into the cytosol (148), these investigators proposed that attachment of a particle to appropriate molecules on the macrophage plasma membrane causes ABP to leave the plasma membrane and bind to subplasmalemmal actin in the region of the bound particle, promoting the assembly of G-actin into F-actin and cross-linking the filaments to form a gel; myosin then contracts the filaments. If filaments anchored by the plasma membrane are normally randomly arranged but become oriented in parallel during contraction of the gel, then the net result of this sequence of events would be extrusion of the plasma membrane and the underlying cellular contents around the bound particle, i.e., pseudopod extension.

These biochemical mechanisms constitute a plausible explanation for at least the initiation of pseudopod extension during phagocytosis. However, in order for pseudopod extension to continue and for contractile elements to be able to return to their resting state, a mechanism for the disassembly of the gelled complex must exist. Such a mechanism has been recently identified. Yin and Stossel (172) isolated from alevolar macrophages another protein that they called gelsolin. When soluble actin was incubated with gelsolin alone, no change in the physical state of actin occurred. When actin was incubated with ABP alone, actin gelation occurred. When all three proteins were incubated together in the presence of micromolar quantities of Ca^{2+}, gelsolin prevented the gelation of actin by ABP. When Ca^{2+} was absent, gelsolin had no effect on the interaction of actin with ABP. These investigators further found that gelsolin did not prevent ABP from binding to actin, that the sol-gel transformations could be reversed by altering the Ca^{2+} content of the incubation medium, and that gelsolin could cause the gel-sol transformation at a ratio of 1 gelsolin molecule to 166 actin molecules. Studies in polymer chemistry have revealed that near a critical point small changes in the polymer:cross-linker ratio can result in an abrupt phase shift of the polymer (43). Yin and Stossel (172) therefore proposed that the physical state of the filament complex is regulated by the ratio of polymer (actin) to cross-linker (ABP) and that gelsolin breaks actin at only a few cross-linking sites, causing a small but significant increase in the ratio of polymer to cross-linker molecules, thereby solubilizing the gel. Regional variations in subcellular Ca^{2+} concentration, which may be governed by cell-surface events such as receptor-ligand binding, would determine the physical state of actin in various regions of the cell and could regulate the flow of pseudopods around the cell's particulate meal. These findings provide a reasonable explanation for the mechanism by which actin filaments and their regulatory proteins provide the motive force for phagocytosis and also demonstrate a critical role for Ca^{2+} in that process.

COOPERATIVE ROLES OF Fc RECEPTORS AND COMPLEMENT RECEPTORS IN HOST DEFENSE AGAINST MICROBIAL INFECTION

It has been known for many years that coating most microorganisms with either IgG or C3b enhances the rate at which they are ingested by phagocytic cells *in vitro* (77,117,136,140,162), and the importance of these molecules in host defense against infection has been apparent from the markedly increased rate of bacterial infection in patients who lack either opsonin (1,125). It had been assumed that both IgG and C3b ligands enhance both the rate of attachment and the rate of ingestion of the opsonized microbes (48,54,74,107,111,117,135,136,146). However, results of several recent studies, which reveal that these ligands do not always promote ingestion have raised serious questions about the availability of the ligands to the cell's Fc and C3b receptors at sites of inflammation *in vivo* and suggest that receptor cooperation may be necessary for optimal host defense.

When studied in tissue culture medium *in vitro*, Fc receptors of all phagocytic cells mediate particle attachment, generate a phagocytic signal, and promote ingestion of IgG-coated particles (14,54,60,95,96,117,118,135,137). Several lines of evidence indicate, however, that phagocytic cells may have difficulty in phagocytizing via their Fc receptors at sites of infection *in vivo*. Uptake of IgG-coated particles by phagocytic cells of both experimental animals and patients with circulating immune complexes is impaired both *in vitro* (64) and *in vivo* (45,61). Macrophages that have either bound immobilized immune complexes (36,78,102,120,121) or ingested soluble immune complexes (52,53) *in vitro* are strikingly defective in their ability to phagocytize either IgG-coated erythrocytes or IgG-coated yeasts of *Cyptococcus neoformans*. Since many microorganisms shed substantial quantities of their surface antigens, immune complexes composed of these antigens and host antibody are probably plentiful at sites of infection in the immune host. Ingestion of these complexes may block the phagocytic cells' Fc receptors and impair their ability to ingest IgG-coated microorganisms. In addition, the Fc portion of microbe-bound IgG may be unavailable to the phagocytic cell's Fc receptors, for the deposition of complement components on antigen-IgG complexes can, under certain conditions, mask the Fc portion of IgG (102,133). If complement were to mask these ligands *in vivo*, then particle-bound IgG would be useless as an opsonin.

It appears as if complement-mediated opsonization may also be inadequate to ensure microbial ingestion. When C3b is generated by activation of the alternative complement pathway by constituents of encapsulated microorganisms, C3b is deposited beneath the microbes' capsules at sites inaccessible to the C3b receptors of phagocytic cells (53,164,169). In contrast, C3b appears to be deposited on the capsules of these microorganisms and is available to cells' C3b receptors when complement is activated by anticapsular immunoglobulin (53). These results strongly suggest that activation of the alternative complement pathway may by itself be an inadequate host-defense mechanism against disease caused by encapsulated microorganisms and indicate that cooperative effects of complement and immunoglobulin may be necessary in order to achieve optimal opsonization.

Even when C3b is available to the cells' C3b receptors, it may not enhance particle ingestion, however, for the C3b receptors of both neutrophils and mononuclear phagocytes mediate only attachment of erythrocytes (14,39,52,54, 55,60,95,96,108,137), staphylococci (136), pneumococci (162), and cryptococci (53) coated with C3b; they appear to be incapable of generating the phagocytic signal and promoting particle ingestion.

How then do Fc and C3b receptors enhance particle uptake? Several investigators found that erythrocytes coated with sufficient quantities of IgG were both bound and ingested by neutrophils and monocytes, whereas erythrocytes coated with C3b were bound but not ingested (39,95,136). When erythrocytes were coated with both ligands, the concentration of IgG on the erythrocyte surface required to promote ingestion was reduced nearly 100-fold, to a level that was insufficient to promote even attachment of erythrocytes coated with that quantity of IgG alone. These investigators proposed that the chief role of C3b and its receptors is to promote particle binding; the chief role of IgG and its receptors is to promote particle ingestion; and, the enhanced particle binding by C3b and its receptors serves to facilitate engagement of the cell's phagocytic signal-generating Fc receptors by IgG. Ehlenberger and Nussenzweig (39) obtained support for this hypothesis by showing that erythrocytes coated with quantities of IgG insufficient to promote their attachment were ingested when physical and chemical means other than C3b were used to bind the erythrocytes to the cell surface.

These findings demonstrate the importance of Fc and C3b receptor cooperation in phagocytosis. They also explain how C3b can opsonize some microorganisms even in the absence of IgG. The microbes that C3b can opsonize alone are those that are nonencapsulated and ingestible, at least to a moderate degree, in their native states, presumably because they display on their surfaces intrinsic ligands that can engage the appropriate cellular "receptors" and thereby generate the phagocytic signal. Since these microbes are nonencapsulated, C3b is presumably deposited at a site accessible to the phagocytic cell's C3b receptors even when it is generated via the alternative complement pathway by components of the microbes themselves. Therefore, the deposition of C3b on the microorganisms would enhance their rate of binding to the phagocytic cell's surface and thereby increase the efficiency with which their own intrinsic ligands bind to appropriate signal-generating receptors. The result would be to increase their phagocytic rate.

In addition to facilitating the engagement of phagocytic signal-generating receptors by their ligands, under some conditions macrophage complement receptors are able to promote ingestion directly (14,52,53,55,60). Mouse peritoneal macrophages elicited by certain inflammatory stimuli, such as the injection into the peritoneal cavity of Brewer's thioglycollate medium, not only bind but also ingest C3b-coated particles (14). This finding suggests that, in certain conditions, the inflammatory response per se may be sufficient to alter the macrophages' physiology or to cause them to mature or to differentiate to a stage at which their complement receptors are capable of promoting particle ingestion. This finding may not be pertinent to host defense against microbial infection, however, for we have been unable to elicit macrophages capable of phagocytizing via their complement receptors when we have used either microorganisms or microbial products as inflammatory stimuli in nonimmunized animals (Shaw and Griffin, Jr., *unpublished observation*).

However, we have recently discovered that, under conditions likely to prevail at sites of microbial infection *in vivo*, macrophage complement receptors can be converted *in vitro* from nonphagocytic to phagocytic receptors by a T lymphocyte product (52,53,55,60). The lymphokine responsible for this effect appears to be different from any previously described lymphokine and cannot be elicited by the classical mechanisms of lymphokine production, i.e., antigenic stimulation of appropriate clones of T lymphocytes (60). Thus, this lymphokine is not a product of classical delayed hypersensitivity reactions; rather, elaboration of the product requires a unique series of cellular interactions. Macrophages must first phagocytize IgG-containing immune complexes; these cells thereby acquire the ability to trigger, by a cell contact-dependent mechanism, T lymphocytes to elaborate a product that imparts to freshly explanted macrophages the ability to phagocytize via their complement receptors (60). The product itself appears to be a small (less than 10,000 daltons) polypeptide (55).

The effect of the lymphokine on the phagocytic capability of the macrophage is selective and specific for the cell's complement receptors, for it does not enhance either Fc receptor-mediated or nonimmunologically mediated phagocytosis (55). Although we do not yet know the precise mechanism by which it acts, it seems most likely that it somehow connects the macrophage's complement receptors with the intercellular phagocytic machinery, i.e., that it permits complement receptor engagement to generate a phagocytic signal.

These findings suggest a second means by which Fc and C3b receptors may cooperate in phagocytosis of pathogenic microorganisms. Microorganisms become coated with both IgG and C3b in the immune host. Many of these offenders also shed antigens that become bound by host antibody. Macrophages present at sites of immunologically mediated inflammation are therefore exposed to large quantities of immune complexes composed of IgG and microbial antigens. Ingestion of these complexes may block or saturate the cells' Fc receptors, rendering macrophages unable to phagocytize via these receptors the offenders they are invited to destroy. In their normal physiologic state, macrophages can bind the microbe via their C3b receptors but cannot ingest it and likely release it when C3b inactivator and proteases destroy C3b; the offender is probably unharmed after such an encounter (54,135). However, ingestion of immune complexes, although it paralyzes macrophages' Fc receptor function, at the same time permits the cells to interact with T lymphocytes, thereby triggering the lymphocytes to elaborate the lymphokine that enhances macrophages' complement receptor function (55,60). Macrophages may then be able to circumvent the immune complex-induced phagocytic blockade and ingest immunologically coated particles via their C3b receptors.

That cooperative effects of macrophages' Fc and C3b receptors are required for eradication of pathogens *in vivo* is suggested by recent studies by Brown and coworkers (19). These investigators found that guinea pigs depleted of complement by cobra venom factor were unable to clear intravenously injected, IgG-coated, encapsulated pneumococci from the circulation and died with pneumococcal bacteremia. In contrast, animals with normal complement levels, in which the pneumococci presumably became coated with complement, efficiently cleared the bacteremia and survived. Since the strain of pneumococcus used was not susceptible to complement-mediated killing, it is probable that complement was required to facilitate microbial ingestion. It may be that ingestion of either pneumococci-IgG complexes or soluble pneumococcal capsular antigen-IgG complexes by macrophages triggered the cells to signal T lymphocytes to elaborate the lymphokine that permitted macrophages to ingest the pneumococci via their complement receptors. Alternatively, C3b on the pneumococcal surface may have served only to enhance the affinity with which macrophages and neutrophils bound the microorganisms and thereby increased the efficiency with which the cells ingested pneumococci via their Fc receptors, as in the previously cited studies by Ehlenberger and Nussenzweig (39). Whatever the exact mechanism, these results emphasize the importance of complement and of complement receptors in host defense against a microorganism that has long been the prototype of microbes that are defended against chiefly by IgG antibody.

AN HYPOTHESIS FOR THE ROLES OF MACROPHAGE Fc AND C3b RECEPTORS IN HOST DEFENSE AGAINST *CRYPTOCOCCUS NEOFORMANS*

Although the model proposed for the physiologic relevance of the lymphokine that augments macrophage complement receptor function is a general model applying to host defense against many pathogens, it may be especially applicable to, and may explain some of the apparent paradoxes of, host defense against *C. neoformans*. Cryptococci are heavily encapsulated yeasts that completely resist phagocytosis by neutrophils and macrophages (20,35,83,84,103). When coated with anticapsular IgG antibody, they are readily ingested *in vitro* (84) and may be rapidly killed intracellularly (35,103,152). In one study (35), phagocytosis and intracellular killing curves were superimposable, indicating that all ingested yeasts were rapidly killed and suggesting that cryptococci are ill-equipped to survive as intracellular parasites within phagocytic cells. Their chief virulence factor appears from these studies to be their capsule, which enables them to escape phagocytosis; the chief host-defense mechanism would appear to be opsonization with anticapsular IgG, which permits phagocytes to ingest the yeasts. Complement-mediated opsonization may also be important in defense against cryptococcosis, since depletion of either classical or alternative complement pathway components renders serum less opsonic for cyptococci (34,103,151) and since guinea pigs depleted of complement by cobra venom factor are more susceptible than guinea pigs with normal complement levels to death from experimental cyptococcal infection (33). In these respects cryptococci resemble encapsulated bacteria such as *Streptococcus pneumoniae* (162).

However, clinically it is not patients with immunoglobulin deficiencies, but those with disorders of the T lymphocyte-macrophage system, who are at greatest risk of developing cryptococcal disease (11,30,49,134,165). Some experimental evidence also suggests that cellular immunity is important in defense against cryptococcosis. For example, athymic mice are highly susceptible to disease and death from *C. neoformans* (50, 51). In one study (46), mice chronically infected with either *Besnoitia jellisoni*, *Listeria monocytogenes*, or *Toxoplasma gondii* were resistant to lethal infection with cryptococci, whereas control mice were not. *In vitro*, peritoneal macrophages from mice infected with either *Besnoitia* or *Listeria* survived cryptococcal infection, whereas macrophages from control mice were destroyed (46). Likewise, normal human macrophages were unable to destroy ingested cryptococci (31). Diamond (29) has found that guinea pigs that received either lymphocytes or transfer factor (but not those that received serum) from animals that had been previously immunized with cryptococci survived cryptococcal infection longer than did their nontreated counterparts. In these respects cryptococcal infections resemble infections due to intracellular parasites, such as *Mycobacterium tuberculosis* (7) and *T. gondii* (76).

These findings indicate that host defense against cryptococcosis probably depends on complex interactions between the humoral and cellular immune systems. In our studies of the lymphokine that enhances macrophage complement receptor function (55,60), we have described *in vitro* conditions wherein these limbs are tightly interwoven in a cyclic amplification of the function of each by the other. Based on our findings and on the findings of others regarding cryptococci, I propose the following model of immunologic events that may occur in response to cryptococcal infection.

At the time of initial infection with *C. neoformans*, the yeasts cannot be ingested by macrophages because their capsules do not bear recognition sites to which the macrophage can bind. The organisms therefore replicate in tissues and shed substantial quantities of capsular polysaccharide antigen (32). As the level of anticapsular IgG increases, some of the yeasts become coated with IgG, are ingested via the macrophage's Fc receptors, and may be rapidly killed within the cell. However, much of the anticapsular antibody is bound by shed capsular antigen, thereby diminishing the quantity of IgG available to opsonize the microbes and also forming soluble immune complexes which the macrophage ingests. Ingestion of these complexes selectively blocks the macrophage's Fc receptors, thereby impairing the cell's ability to ingest the IgG-coated yeasts. Although the microbes are probably heavily coated with C3b, deposited via both the classical and alternative complement pathways (87), and although the macrophage's complement receptors are not blocked by ingestion of the complexes (52,53), the cell cannot, in its natural state, ingest the yeasts via its complement receptors. Thus, the deposition of both IgG and C3b on the microbe's surface is insufficient to promote the ingestion of cryptococci by macrophages.

Appropriate clones of T lymphocytes also respond to cryptococcal antigens (30) and elaborate lymphokines, such as macrophage activating factor, that enhance the macrophage's ability to kill the yeasts intracellularly but have no effect on its ability to phagocytize the microbes (60). This enhanced fungicidal capacity may by itself be of minimal aid to the host, for the ineffectiveness of opsonizing antibody and complement may make ingestion, not intracellular killing, the limiting step in eradication of the microorganism.

Uptake of immune complexes, although it paralyzes the macrophage's Fc receptors, at the same time initiates the series of cellular interactions described above, resulting in elaboration of the lymphokine that enables macrophages to phagocytize via their complement receptors (55,60). Macrophages that have been acted on by the lymphokine can then ingest immunologically coated cryptococci via their complement receptors (53).

A central concept of the model is that complement receptor-mediated phagocytosis is of paramount importance in host defense against cryptococcosis. Since an intact T lymphocyte-macrophage system is necessary to generate the lymphokine that augments macrophage complement receptor function (60), the model predicts that disorders of the T lymphocyte-macrophage system predispose patients to cryptococcosis by impairing either the ability of their lymphocytes to elaborate the lymphokine or the ability of their macrophages to respond to it and phagocytize cryptococci via their complement receptors.

I have found that treatment of macrophages and lymphocytes with pharmacologically achievable concentrations of either hydrocortisone or cyclophosphamide had no effect on the generation of the lymphokine but severely impaired the macrophages' ability to respond to it and to ingest immunologically coated cryptococci via their complement receptors (53). Therefore, the major factor predisposing immunosuppressed patients to cryptococcosis may be the inability of their macrophages to respond to the lymphokine that enables them to ingest cryptococci via their complement receptors.

ACKNOWLEDGMENTS

The author's work cited herein was supported by grants AI-08697 from the National Institutes of Health, PCM 75-17106 from the National Science Foundation, IM-173 from the American Cancer Society, Inc., a grant from the Veterans Administration, and Research Career Development Award AI-00135 from the National Institutes of Health. I am very grateful to Ms. Susan Lamb for superb secretarial assistance.

REFERENCES

1. Agnello, V. (1978): Complement deficiency states. *Medicine*, 57:1–23.

2. Alexander, E. L., Titus, J. A., and Segal, D. M. (1979): Human leukocyte Fc (IgG) receptors: Quantitation and affinity with radiolabeled affinity cross-linked rabbit IgG. *J. Immunol.*, 123:295–302.
3. Allison, A. C., and Davies, P. (1974): Mechanisms of endocytosis and exocytosis. Transport at the cellular level. *Symp. Soc. Exp. Biol.*, 28:419–446.
4. Allison, A. C., Davies, P., and dePetris, S. (1971): Role of contractile microfilaments in macrophage movement and endocytosis. *Nature (New Biol.)*, 232:153–155.
5. Anderson, C. L., and Grey, H. M. (1977): Solubilization and partial characterization of cell membrane Fc receptors. *J. Immunol.*, 118:819–825.
6. Arend, W. P., and Mannik, M. (1973): The macrophage receptor for IgG: Number and affinity of binding sites. *J. Immunol.*, 110:1455–1463.
7. Armstrong, J. A., and D'Arcy Hart, P. (1971): Response of cultured macrophages to *Mycobacterium tuberculosis*, with observations on fusion of lysosomes with phagosomes. *J. Exp. Med.*, 134:713–740.
8. Axline, S. G., and Reaven, E. P. (1974): Inhibition of phagocytosis and plasma membrane mobility of the cultivated macrophage by cytochalasin B. Role of subplasmalemmal microfilaments. *J. Cell Biol.*, 62:647–659.
9. Barnett Foster, D. E., Dorrington, K. J., and Painter, R. H. (1980): Structure and function of immunoglobulin domains. VIII. An analysis of the structural requirements in human IgG1 for binding to the Fc receptor of human monocytes. *J. Immunol.*, 124:2186–2190.
10. Bar-Shavit, Z., Ofek, I., Goldman, R., Mirelman, D., and Sharon, N. (1977): Mannose residues on phagocytes as receptors for the attachment of *Escherichia coli* and *Salmonella typhi*. *Biochem. Biophys. Res. Commun.*, 78:455–460.
11. Bennett, J. E., Disnukes, W. E., Duma, R. J., Medoff, G., Sande, M. A., Gallis, H., Leonard, J., Fields, B. T., Bradshaw, M., Haywood, H., McGee, Z. A., Cate, T. R., Cobbs, C. G., Warner, J. F., and Alling, D. W. (1979): A comparison of amphotericin B alone and combined with flucytosine in the treatment of cryptococcal meningitis. *N. Engl. J. Med.*, 301:126–131.
12. Bergman, M. J., Guerrant, R. L., Murad, F., Richardson, S. H., Weaver, D., and Mandell, G. L. (1978): Interaction of polymorphonuclear neutrophils with *Escherichia coli*. Effect of enterotoxin on phagocytosis, killing, chemotaxis, and cyclic AMP. *J. Clin. Invest.*, 61:227–234.
13. Berken, A., and Benacerraf, B. (1966): Properties of antibodies cytophilic for macrophages. *J. Exp. Med.*, 123:119–144.
14. Bianco, C., Griffin, F. M., Jr., and Silverstein, S. C. (1975): Studies of the macrophage complement receptor. Alteration of receptor function upon macrophage activation. *J. Exp. Med.*, 141:1278–1290.
15. Bourne, H. R., Lehrer, R. I., Cline, M. J., and Melmon, K. L. (1971): Cyclic 3',5'-adenosine monophosphate in the human leukocyte: Synthesis, degradation, and effects on neutrophil candidacidal activity. *J. Clin. Invest.*, 50:920–929.
16. Boxer, L. A., Baehner, R. L., and Davis, J. (1977): The effect of 2-deoxyglucose on guinea pig polymorphonuclear leukocyte phagocytosis. *J. Cell. Physiol.*, 91:89–102.
17. Boxer, L. A., Hedley-White, E. T., and Stossel, T. P. (1974): Neutrophil actin dysfunction and abnormal neutrophil behavior. *N. Engl. J. Med.*, 291:1093–1099.
18. Boxer, L. A., and Stossel, T. P. (1976): Interactions of actin, myosin, and an actin-binding protein of chronic myelogenous leukemia leukocytes. *J. Clin. Invest.*, 57:964–976.
19. Brown, E. J., Hosea, S. W., and Frank, M. M. (1980): Complement-mediated reticuloendothelial clearance in pneumococcal bacteremia. *Fed. Proc.*, 39:1204.
20. Bulmer, G. S., and Sans, M. D. (1968): *Cryptococcus neoformans*. III. Inhibition of phagocytosis. *J. Bacteriol.*, 95:5–8.
21. Carlo, J. R., Ruddy, S., Studer, E. J., and Conrad, D. H. (1979): Complement receptor binding of C3b-coated cells treated with C3b inactivator, β1H globulin and trypsin. *J. Immunol.*, 123:523–528.
22. Chasin, M., and Harris, D. N. (1976): Inhibitors and activators of cyclic nucleotide phosphodiesterases. *Adv. Cyclic Nucleotide Res.*, 7:225–264.
23. Ciccimarra, F., Rosen, F. S., and Merler, E. (1975): Localization of the IgG effector site for monocyte receptors. *Proc. Natl. Acad. Sci. U.S.A.*, 72:2081–2083.
24. Cox, J. P., and Karnovsky, M. L. (1973): The depression of phagocytosis by exogenous cyclic nucleotides, prostaglandins, and theophylline. *J. Cell Biol.*, 59:480–490.
25. Czop, J. K., and Austen, K. F. (1980): Functional discrimination by human monocytes between their C3b receptors and their recognition units for particulate activators of the alternative complement pathway. *J. Immunol.*, 125:124–128.

26. Czop, J. K., Fearon, D. T., and Austen, K. F. (1978): Membrane sialic acid on target particles modulates their phagocytosis by a trypsin-sensitive mechanism on human monocytes. *Proc. Natl. Acad. Sci. U.S.A.*, 75:3831–3835.
27. Czop, J. K., Fearon, D. T., and Austen, K. F. (1978): Opsonin-independent phagocytosis of activators of the alternative complement pathway by human monocytes. *J. Immunol.*, 120:1132–1138.
28. Densen, P., and Mandell, G. L. (1978): Gonococcal interactions with polymorphonuclear neutrophils. Importance of the phagosome for bactericidal activity. *J. Clin. Invest.*, 62:1161–1171.
29. Diamond, R. D. (1977): Effects of stimulation and suppression of cell-mediated immunity on experimental cryptococcosis. *Infect. Immun.*, 17:187–194.
30. Diamond, R. D., and Bennett, J. E. (1973): Disseminated cryptococcosis in man: Decreased lymphocyte transformation in response to *Cryptococcus neoformans. J. Infect. Dis.*, 127:694–697.
31. Diamond, R. D , and Bennett, J. E. (1973): Growth of *Cryptococcus neoformans* within human macrophages *in vitro. Infect. Immun.*, 7:231–236.
32. Diamond, R. D., and Bennett, J. E. (1974): Prognostic factors in cryptococcal meningitis. A study in 111 cases. *Ann. Intern. Med.*, 80:176–181.
33. Diamond, R. D., May, J. E., Kane, M. A., Frank, M. M., and Bennett, J. E. (1973): The role of late complement components and the alternate complement pathway in experimental cryptococcosis. *Proc. Soc. Exp. Biol. Med.*, 144:312–315.
34. Diamond, R. D., May, J. E., Kane, M. A., Frank, M. M., and Bennett, J. E. (1974): The role of the classical and alternate complement pathways in host defenses against *Cryptococcus neoformans* infection. *J. Immunol.*, 112:2260–2270.
35. Diamond, R. D., Root, R. K., and Bennett, J. E. (1972): Factors influencing killing of *Cryptococcus neoformans* by human leukocytes *in vitro. J. Infect. Dis.*, 125:367–376.
36. Douglas, S. D. (1976): Human monocyte spreading *in vitro*–inducers and effects on Fc and C3 receptors. *Cell. Immunol.*, 21:344–349.
37. Douglas, S. D. (1978): Alterations in intramembrane particle distribution during interaction of erythrocyte-bound ligands with immunoprotein receptors. *J. Immunol.*, 120:151–157.
38. D'Urso-Coward, M., and Cone, R. E. (1978): Membrane proteins of the P388D₁ macrophage cell line: Isolation of membrane polypeptides that bind to the Fc portion of aggregated IgG. *J. Immunol.*, 121:1973–1980.
39. Ehlenberger, A. G., and Nussenzweig, V. (1977): The role of membrane receptors for C3b and C3d in phagocytosis. *J. Exp. Med.*, 145:357–371.
40. Fearon, D. T. (1980): Identification of the membrane glycoprotein that is the C3b receptor of the human erythrocyte, polymorphonuclear leukocyte, B lymphocyte, and monocyte. *J. Exp. Med.*, 152:20–30.
41. Fenn, W. O. (1921): The phagocytosis of solid particles. III. Carbon and quartz. *J. Gen. Physiol.*, 3:575–593.
42. Fine, D. P., Harper, B. L., Carpenter, E. D., Davis, C. P., Cavallo, T., and Guckian, J. C. (1980): Complement-independent adherence of *Escherichia coli* to complement receptors in vitro. *J. Clin. Invest.*, 66:465–472.
43. Flory, P. J. (1941): Molecular size distribution in three dimensional polymers. III. Tetrafunctional branching units. *Am. Chem. Soc. J.*, 63:3096–3100.
44. Frank, M. M. (1979): The complement system in host defense and inflammation. *Rev. Infect. Dis.*, 1:483–501.
45. Frank, M. M., Hamburger, M. I., Lawley, T. J., Kimberly, R. P., and Plotz, P. H. (1979): Defective reticuloendothelial system Fc-receptor function in systemic lupus erythematosus. *N. Engl. J. Med.*, 300:518–523.
46. Gentry, L. O., and Remington, J. S. (1971): Resistance against *Cryptococcus* conferred by intracellular bacteria and protozoa. *J. Infect. Dis.*, 123:22–31.
47. Gibbs, D. L., and Roberts, R. B. (1975): The interactions in vitro between human polymorphonuclear leukocytes and *Neisseria gonorrhoeae* cultivated in the chick embryo. *J. Exp. Med.*, 141:155–171.
48. Gigli, I., and Nelson, R. A. (1968): Complement dependent immune phagocytosis. I. Requirements for C'1, C'4, C'2, C'3. *Exp. Cell Res.*, 51:45–67.
49. Graybill, J. R., and Alford, R. H. (1974): Cell-mediated immunity in cryptococcosis. *Cell. Immunol.*, 14:12–21.
50. Graybill, J. R., Craven, P. C., Mitchell, L. F., and Drutz, D. J. (1978): Interaction of chemotherapy and immune defenses in experimental murine cryptococcosis. *Antimicrob. Agents Chemother.*, 14:659–667.

51. Graybill, J. R., and Drutz, D. J. (1978): Host defense in cryptococcosis. II. Cryptococcosis in the nude mouse. *Cell. Immunol.*, 40:263–274.
52. Griffin, F. M., Jr. (1980): Effects of soluble immune complexes on Fc receptor- and C3b receptor-mediated phagocytosis by macrophages. *J. Exp. Med.*, 152:905–919.
53. Griffin, F. M., Jr. (1981): Roles of macrophage Fc and C3b receptors in phagocytosis of immunologically coated *Cryptococcus neoformans*. *Proc. Natl. Acad. Sci. USA*. 78:3853–3857.
54. Griffin, F. M., Jr., Bianco, C., and Silverstein, S. C. (1975): Characterization of the macrophage receptor for complement and demonstration of its functional independence from the receptor for the Fc portion of immunoglobulin G. *J. Exp. Med.*, 141:1269–1277.
55. Griffin, F. M., Jr., and Griffin, J. A. (1980): Augmentation of macrophage complement receptor function *in vitro*. II. Characterization of the effects of a unique lymphokine upon the phagocytic capabilities of macrophages. *J. Immunol.*, 125:844–849.
56. Griffin, F. M., Jr., Griffin, J. A., Leider, J. E., and Silverstein, S. C. (1975): Studies on the mechanism of phagocytosis. I. Requirements for circumferential attachment of particle-bound ligands to specific receptors on the macrophage plasma membrane. *J. Exp. Med.*, 142:1263–1282.
57. Griffin, F. M., Jr., Griffin, J. A., and Silverstein, S. C. (1976): Studies on the mechanism of phagocytosis. II. The interaction of macrophages with antiimmunoglobulin IgG-coated bone marrow-derived lymphocytes. *J. Exp. Med.*, 144:788–809.
58. Griffin, F. M., Jr., and Mullinax, P. J. (1981): Augmentation of macrophage complement receptor function *in vitro*. III. C3b receptors that promote phogocytosis migrate within the plane of the macrophage plasma membrane. *J. Exp. Med.*, 154:291–305.
59. Griffin, F. M., Jr., and Silverstein, S. C. (1974): Segmental response of the macrophage plasma membrane to a phagocytic stimulus. *J. Exp. Med.*, 139:323–336.
60. Griffin, J. A., and Griffin, F. M., Jr. (1979): Augmentation of macrophage complement receptor function *in vitro*. I. Characterization of the cellular interactions required for the generation of a T-lymphocyte product that enhances macrophage complement receptor function. *J. Exp. Med.*, 150:653–675.
61. Haakenstad, A. O., and Mannik, M. (1974): Saturation of the reticuloendothelial system with soluble immune complexes. *J. Immunol.*, 112:1939–1948.
62. Haeffner- Cavaillon, N., Dorrington, K. J., and Klein, M. (1979): Studies on the Fc$_\gamma$ receptor of the murine macrophage-like cell line P388D$_1$. II. Binding of human IgG subclass proteins and their proteolytic fragments. *J. Immunol.*, 123:1914–1919.
63. Haeffner-Cavaillon, N., Klein, M., and Dorrington, K. J. (1979): Studies on the Fc$_\gamma$ receptor of the murine macrophage-like cell line P388D$_1$. I. The binding of homologous and heterologous immunoglobulin G. *J. Immunol.*, 123:1905–1913.
64. Hallgren, R., Hakanssen, L., and Venge, P. (1978): Kinetic studies of phagocytosis. I. The serum independent particle uptake of PMN from patients with rheumatoid arthritis and systemic lupus erythematosus. *Arthritis Rheum.*, 21:107–113.
65. Hardman, J. G., Robinson, G. A., and Sutherland, E. W. (1971): Cyclic nucleotides. *Annu. Rev. Physiol.*, 33:311–336.
66. Hartwig, J. H., and Stossel, T. P. (1975): Isolation and properties of actin, myosin, and a new actin-binding protein in rabbit alveolar macrophages. *J. Biol. Chem.*, 250:5696–5705.
67. Hartwig, J. H., and Stossel, T. P. (1976): Cytochalasin B dissolves macrophage cytoplasmic gels. *Fed. Proc.*, 35:717.
68. Hellio, R., and Ryter, A. (1980): Relationships between anionic sites and lectin receptors in the plasma membrane of *Dictyostelium discoideum* and their role in phagocytosis. *J. Cell Sci.*, 41:89–104.
69. Heusser, C. H., Anderson, C. L., and Grey, H. M. (1977): Receptors for IgG: Subclass specificity of receptors on different mouse cell types and the definition of two distinct receptors on a macrophage cell line. *J. Exp. Med.*, 145:1316–1327.
70. Holland, P., Holland, N. H., and Cohn, Z. A. (1972): The selective inhibition of macrophage phagocytic receptors by anti-membrane antibodies. *J. Exp. Med.*, 135:458–475.
71. Huber, H., and Douglas, S. D. (1970): Receptor sites on human monocytes for complement: Binding of red cells sensitized by cold auto-antibodies. *Br. J. Haematol.*, 19:19–26.
72. Huber, H., Douglas, S. D., and Fudenberg, H. H. (1969): The IgG receptor: An immunological marker for the characterization of mononuclear cells. *Immunology*, 17:7–21.
73. Huber, H., and Fudenberg, H. H. (1968): Receptor sites of human monocytes for IgG. *Int. Arch. Allergy Appl. Immunol.*, 34:18–31.

74. Huber, H., Polley, M. J., Linscott, W. D., Fudenberg, H. H., and Müller-Eberhard, H. J. (1968): Human monocytes: Distinct receptor sites for the third component of complement and for immunoglobulin G. *Science*, 162:1281–1283.
75. Inchley, C., Grey, H. M., and Uhr, J. W. (1970): The cytophilic activity of human immunoglobulins. *J. Immunol.*, 105:362–369.
76. Jones, T. C., Len, L., and Hirsch, J. G. (1975): Assessment in vitro of immunity against *Toxoplasma gondii*. *J. Exp. Med.*, 141:466–482.
77. Jones, T. C., Yeh, S., and Hirsch, J. G. (1972): Studies on attachment and ingestion phases of phagocytosis of *Mycoplasma pulmonis* by mouse peritoneal macrophages. *Proc. Soc. Exp. Biol. Med.*, 139:464–470.
78. Kaplan, G., Eskeland, T., and Seljelid, R. (1978): Difference in the effect of immobilized ligands on the Fc and C3 receptors of mouse peritoneal macrophages in vitro. *Scand. J. Immunol.*, 7:19–24.
79. Karnovsky, M. L. (1962): Metabolic basis of phagocytic activity. *Physiol. Rev.*, 42:143–168.
80. Karnovsky, M. L., Lazdins, J., and Simmons, S. R. (1975): Metabolism of activated mononuclear phagocytes at rest and during phagocytosis. In: *Mononuclear Phagocytes in Immunity, Infection and Pathology*, edited by R. van Furth, pp. 423–439. Blackwell Publishing Co. Ltd., Oxford, England.
81. Karnovsky, M. L., Simmons, S., Glass, E. A., Shale, A. W., and D'Arcy Hart, P. (1970): Metabolism of macrophages. In: *Mononuclear Phagocytes*, edited by R. van Furth, pp. 103–120. Blackwell Publishing Co. Ltd., Oxford, England.
82. Koopman, W. J., Gillis, M. H., and David, J. R. (1973): Prevention of MIF activity by agents known to increase cellular cyclic GMP. *J. Immunol.*, 110:1609–1614.
83. Kozel, T. R. (1977): Non-encapsulated variant of *Cryptococcus neoformans*. II. Surface receptors for cryptococcal polysaccharide and their role in inhibition of phagocytosis by polysaccharide. *Infect. Immun.*, 16:99–106.
84. Kozel, T. R., and McGaw, T. G. (1979): Opsonization of *Cryptococcus neoformans* by human immunoglobulin G: Role of immunoglobulin G in phagocytosis by macrophages. *Infect. Immun.*, 25:255–261.
85. Kozel, T. R., Reiss, E., and Cherniak, R. (1980): Concomitant but not causal association between surface charge and inhibition of phagocytosis by cryptococcal polysaccharide. *Infect. Immun.*, 29:295–300.
86. Kulczycki, A., Jr., Krause, V., Chew Killion, C., and Atkinson, J. P. (1980): Purification of Fc receptor from rabbit alveolar macrophages that retains ligand-binding activity. *J. Immunol.*, 124:2772–2779.
87. Laxalt, K. A., and Kozel, T. R. (1979): Chemotaxigenesis and activation of the alternative complement pathway by encapsulated and non-capsulated *Cryptococcus neoformans*. *Infect. Immun.*, 26:435–440.
88. Lay, W. H., and Nussenzweig, V. (1968): Receptors for complement on leukocytes. *J. Exp. Med.*, 128:991–1009.
89. Leonard, E. J., and Skeel, A. (1978): The action of the adenosylhomocysteine hydrolase inhibitor, 3-deazaadenosine, on phagocytic function of mouse macrophages and human monocytes. *Biochem. Biophys. Res. Commun.*, 84:102–109.
90. LoBuglio, A. F., Cotran, R. S., and Jandl, J. H. (1967): Red cells coated with immunoglobulin G: Binding and sphering by mononuclear cells in man. *Science*, 158:1582–1585.
91. Loike, J. D., Kozler, V. F., and Silverstein, S. C. (1979): Increased ATP and creatine phosphate turnover in phagocytosing mouse peritoneal macrophages. *J. Biol. Chem.*, 254:9558–9564.
92. Loube, S. R., and Dorrington, K. J. (1980): Isolation of biosynthetically-labeled Fc-binding proteins from detergent lysates and spent culture fluid of a macrophage-like cell line (P388D₁). *J. Immunol.*, 125:970–975.
93. Loube, S. R., McNabb, T. C., and Dorrington, K. J. (1978): Isolation of an Fcᵧ-binding protein from the cell membrane of a macrophage-like cell line (P388D₁) after detergent solubilization. *J. Immunol.*, 120:709–715.
94. Manganiello, V., Evans, W. H., Stossel, T. P., Mason, R. J., and Vaughan, M. (1971): The effect of polystyrene beads on cyclic 3′,5′-adenosine monophosphate concentration in leukocytes. *J. Clin. Invest.*, 50:2741–2744.
95. Mantovani, B. (1975): Different roles of IgG and complement receptors in phagocytosis by polymorphonuclear leukocytes. *J. Immunol.*, 115:15–17.

96. Mantovani, B., Rabinovitch, M., and Nussenzweig, V. (1972): Phagocytosis of immune complexes by macrophages. Different roles of the macrophage receptor sites for complement (C3) and for immunoglobulin (IgG). *J. Exp. Med.*, 135:780–792.
97. Mason, R. J., Stossel, T. P., and Vaughan, M. (1973): Quantitative studies of phagocytosis by alveolar macrophages. *Biochim. Biophys. Acta*, 304:864–874.
98. Mellman, I. S., and Unkeless, J. C. (1980): Purification of a functional mouse Fc receptor through the use of a monoclonal antibody. *J. Exp. Med.*, 152:1048–1069.
99. Messner, R. P., and Jelinek, J. (1970): Receptors for human γG globulin on human neutrophils. *J. Clin. Invest.*, 49:2165–2171.
100. Michl, J., Ohlbaum, D. J., and Silverstein, S. C. (1976): 2-Deoxyglucose selectively inhibits Fc and complement receptor-mediated phagocytosis in mouse peritoneal macrophages. I. Description of the inhibitory effect. *J. Exp. Med.*, 144:1465–1483.
101. Michl, J., Ohlbaum, D. J., and Silverstein, S. C. (1976): 2-Deoxyglucose selectively inhibits Fc and complement receptor-mediated phagocytosis in mouse peritoneal macrophages. II Dissociation of the inhibitory effects of 2-deoxyglucose on phagocytosis and ATP generation. *J. Exp. Med.*, 144:1484–1493.
102. Michl, J., Pieczonka, M. M., Unkeless, J. C., and Silverstein, S. C. (1979): Effects of immobilized immune complexes on Fc- and complement-receptor function in resident and thioglycollate-elicited mouse peritoneal macrophages. *J. Exp. Med.*, 150:607–621.
103. Mitchell, T. G., and Friedman, L. (1972): *In vitro* phagocytosis and intracellular fate of variously encapsulated strains of *Cryptococcus neoformans*. *Infect. Immun.*, 5:491–498.
104. Mudd, S., McCutcheon, M., and Lucké, B. (1935): Phagocytosis. *Physiol. Rev.*, 14:210–275.
105. Muschel, R. J., Rosen, N., and Bloom, B. R. (1977): Isolation of variants in phagocytosis of a macrophage-like continuous cell line. *J. Exp. Med.*, 145:175–186.
106. Muschel, R. J., Rosen, N., Rosen, O. M., and Bloom, B. R. (1977): Modulation of Fc-mediated phagocytosis by cyclic AMP and insulin in a macrophage-like cell line. *J. Immunol.*, 119:1813–1820.
107. Musson, R. A., and Becker, E. L. (1977): The role of an activatable esterase in immune-dependent phagocytosis by human neutrophils. *J. Immunol.*, 118:1354–1365.
108. Newman, S. L., and Johnston, R. B., Jr. (1979): Role of binding through C3b and IgG in polymorphonuclear neutrophil function: Studies with trypsin-generated C3b. *J. Immunol.*, 123:1839–1846.
109. Oren, R., Farnham, A. W., Saito, K., Milofsky, E., and Karnovsky, M. L. (1963): Metabolic patterns in three types of phagocytizing cells. *J. Cell Biol.*, 17:487–501.
110. Park, B. H., Good, R. A., Beck, N. P., and Davis, B. B. (1971): Concentration of cyclic adenosine 3',5'-monophosphate in human leukocytes during phagocytosis. *Nature (New Biol.)*, 229:27–29.
111. Pearlman, D. S., Ward, P. A., and Becker, E. L. (1969): The requirement of serine esterase function in complement-dependent erythrophagocytosis. *J. Exp. Med.*, 130:745–764.
112. Phillips-Quagliata, J. M., Levine, B. B., Quagliata, F., and Uhr, J. W. (1971): Mechanisms underlying binding of immune complexes to macrophages. *J. Exp. Med.*, 133:589–601.
113. Pike, M. C., Kredich, N. M., and Snyderman, R. (1978): Requirement of S-adenosyl-L-methionine-mediated methylation for human monocyte chemotaxis. *Proc. Natl. Acad. Sci. U.S.A.*, 75:3928–3932.
114. Pike, M. C., Kredich, N. M., and Snyderman, R. (1979): Phospholipid methylation in macrophages is inhibited by chemotactic factors. *Proc. Natl. Acad. Sci. U.S.A.*, 76:2922–2926.
115. Pollard, T. D., and Weihing, R. R. (1974): Actin and myosin and cell movement. *CRC Crit. Rev. Biochem.*, 2:1–65.
116. Ponder, E. (1928): The influence of surface charge and of cytoplasmic viscosity on the phagocytosis of a particle. *J. Gen. Physiol.*, 11:757–777.
117. Quie, P. G., Messner, R. P., and Williams, R. C. (1968): Phagocytosis in subacute bacterial endocarditis. Localization of the primary opsonic site to Fc fragment. *J. Exp. Med.*, 128:553–570.
118. Rabinovitch, M. (1967): Studies on the immunoglobulins which stimulate the ingestion of glutaraldehyde-treated red cells attached to macrophages. *J. Immunol.*, 99:1115–1120.
119. Rabinovitch, M. (1968): Phagocytosis: The engulfment stage. *Semin. Hematol.*, 5:134–155.
120. Rabinovitch, M., Manejias, R. E., and Nussenzweig, V. (1975): Selective phagocytic paralysis induced by immobilized immune complexes. *J. Exp. Med.*, 142:827–838.
121. Ragsdale, C. G., and Arend, W. P. (1980): Loss of Fc receptor activity after culture of human monocytes on surface-bound immune complexes. Mediation by cyclic nucleotides *J. Exp. Med.*, 151:32–44.

122. Reaven, E. P., and Axline, S. G. (1973): Subplasmalemmal microfilaments and microtubules in resting and phagocytizing cultivated macrophages. *J. Cell Biol.*, 59:12–27.
123. Roberts, J., and Quastel, J. H. (1963): Particle uptake by polymorphonuclear leukocytes and Ehrlich ascites-carcinoma cells. *Biochem. J.*, 89:150–156.
124. Romans, D. G., Pinteric, L., Falk, R. E., and Dorrington, K. J. (1976): Redistribution of the Fc receptor on human blood monocytes and peritoneal macrophages induced by immunoglobulin G-sensitized erythrocytes. *J. Immunol.*, 116:1473–1481.
125. Rosen, F. S., and Janeway, C. A. (1966): The gamma globulins. III. The antibody deficiency syndromes. *N. Engl. J. Med.*, 275:709–715, 769–775.
126. Ross, G. D., and Rabellino, E. M. (1979): Identification of a neutrophil and monocyte complement receptor (CR3) that is distinct from lymphocyte CR1 and CR2 and specific for a site contained within C3bi. *Fed. Proc.*, 38:1467.
127. Rottini, G., Cian, F., Soranzo, M. R., Albrigo, R., and Patriarca, P. (1979): Evidence for the involvement of human polymorphonuclear leukocyte mannose-like receptors in the phagocytosis of *Escherichia coli*. *FEBS Letters*, 105:307–312.
128. Ruch, T. C., and Fulton, J. F. (1960): *Medical Physiology and Biophysics*, p. 63. W. B. Saunders Co., Ltd., London.
129. Ryter, A., and Hellio, R. (1980): Electron-microscope study of *Dictyostelium discoideum* plasma membrane and its modifications during and after phagocytosis. *J. Cell Sci.*, 41:75–88.
130. Sandler, J. A., Smith, T. K., Manganiella, V. C., and Kirkpatrick, C. H. (1975): Stimulation of monocyte cGMP by leukocyte dialysates. An antigen-independent property of dialyzable transfer factor. *J. Clin. Invest.*, 56:1271–1279.
131. Sbarra, A. J., and Karnovsky, M. L. (1959): The biochemical basis of phagocytosis. I. Metabolic changes during the ingestion of particles by polymorphonuclear leukocytes. *J. Biol. Chem.*, 234:1355–1362.
132. Sbarra, A. J., and Shirley, W. (1963): Phagocytosis inhibition and reversal. I. Effect of glycolytic intermediates and nucleotides on particle uptake. *J. Bacteriol.*, 86:259–265.
133. Scharfstein, J., Correa, E. B., Gallo, G. R., and Nussenzweig, V. (1979): Human C4-binding protein. Association with immune complexes in vitro and in vivo. *J. Clin. Invest.*, 63:437–442.
134. Schimpff, S. C., and Bennett, J. E. (1975): Abnormalities in cell-mediated immunity in patients with *Cryptococcus neoformans* infection. *J. Allergy Clin. Immunol.*, 55:430–441.
135. Schreiber, A. D., and Frank, M. M. (1972): Role of antibody and complement in the immune clearance and destruction of erythrocytes. I. In vivo effects of IgG and IgM complement-fixing sites. *J. Clin. Invest.*, 51:575–582.
136. Scribner, D. J., and Fahrney, D. (1976): Neutrophil receptors for IgG and complement: Their roles in the attachment and ingestion phases of phagocytosis. *J. Immunol.*, 116:892–897.
137. Shaw, D. R., and Griffin, F. M., Jr. (1981): Phagocytosis requires repeated triggering of macrophage phagocytic receptors during particle ingestion. *Nature (London)*, 289:409–411.
138. Silverstein, S. C., Steinman, R. M., and Cohn, Z. A. (1977): Endocytosis. *Annu. Rev. Biochem.*, 46:669–772.
139. Skosey, J. L., Chow, D., Damgaard, E., and Sorensen, L. B. (1973): Effect of cytochalasin B on response of human polymorphonuclear leukocytes to zymosan. *J. Cell Biol.*, 57:237–240.
140. Smith, M. R., Shin, H. S., and Wood, W. B. (1969): Natural immunity to bacterial infections: The relation of complement to heat-labile opsonins. *Proc. Natl. Acad. Sci. U.S.A.*, 63:1151–1156.
141. Spudich, J. A. (1972): Effects of cytochalasin B on actin filaments. *Cold Spring Harbor Symp. Quant. Biol.*, 37:585–593.
142. Spudich, J. A., and Lin, S. (1972): Cytochalasin B, its interaction with actin and actomyosin from muscle. *Proc. Natl. Acad. Sci. U.S.A.*, 69:442–446.
143. Stendahl, O. I., Hartwig, J. H., Brotschi, E. A., and Stossel, T. P. (1980): Distribution of actin-binding protein and myosin in macrophages during spreading and phagocytosis. *J. Cell Biol.*, 84:215–224.
144. Stolc, V. (1974): Restrained adenyl cyclase in human neutrophils: Stimulation of cyclic adenosine 3′:5′-monophosphate formation and adenyl cyclase activity by phagocytosis and prostaglandins. *Blood*, 43:743–748.
145. Stossel, T. P. (1977): Contractile proteins in phagocytosis: An example of cell surface-to-cytoplasm communication. *Fed. Proc.*, 36:2181–2184.
146. Stossel, T. P., Alper, C. A., and Rosen, F. S. (1973): Serum-dependent phagocytosis of paraffin oil emulsified with bacterial lipopolysaccharide. *J. Exp. Med.*, 137:690–705.

147. Stossel, T. P., and Hartwig, J. H. (1975): Interactions between actin, myosin, and a new actin-binding protein of rabbit alveolar macrophages. Macrophage myosin Mg^{2+}-adenosine triphosphatase requires a cofactor for activation by actin. *J. Biol. Chem.*, 250:5706–5712.

148. Stossel, T. P., and Hartwig, J. H. (1976): Interactions of actin, myosin, and a new actin-binding protein of rabbit pulmonary macrophages. II. Role in cytoplasmic movement and phagocytosis. *J. Cell Biol.*, 68:602–619.

149. Stossel, T. P., Mason, R. J., Hartwig, J., and Vaughan, M. (1972): Quantitative studies of phagocytosis by polymorphonuclear leukocytes: Use of emulsions to measure the initial rate of phagocytosis. *J. Clin. Invest.*, 51:615–624.

150. Sung, S-S. J., Raker, J. H., and Silverstein, S. C. (1980): Phagocytosis inhibition of mouse peritoneal macrophages by methylation inhibitors. *Fed. Proc.*, 39:1820.

151. Swenson, F. J., and Kozel, T. R. (1978): Phagocytosis of *Cryptococcus neoformans* by normal and thioglycollate-activated macrophages. *Infect. Immun.*, 21:714–720.

152. Tacker, J. R., Farhi, F., and Bulmer, G. S. (1972): Intracellular fate of *Cryptococcus neoformans*. *Infect. Immun.*, 6:162–167.

153. Tsan, M. F., and Berlin, R. D. (1972): Effect of phagocytosis on membrane transport of nonelectrolytes. *J. Exp. Med.*, 134:1016–1035.

154. Uhr, J. W., and Phillips, J. M. (1966): *In vitro* sensitization of phagocytes and lymphocytes by antigen-antibody complexes. *Ann. N.Y. Acad. Sci.*, 129:793–798.

155. Unkeless, J. C. (1977): The presence of two Fc receptors on mouse macrophages: Evidence from a variant cell line and differential trypsin sensitivity. *J. Exp. Med.*, 145:931–945.

156. Unkeless, J. C. (1979): Characterization of a monoclonal antibody directed against mouse macrophage and lymphocyte Fc receptors. *J. Exp. Med.*, 150:580–596.

157. Unkeless, J. C., Kaplan, G., Plutner, H., and Cohn, Z. A. (1979): Fc-receptor variants of a mouse macrophage cell line. *Proc. Natl. Acad. Sci. U.S.A.*, 76:1400–1404.

158. Vogel, G., Thilo, L., Schwarz, H., and Steinhart, R. (1980): Mechanism of phagocytosis in *Dictyostelium discoideum*: Phagocytosis is mediated by different recognition sites as disclosed by mutants with altered phagocytic properties. *J. Cell Biol.*, 86:456–465.

159. Walker, W. S. (1976): Separate Fc-receptors for immunoglobulins IgG2a and IgG2b on an established cell line of mouse macrophages. *J. Immunol.*, 116:911–914.

160. Walker, W. S. (1977): Mediation of macrophage cytolytic and phagocytic activities by antibodies of different classes and class-specific Fc-receptors. *J. Immunol.*, 119:367–373.

161. Walter, R. J., Berlin, R. D., Pfeiffer, J. R., and Oliver, J. M. (1980): Polarization of endocytosis and receptor topography on cultured macrophages. *J. Cell Biol.*, 86:199–211.

162. Ward, H. K., and Enders, J. F. (1933): An analysis of the opsonic and tropic action of normal and immune sera based on experiments with the pneumococcus. *J. Exp. Med.*, 57:527–547.

163. Weissmann, G., Dukor, P., and Zurier, R. B. (1971): Effect of cyclic AMP on release of lysosomal enzymes from phagocytes. *Nature (New Biol.)*, 231:131–135.

164. Wilkinson, B. J., Sisson, S. P., Kim, Y., and Peterson, P. K. (1979): Localization of the third component of complement on the cell wall of encapsulated *Staphylococcus aureus* M: Implications for the mechanism of resistance to phagocytosis. *Infect. Immun.*, 26:1159–1163.

165. Williams, D. M., Krick, J. A., and Remington, J. S. (1976): Pulmonary infection in the compromised host. *Am. Rev. Resp. Dis.*, 114:359–394, 593–627.

166. Willinger, M., and Frankel, F. R. (1979): Fate of surface proteins of rabbit polymorphonuclear leukocytes during phagocytosis. I. Identification of surface proteins. *J. Cell Biol.*, 82:32–44.

167. Willinger, M., Gonatas, N., and Frankel, F. R. (1979): Fate of surface proteins of rabbit polymorphonuclear leukocytes during phagocytosis. II. Internalization of proteins. *J. Cell Biol.*, 82:45–56.

168. Willingham, M. C. (1976): Cyclic AMP and cell behavior in cultured cells. *Int. Rev. Cytol.*, 44:319–363.

169. Winklestein, J. A., Abramovitz, A. S., and Tomasz, A. (1980): Activation of C3 via the alternative complement pathway results in fixation of C3b to the pneumococcal cell wall. *J. Immunol.*, 124:2502–2506.

170. Wright, A. E., and Douglas, S. R. (1903): An experimental investigation of the role of the body fluids in connection with phagocytosis. *Proc. Roy. Soc. Lond.*, 72:357–370.

171. Yagawa, K., Onoue, K., and Aida, Y. (1979): Structural studies of Fc receptors. I. Binding properties, solubilization, and partial characterization of Fc receptors of macrophages. *J. Immunol.*, 122:366–373.

172. Yin, H. L., and Stossel, T. P. (1979): Control of cytoplasmic actin gel-sol transformation by gelsolin, a calcium-dependent regulatory protein. *Nature (London)*, 281:583–586.
173. Zigmond, S. H., and Hirsch, J. G. (1972): Effects of cytochalasin B on polymorphonuclear leucocyte locomotion, phagocytosis and glycolysis. *Exp. Cell Res.*, 73:383–393.

Advances in Host Defense Mechanisms, Vol. 1,
edited by John I. Gallin and Anthony S. Fauci,
Raven Press, New York © 1982.

Human Pyrogen: A Monocyte Product Mediating Host Defenses

Charles A. Dinarello

Division of Experimental Medicine, Department of Medicine, Tufts University School of Medicine—New England Medical Center, Boston, Massachusetts 02111

Fever is a highly integrated biological response to a large number of external agents and internal dysfunctions. Clinically, fever is recognized as a hallmark of disease. From a physiological standpoint, fever includes elevated temperature, several metabolic changes, and functional alterations in neural as well as nonneural tissues. From an evolutionary standpoint, investigators have reasoned that fever is most likely a beneficial adaptive response, in that it has provided a mechanism which aids the host in surviving infections and other potentially fatal disease conditions. In fact, there is experimental evidence to suggest that in mammals and nonmammals a relationship exists between the magnitude of the febrile response and survival from gram-negative bacteremia (63,64). However, it should be noted that although survival rate increases at moderate febrile levels, there is a decrease in the number of surviving animals at higher temperatures (64). The adverse effect of high temperature has also been demonstrated in rabbits given endotoxin (5). Similar disagreement between the beneficial and deleterious effects of fever in humans has been demonstrated in several large clinical reviews (10,38,67), and the question of any ameliorating aspect of fever remains unresolved (60). One difficulty rests in the fact that fever cannot be equated with hyperthermia; whereas hyperthermia is the result of heating (usually exogenously), fever is an endogenously controlled process of which hyperthermia is only a part.

The difference between fever and hyperthermia is best understood at the hypothalamic level, and the home thermostat can be used as an analogy for hypothalamic control of body temperature. The thermoregulatory center located in the anterior and posterior hypothalmus regulates internal temperatures at about 37°C, primarily by its ability to balance heat production and peripheral heat loss. During fever, the thermostat setting in the hypothalamus shifts upward, for example from 37° to 39°C. This results in signals from the posterior hypothalamus to increase heat production and decrease peripheral heat loss. Heat production from shivering muscles and heat conservation from peripheral vasoconstriction continue until the temperature of the blood supplying the hypothalamus matches the higher thermostat setting. In contradistinction to fever, the setting of the thermoregulator center during hyperthermia remains unchanged at its normothermic level while, in an uncontrolled fashion, body temperature increases and overrides the ability to lose heat.

There is currently considerable interest in the use of hyperthermia as adjunct therapy for cancer patients (26,109). However, the use of hyperthermia as a therapeutic agent in clinical situations predates the present interest in cancer therapy (43). During the 19th century and well into the first two decades of the 20th century, hyperthermia was used for treating such diseases as syphilis, gonorrhea, and a variety of inflammatory diseases. Some physicians used a "hot box" to induce hyperthermia, whereas others infused endotoxins (commonly typhoid vaccine) and induced fever. In fact, a Nobel Prize in Physiology or Medicine was awarded to Wagner-Jauregg for using malaria to treat tertiary syphilis (108). Although the use of fever therapy and hyperthermia was associated with some ameliorating effects, it was quickly displaced with the dawn of specific antimicrobial agents. Only recently has the concept of using differential thermosensitivity, particularly for neoplastic cells, but also for several viruses been reintroduced as a useful therapy. However, at this time hyperthermia and not fever therapy has predominated. On the other hand, the use of immunopotentiation for cancer therapy using such agents as polynucleotides, endotoxin, and mycobacterial immunization carries the distinct association with fever (81,89).

An important question emerges: Can the functional alterations in a variety of cells observed during fever be beneficial as a host-defense mechanism apart from the theromodynamic effects of elevated temperature during the febrile response? Clearly the role of leukocytic pyrogen (LP) is critical in understanding the physiologic parameters of fever; for in addition to the initiating of the hypothalamic mechanisms leading to an elevated thermostat setting, LP may regulate certain cellular functions. Some of these cellular changes could be viewed as beneficial for the host in defending itself against disease processes, particularly invading microorganisms. The purpose of this chapter is to examine the role of LP as a possible mediator of host defense.

PRODUCTION OF LEUKOCYTIC PYROGEN

Although current data implicate pyrogen as a mediator of fever as well as certain parameters of the acute inflammatory response, the history of its discovery, production from phagocytic cells, and physical characteristics is derived almost exclusively from the study of its pyrogenic effects. The discovery over 30 years ago that the host produced its own pyrogenic substance was one of the most important observations in over two millenia of speculation about fever. This material, first described in sterile, endotoxin-free peritoneal exudates (7) has been called granulocyte, endogenous (3) or leukocytic pyrogen. It is this latter term, LP, which is most commonly used, since it is a description of the source of the molecule without the limitations of a specific cell type. At first, most research on the property of this molecule was focused on the peritoneal exudate granulocyte and later, the blood granulocyte. These cells accounted for the overwhelming majority of cells in any particular cell preparation studied. In addition, granulocytes were most often associated with febrile diseases.

In the late 1960s, attention shifted to the mononuclear phagocyte as a source of LP. This interest came about primarily because of the availability of methods to isolate mononuclear cells. By 1968, it became clear that human blood monocytes (16), the rabbit peritoneal macrophage (47), and the rabbit alveolar macrophage (4) were important sources of LP. It was not long after this observation that research into the characteristics of this molecule was directed toward factors recovered from stimulated monocytes. Most recently, the death knell has been struck for the granulocyte as an important source of LP (48). This had been anticipated when studies demonstrated that the human blood monocyte produces 40 to 60 times more LP than the human blood neutrophil (33). It now appears that most of the early characterizations of rabbit and human LP were conducted on pyrogen produced from contaminating monocytes. For humans, there has been considerable interest in the blood monocyte as a source of pyrogen. However, the human fixed macrophage pool has also been shown to produce LP. These cells include the hepatic Kupffer cell, synovial cells, and the alveolar macrophage (17,19). In rabbits, these fixed macrophages have been well characterized as important sources of LP (4,32,46). For humans, however, the fixed macrophage pool may play an important role in mediating fever in patients with depleted peripheral and bone marrow mononuclear phagocytes secondary to chemotherapy, since the fixed macrophage pool seems less susceptible to several antineoplastic agents.

Leukocytic pyrogen is not preformed but rather synthesized *de novo*. This fact has been shown using inhibitors of mRNA synthesis (13,88), protein synthesis (13,88), and intrinsic labeling with amino acids (85). Once synthesized, LP is released into the supernatant medium without appreciable intracellular accumulation (14). The signal for LP synthesis in the resting mononuclear phagocyte is unclear. However, most if not all agents which induce LP either *in vivo* or *in vitro* are themselves pyrogenic when injected into animals or humans (30,31). Generally, phagocytosis is one of the most well described stimulators of LP synthesis, and this has also been shown using dead organisms (98). Bacterial products from a large number of gram-negative as well as gram-positive organisms also induce LP synthesis (28). Of these, endotoxin is perhaps the most potent soluble agent known that activates phagocytes for pyrogen production. These and other soluble agents that stimulate pyrogen release most likely activate cells through membrane receptors. There is evidence that such membrane activation using phagocytic particles does not require the formation of a phagolysozome in order to signal LP synthesis (82).

Recently, a new class of stimulators of LP production have been described. These are soluble products of human lymphocytes (most likely T lymphocytes), which are released under antigenic or mitogenic stimulation (11,34). Of the methods used to produce these pyrogen-inducing lymphokines, the human mixed leukocyte reaction (MLR) (34) seems to be clinically relevant. The production of this factor in the mixed leukocyte reaction can be viewed as an experimental model to study graft-rejection fever and the fever associated with several autoimmune diseases. The identification or characteristics of the pyrogen-inducing lymphokine is presently unknown. However, there is some evidence that lymphokines such as macrophage-activating factor and colony-stimulating factor (CSF) may stimulate pyrogen production. Finally, several other agents have been described which induce LP release from human cells *in vitro* and which may be relevant in augmenting host-defense mechanisms. These include etiocholanolone and synthetic polynucleotides such as poly I:C. A summary of agents which induce synthesis of LP from human cells is presented in Table 1.

HOST-DEFENSE FUNCTIONS OF PYROGEN

Elevated Temperature

Prior to the current interest in pyrogen as a soluble mediator of host defense, the role of pyrogen as the endogenous initiator of elevated temperature had already been established. With few exceptions, it can be assumed that during infections, the synthesis and release of LP into the circulation results in an upward shift of the hypothalamic thermostat. These exceptions are a) patients with cervical cord injuries in whom sympathetic efferents have been destroyed, b) patients receiving high doses of antipyretics, and c) patients with anatomical or drug-induced hypothalamic dysfunction. In the first example, the ability to vasoconstrict and reduce significant peripheral heat loss is impaired. In the second situation, pyrogen is produced from phagocytes, but antipyretics block important hypothalamic mediators such as prostaglandins. In the third example, hypothalamic neurotransmission may be altered. Thus, in these situations, pyrogen production is not impaired, but rather, a recognized defect in thermoregulation prevents the raising of body temperature. It should be noted, however, that antipyretics such as aspirin and other inhibitors of cyclooxygenase do not interfere with the synthesis and release of LP (20,90). However, patients on high-dose corticosteroid therapy frequently do not develop fever when infected, because several mechanisms involving the recruitment and

TABLE 1. *Agents that induce human LP synthesis*

Microbial Agents	Pyrogenic Steroids
Viruses	Etiocholanolone
Bacteria	Lithocholic acids
Fungi	
Microbial Products	Lymphokines
Endotoxins	From concanavalin A-stimulated lymphocytes
Erythrogenic toxins	Released in the mixed leukocyte reaction
Staphylococcal exotoxins	
Cryptococcal polysaccharides	
Synthetic Agents	
Polynucleotides	
Muramyl dipeptides	

activation of phagocytic cells may be impaired; these defects can lead to decreased pyrogen production.

Another group of patients who rarely develop fever deserve to be mentioned. These are malnourished individuals who demonstrate both a certain thermolability to their environment as well as failure to develop fever in the presence of over-whelming infection. Although there are no studies concerning the ability of these malnourished individuals to produce LP, studies on an animal protein-deprivation model have investigated the role of malnutrition in the development of the febrile response. After 56 days of dietary protein restriction, rabbits fail to develop fever when injected with gram-negative bacteria but do respond to LP that had been produced by healthy rabbits (49). In addition, peritoneal exudate cells from mal-nourished rabbits produce less LP on a cell-to-cell basis when compared to cells from normal rabbits. What is unclear from these studies is whether the amount of LP is decreased from malnourished rabbits or whether it is released without an essential co-factor. Co-factor depletion as a result of the malnutrition could account for these differences, whereas decreased protein synthesis is unlikely.

On the assumption that the vast majority of patients synthesizing LP have a functional thermoregulatory system, core temperature increases, within certain lim-its, in proportion to the amount of LP released. It is important to independently examine the role that elevated temperature plays as a host-defense mechanism. This area of interest has been the subject of intense investigation for many years. Two major points of interest need to be considered: a) the effect of elevated temperature on the growth and virulence of microorganisms and b) the effect of elevated tem-perature on host cells. Before considering either situation, it is important to view both these effects with respect to the actual level of temperature elevations observed in various disease states. Although there are reports of exogenous hyperthermia (heat stroke) reaching levels as high as 110°F, temperature in humans rarely exceeds 106°F during fever associated with severe bacterial infections (37). This has led to the concept of a "thermal ceiling" in hypothalamic mechanisms controlling body temperature (24). At temperature elevations obtainable during fever, the growth rate for certain viruses, bacteria, or fungi significantly decreases. For viruses, growth of polio, and other enteroviruses is inhibited at temperatures of 40°C, and this mechanism seems to be related to decreased viral replication as shown by *in vitro* studies (74). However, comparable *in vivo* temperature elevations induced with hyperthermia in animals often increases resistance to certain viral infections by mechanisms related to host defenses rather than viral replication (8).

There is a large body of evidence to suggest that bacterial growth and virulence is adversely affected at temperature elevations associated with fever. Although microbiologists recognize three types of bacteria with regard to their optimal tem-perature for growth (thermophiles, mesophiles, and psychrophiles), there are only a few bacteria in the mesophilic class that are associated with human disease. Of these, the most studied is the pneumococcus. Several laboratory and clinical studies have established that growth of pneumococci is dramatically inhibited at temper-atures produced during fever in humans (41,102). Type III pneumococci are particularly sensitive to temperature elevation. Thus, it is not surprising that studies have established the fact that hypothermia increases mortality rates from pneumococcal infections (103). *Neisseriae gonorrhea* also falls into the category of highly thermosensitive bacteria. Thus, hyperthermia and fever therapy for this infection was standard practice in the preantibiotic era (95). For syphilis, there is doubt that the beneficial effect of high-temperature therapy was related to the thermosensitivity of *Treponema pallidum*, since this organism requires temperatures above 41°C to significantly reduce growth (22,75).

Other direct effects of temperature elevations on bacteria include changes in bacterial morphology, changes in cell wall and cell membrane components, decreased production of virulence factors (for example, penicillinase and toxins), increased antibiotic susceptibility and altered bacterial metabolism (2,27). Of these, the most interesting and perhaps most relevant to host-defense mechanisms is the decreased production, at higher temperatures, of phenolate iron transport compounds (siderophores). The role of iron in bacterial growth has received considerable attention (110). In brief, at temperature elevations easily attainable during most fevers, the iron requirement of several bacteria drastically increases. Bacteria synthesize and release siderophores for transporting iron back into the organisms. At elevated temperatures, there is decreased production of these siderophores and, in addition, coupled to increase nutritional requirement for iron, bacterial replication slows and may cease. Thus, this mechanism may account for the thermosensitivity of several bacteria. This relationship between iron, temperature, and bacterial replication has been shown using an *in vivo* model of survival from gram-negative bacteremia (45). Moreover, the role of iron as a host-defense mechanism in nonspecific resistance to infection has also been suggested (40).

The effect of temperature elevations on host-defense functions is less obvious than that shown for microbial growth. There seems to be some evidence that human neutrophil motility increases at temperatures of approximately 40°C (23,87). In one report (87), the Q_{10}[1] for human neutrophil motility between 32° and 42°C was 5.2. This finding is dubious since, with the exception of thermosensitive neurons, most cellular and biochemical functions have a Q_{10} of 2.2. However, as expected, other investigators have not been able to demonstrate increased motility at high temperatures using Boyden chambers (6,93). The uptake of *Staphylococcus aureus* by human neutrophils was reported to be increased at 43°C (73), but clearly, this degree of temperature elevation is too great to play a feasible role in influencing host-defense mechanisms in pyrogen-induced fever. Using temperature levels of 40° and 41°C, other investigators noted no effect on phagocytosis or killing (76,92). However, still other studies demonstrated small but significant bactericidal activity of human neutophils for gram-negative organisms and *Listeria monocytogenes* at these levels (97). There was no increased killing for *S. aureus* at 40°C.

---

[1]Q_{10} is an expression for the relationship of a temperature increase of 10° C to certain biological functions.

Differences in killing at hyperthermic temperatures may also be affected by serum components (104). Generally, there is no consistent pattern, and it is likely that if elevated temperature increases human phagocytic function, this effect is minimal at best and should not be considered a major host-defense mechanism.

The effect of elevated temperature on human lymphocyte function seems to be less controversial. Several investigators have established that human lymphocyte responses to mitogens and antigens is significantly enhanced at mildly febrile temperatures of 38.5° and 39°C (77,97). In addition, the production of lymphokines from stimulated and unstimulated human lymphocytes is augmented at temperatures of 38.5°C (96). Despite the seemingly beneficial effect of hyperthermia on human lymphocyte function, there is little or no evidence that elevated temperatures result in increased antibody production *in vivo* (10). However, there are no studies on the effect of elevated temperatures on *in vitro* antibody production.

Ability of Human LP to Alter Neutrophil Function

Several studies have reported the association between fever and altered neutrophil function (68). Experiments have now investigated the specific role of LP in mediating some of these changes by examining the direct *in vitro* effect of LP on the human neutrophil (61,62). The intravenous injection of unfractionated, crude supernatants from activated phagocytic cells into animals results in fever and hypoferremia; but, in neutropenic animals, there is no significant reduction in iron levels (53). Therefore, it has been proposed that there is a relationship between fever produced by LP, the requirement for neutrophils, and a decrease in plasma iron. To examine this relationship, preparations of semipurified human LP were incubated with human neutrophils. The release of lactoferrin and lysozyme was observed, and the ability of human LP to induce release of specific granule contents from human neutrophils was demonstrated (61). These experiments also demonstrated that release of granule contents occurred in the absence of cytochalasin B, was Ca^{2+} and Mg^{2+} dependent, and that release was not a result of cell death. In addition, the use of two cyclooxygenase inhibitors, indomethacin and naproxen failed to alter the ability of LP to induce specific granule release.

Further extension of these studies sought to relate fever, LP, and changes in neutrophil oxygen-dependent metabolism. Human neutrophils exposed to human LP *in vitro* showed an increase in the percentage of cells reducing nitroblue tetrazolium (NBT), an increase in superoxide dismutase inhibitable reduction of ferricytochrome C, and an increase in hexose monophosphate shunt activity (62). Using semipurified LP injected into rabbits, increases in the percentage of NBT-positive neutrophils in the circulation were observed 2 hr after the injection of pyrogen. However, LP had no effect on the ingestion of bacteria by neutrophils *in vitro*. Studies on the effect of LP on neutrophil oxygen metabolism have recently been confirmed using partially purified rabbit LP injected into rats. Chemiluminescence increased 10-fold in blood neutrophils 24 hr following LP injection, and enhanced chemiluminescence was observed following *in vitro* exposure of cells to LP (105).

The clinical implication for the direct effect of LP on neutrophil function *in vitro* is that LP is a possible direct mediator of host defense. Since *in vitro* studies have been conducted at 37°C, they do not take into account the effect of LP on neutrophil function at temperature levels comparable to those observed in fever. There are two mechanisms by which LP could aid the host in defense against infection: a) LP releases lactoferrin which, by its ability to bind iron, plays a role in host defense, and b) LP stimulates the killing ability of neutrophils.

The evidence that lactoferrin is an important factor in host defense derives primarily from several years of experimentation, which suggest that reduced iron levels are beneficial to the host during certain infections (40,65). Certainly, bacterial siderophores and lactoferrin compete for the same plasma-transferrin-bound Fe^{2+}. The ability of lactoferrin to bind Fe^{2+} preferentially from transferrin and deposit Fe^{2+} in the reticuloendothelial cells is an efficient host mechanism for reducing plasma iron during infection. In experimental models, *in vitro* bacterial growth is markedly reduced at comparable concentrations of plasma iron and at levels of temperature elevation which occur during fever (45). There are comparable experiments in humans. The level of hypoferremia and relative temperature elevation, which occur following the injection of certain pyrogens such as endotoxin (111), is similar to those in rabbit experiments.

In addition to decreased iron levels which possibly result from LP-induced release of lactoferrin, human apolactoferrin has a direct bactericidal activity for a variety of bacteria including *Streptococcus mutans*, *Streptococcus pneumoniae*, and *Vibro cholerae* (1). When lactoferrin is added to bacterial cultures, its effects are reversible by the addition of excess iron. These experiments, like those on the iron requirements of bacteria, demonstrate the ability of the host to defend itself against parasitism from invading organisms by "nutritional immunity" (65).

In addition to LP mediating lactoferrin release, the role of LP in host defense may also be related to a direct effect on neutrophil-bacterial interaction. Two groups of investigators have examined this possibility using an *in vivo* model of protection against lethal infection in rats injected with *Salmonella tryphimurium*. Using crude and semipurified preparations of rabbit LP, there was speculation that the increased survival rate of rats injected with LP 24 hr prior to challenge was due to increased microbicidal activity of neutrophils (105). Others claim that such an *in vivo* protected effect by LP is multifactorial and includes effects on iron and phagocytic function of the reticuloendothelial system (51). At present, it is not possible to define the probable mechanism by which LP-containing preparations protect rats against *Salmonella* infections. However, the ability of LP to directly stimulate oxygen-dependent neutrophil function and induce specific granule release may account for a direct role of LP in augmenting host defenses.

Ability of Human LP to Activate Lymphocytes

Considerable attention has been focused on the potential benefit of immunostimulation (immunotherapy) for cancer treatment. Two agents frequently used to increase nonspecific resistance to infection in mice and rats, bacille Calmette Guérin (BCG) and endotoxin, have also been used in certain cancer patients as immuno-stimulants (81,87). These and similar biologically derived substances are known activators of macrophages. Moreover, some of the adjuvant properties of myco-bacteria have recently been shown to reside in an N-acetyl-muramic dipeptide (MDP), which can be synthesized and still retain its adjuvanticity. The MDP and similar compounds are, like the parent BCG, potent activators of human macro-phages (36,81). Therefore, studies on nonspecific and specific resistance to infection must consider the important role of the macrophage in mediating any beneficial effects for host defenses due to immunostimulants.

Although there is ample evidence that macrophages have a critical if not essential function for the development of cellular and humoral immunocompetence (99), the contribution of soluble factors from macrophages to this immunocompetence is less understood than the role of macrophage-processing for lymphocyte function (107). The activation of macrophages results in an increase in phagocytic, microbicidal, and metabolic activity. In addition, activated macrophages also release a large number of enzymes, complement components, and bioregulatory molecules. Of the various macrophage products, those that alter or regulate cell function in other tissues have attracted considerable attention. The substances include lymphocyte-activating factor (LAF), colony-stimulatory factor (CSF), interferon, and pyrogen. The potential role of interferon in the host-defense mechanism is currently well appreciated, but substances such as LAF have only recently been identified as mediators of host responses to infection and immunological dysfunction (94).

Early characterization of human LAF suggested certain physical similarities to human LP. Human LP produced by monocytes stimulated by phagocytosis of heat-killed staphylococci was shown to exist in two molecular forms: a 15,000-dalton protein with a pI of 6.8 to 6.9 and a larger molecule approximately 38 to 42,000 daltons with a pI of 5.1 to 5.3 (33). Using various gel-filtration media and different stimulants, LAF produced by human monocytes was also shown to exist in two forms: a 15,000-dalton protein with a pI of 6.8 and another larger species with a molecular weight of 50 to 70,000 daltons (12,70,106,112,113). The LAF eluting from gel-filtration media with large-molecular-weight proteins was thought to be 15,000-dalton LAF, which had become absorbed or complexed to albumin or other serum proteins (106). However, LAF production and characterization had been conducted using significant (5%) concentrations of human serum, whereas human LP had been produced and characterized in predominantly serum-free conditions (35). The LAF activity also existed at pI 5.3 (113). Although the large-molecular-weight components of human LAF do not consistently correspond to those of human LP, some investigators report LAF activity at both 35,000 daltons as well as at those molecular weights associated with human serum albumin (9,113).

Despite these minor differences, there was considerable evidence that both human LAF and LP were closely related in several physical and chemical parameters. In addition, most agents reported as stimulators of macrophages and monocytes to release LAF had been established as exogenous pyrogens and stimulators of LP synthesis *in vitro*. However, in some studies, human monocytes apparently released LAF spontaneously without stimulation (69,42). This fact shed considerable doubt on the relationship between LP and LAF, since there is no evidence that LP is spontaneously produced from human cells (28,30,31). It was later shown that spontaneous production of LAF was actually due to minute quantities of contaminating (? endotoxin) materials (71). These studies established that both LP and LAF production can be stimulated by low [picogram (pg)] quantities of endotoxins. With these new observations, the hypothesis that LP and LAF were related substances once again became viable. This hypothesis gained further support from studies on murine cells. Murine cell lines, particularly PD388D, had been shown to produce LAF (83,84) and LP (15). In addition, early characterization of murine LAF revealed physical similarities with preliminary experiments on the molecular weight of LP produced from resident murine peritoneal macrophages (83,84,15). These latter experiments had been carried out by the late Dr. Phyllis Bodel and communicated to the present author.

In the human system, however, studies reported that the human histocytic lymphoma cell line, U937, did not produce LAF (72). This cell line has been well studied as having several characteristics of macrophages, with the notable exception of Ia-like antigens. When this cell line was activated by supernates of the human mixed leukocyte reaction (MLR), cell morphological changes, and augmentation of antibody-dependent cellular cytotoxicity against tumor cells were observed (66). Despite activation by the MLR as well as by endotoxin, U937 does not produce LAF (72). However, there is a report that U937 spontaneously releases human LP (21). This observation was made using a murine pyrogen assay which had been shown to be useful in detecting LP of rabbit, mouse, and human origin (18). Recent evidence on the chemistry of human LP using the mouse assay has revealed the presence of a small peptide breakdown product which produces fever in mice but not in rabbits (44). Thus, the difficulty in determining if U937 produces LP has not been confirmed in the rabbit pyrogen assay. If, in fact, U937 synthesizes LP but not LAF, it would be unlikely that these molecules share identity.

Nevertheless, since there is evidence that LP and LAF are physically similar molecules, experiments were designed to investigate this possibility. The first experiments were conducted using a model of macrophage-dependent murine T-cell antigen recognition (100). Soluble products of cultured adherent cells of macrophage lineage had been shown to partially replace the requirement for the macrophage in T-cell mitogen (25) as well as antigen activation (100). In the experimental system used, mice were immunized with a dinitrophenyl conjugate of egg albumin. Lymph node T-cells stimulated with the specific antigen would undergo blastogenesis only in the presence of macrophages or macrophage supernatants. These supernates were replaced by crude human LP but not crude human monocyte supernates produced in the presence of cycloheximide. Thus, these experiments suggested that proteins synthesized by human monocytes were capable of replacing murine macrophage supernates in this model. When semipurified preparations of human LP were used, similar results were obtained. Further purification of human LP using ^{125}I-labeling as a tracer was carried out, and pyrogen purified to apparent homogeneity, was capable of replacing the property of crude macrophage supernates (101). Hence these experiments suggested that human LP had properties similar to that of LAF.

In the human system, initial observations using murine lymph node T cells were confirmed in the standard LAF assay. This assay involves the stimulation of murine thymocytes with submitogenic levels of phytohemagglutinin (PHA). Supernates containing pyrogen activity at various levels of purity enhanced murine proliferation to PHA (29). Using this LAF assay, a single unit dose of human pyrogen (rabbit pyrogen dose produces 0.6° to 0.9°C peak fever in rabbits) could be diluted 10^{-6} and still produce significant enhancement of PHA responses in murine thymocytes. During sequential purification, all fractions generated during chromatographic separations were tested for their ability to produce fever in rabbits and exhibit LAF activity. In each case, these biological activities coincided in the same fractions or pools of fractions. Therefore, the human pyrogen molecule appears to have lymphocyte-activating properties, or alternatively, LP and LAF are the same molecule. Using rabbit peritoneal macrophages as a source of crude rabbit LP and rabbit LAF prepared from rabbit alveolar macrophages, similar experiments were conducted with identical results (86). Fractions on an isoelectric focusing gradient distinguished between two rabbit LPs with pIs of 4.6 and 4.7, and both peaks of pyrogen activity coincided with LAF activity. In further experiments, specific antisera raised to different preparations of rabbit LP neutralized LAF and pyrogen activity. Similar studies conducted using a sequential purification scheme of rabbit LP prepared from peritoneal exudate cells also confirmed studies by other investigators (Kampschmidt, personal communication).

These studies have considerable importance with regard to the role of fever in host defense. The potential biological consequences of LAF are far reaching. There is ample evidence that LAF and B-cell activating factor (BAF) are the same molecules (112,113); whereas LAF reflects increased T-cell activity, BAF augments antibody (IgM) production from murine B-cells. The activity of BAF seems to be a direct effect on B-cells in that the same responses are observed with splenocytes from nude mice as well as T-depleted splenocytes from normal mice. There can be little doubt that augmentation of antibody production comprises a major host-defense mechanism. Clearly, the ability of LP/LAF/BAF to stimulate cells reflects a similar process on multiple target cells for an apparently single substance. Of course, the issue as to whether LP, LAF, and BAF are identical substances awaits at least partial amino acid sequencing. However, if such sequence studies were to show microheterogeneity of amino acids from these molecules, and that they are, in fact, not identical, there still remains the significant biological mechanism that most natural activators of macrophages induce the synthesis of all three substances. The issue then settles on whether the active sites of LP, LAF, and BAF are the same. Although amino-acid differences between these molecules may exist, the essential question is whether the active site sequence and configuration is shared.

At present, the burden of proof is on the investigator who is charged with purification of these active supernatants. Studies must demonstrate either coincidence or separation of the three activities, namely, fever, T-cell activation, and increased antibody synthesis. Two approaches have been taken: a) assays of all three functions on purified material and b) assays on individual fractions under various chromatographic conditions. The first method is open to critical assessment of the purity of the preparation. Because LP/LAF/BAF are produced in monocyte cultures at pg/ml levels, purification procedures are costly and require a 10^6-fold increase in specific activity. Like the interferons, these biologically active molecules comprise less than 10^{-6} of the total protein release in cell supernatant, following activation. The second method, although producing highly convincing evidence, can only lead to the conclusion that, at the most, these molecules represent a situation of microheterogeneity.

Leukocytic Endogenous Mediator and Leukocytic Pyrogen

This term, leukocyte endogenous mediator (LEM), was introduced 20 years ago by Kampschmidt, and its role in mediating host-defense mechanisms has been suggested by several studies. These include lowering of plasma iron (53,54), lowering of plasma zinc (55), increases in plasma copper (91), release of bone marrow neutrophils (58), stimulation of granulopoiesis (57), and increased hepatic synthesis of fibrinogen (56), haptoglobin (56), alpha-1-macrofetoprotein (39), ceruloplasmin (91), and C-reactive protein (79). Studies demonstrate that LEM stimulates antimicrobial activity in that an intraperitoneal injection of LEM in rats 24 hr prior to bacterial challenge with *Salmonella typhimurium* results in an 87% survival rate (51).

These and previously mentioned studies support the concept that phagocytic cells release materials which, when administered to the same or another species, induce functional changes which can be interpreted as beneficial to the host surviving an infection. As expected, LEM also produces fever, and several studies have tried unsuccessfully to separate LP from LEM activities (59,80). Although the majority of LEM activities have been demonstrated using semipurified and even highly purified rabbit exudate cell supernatants, studies have also been carried out using supernatants from human monocytes stimulated with heat-killed staphylococci (52). In addition to producing fever, there are experiments which demonstrate that semipurified human LP increases hepatic haptoglobin synthesis *in vitro* (50), and SAA-synthesis *in vivo* (78). However, as with LAF and BAF activities being attributed to LP, the same criticism can be extended to LEM studies. Although it is apparent that the LEM molecule or group of molecules is responsible for these various activities in mediating both the acute-phase reaction as well as several parameters of increased host defenses, proof of homogeneity of these preparations comprises the ultimate judication.

CONCLUSIONS

Studies on LP have been very extensive and have established a basic concept: the host produces its own endogenous mediator(s), which is responsible for fever and for some aspect of the acute-phase reaction. Thus, the disease process, whether microbial or immunological, in addition to its direct pathological properties also serves as a stimulator of mononuclear phagocytic secretory function. How much of the acute-phase reaction is due to the direct effect of the invading microbe on the host, and how much is secondary to the release of endogenous mediators from macrophages is presently unknown. However, it is clear that the most consistent property of the endogenous mediator molecule(s) is the production of fever. The ability of LP to raise body temperature and any subsequent benefit that the host derives from this cannot be disputed. Although it is highly likely that LP is also a mediator of neutrophil degranulation, lymphocyte activation or is responsible for the acute phase reaction, the difficulties encountered in the purification of LP requires continued caution. At present, this would involve discerning the possible microheterogeneity of this and similar molecules. At present, there is no method commonly used in protein chemistry that separates these activities. Because of its potential role in mediating host-defense mechanisms during disease, the structure-function relation of LP holds the key to understanding a vital mechanism for host defenses.

ACKNOWLEDGMENTS

The author acknowledges Dr. Sheldon M. Wolff whose helpful advice and support has been indispensable in these and countless other studies on the defense mechanisms of the host.

REFERENCES

1. Arnold, R. R., Brewer, M., and Gauthier, J. J. (1980): Bactericidal activity of human lactoferrin: sensitivity of a variety of microorganisms. *Infect. Immun.*, 28:893–898.
2. Asheshov, E. H. (1966): Loss of antibiotic resistance in *Staphyloccus aureus* resulting from growth at high temperature. *J. Gen. Microbiol.*, 42:403–410.
3. Atkins, E. (1960): Pathogenesis of fever. *Physiol. Rev.*, 40:580–646.
4. Atkins, E., Bodel, P., and Francis, L. (1967): Release of an endogenous pyrogen *in vitro* from rabbit mononuclear cells. *J. Exp. Med.*, 126:357–386.
5. Atwood, R. P., and Kass, E. H. (1977): Relationship of body temperature to the lethal action of bacterial endotoxin. *J. Clin. Invest.*, 43:151–159.
6. Austin, T. W., and Truant, G. (1978): Hyperthermia, antipyretics and function of polymorphonuclear leukocytes. *Can. Med. Assoc. J.*, 118:493–495.
7. Beeson, P. B. (1948): Temperature-elevating effect of a substance obtained from polymorphonuclear leucocytes. *J. Clin. Invest.*, 27:524.
8. Bell, J. F., and Moore, G. J. (1974): Effects of high ambient temperature on various stages of rabies virus infection in mice. *Infect. Immun.*, 10:510–515.
9. Beller, D. I., and Unanue, E. R. (1977): Thymic maturation *in vitro* by a secretory product from macrophages. *J. Immunol.*, 118:1780.
10. Bennet, I. L., Jr., and Nicastri, A. (1960): Fever as a mechanism of resistance. *Bacteriol. Rev.*, 24:16–34.
11. Bernheim, H. A., Block, L. H., Francis, L., and Atkins, E. (1980): Release of endogenous pyrogen-activating factor from concanavalin A-stimulated human lymphocytes. *J. Exp. Med.*, 152:1811–1816.
12. Blyden, G., and Handschumacker, R. E. (1977): Purification and properties of human lymphocyte activating factor (LAF). *J. Immunol.*, 118:1631–1638.

13. Bodel, P. (1970): Studies on the mechanism of endogenous pyrogen production. I. Investigation of new protein synthesis in stimulated human blood leukocytes. *Yale J. Biol. Med.*, 43:145–163.
14. Bodel, P. (1974): Studies on the mechanism of endogenous pyrogen production. II. Role of cell products in the regulation of pyrogen release from blood leukocytes. *Infect. Immun.*, 10:451–457.
15. Bodel, P. (1978): Spontaneous pyrogen production by mouse histiocytic and myelomonocytic tumor cell lines *in vitro. J. Exp. Med.*, 147:1503–1516.
16. Bodel, P., and Atkins, E. (1967): Release of endogenous pyrogen by human monocytes. *N. Engl. J. Med.*, 276:1002–1008.
17. Bodel, P. T., and Hollingsworth, J. W. (1968): Pyrogen release from human synovial exudate cells. *Br. J. Exp. Pathol.*, 49:11–19.
18. Bodel, P., and Miller, H. (1976): Pyrogen from mouse macrophages causes fever in mice. *Proc. Soc. Exp. Biol. Med.*, 151:93–96.
19. Bodel, P., and Miller, H. (1978): A new sensitive method from detecting human endogenous (leukocyte) pyrogen. *Inflammation*, 3:103–110.
20. Bodel, P., Reynolds, C. F., and Atkins, E. (1973): Lack of effect of salicylate on pyrogen release from human blood leukocytes *in vitro. Yale J. Biol. Med.*, 46:190–195.
21. Bodel, P., Ralph, P., Wenc, K., and Long, J. C. (1980): Endogenous pyrogen production by Hodgkin's disease and human histiocytic lymphoma cell lines *in vitro. J. Clin. Invest.*, 65:514–518.
22. Bruetsch, W. L. (1949): Why malaria cures general paralysis. *J. Indiana State Med. Assoc.*, 42:211–216.
23. Bryant, R. E., Des Prez, R. M., Van Way, M. H., and Rogers, D. E. (1966): Studies on human leukocyte motility. I. Effect of alteration in pH, electrolyte concentration and phagocytosis on leukocyte migration, adhesiveness and aggregation. *J. Exp. Med.*, 124:483–499.
24. Bynum, G. D., Pandolf, K. B., Schuette, W. H., Goldman, R. F., Lees, D. E., Whang-Peng, J., Atkison, E. R., and Bull, J. M. (1978): Induced hyperthermia in sedated humans and the concept of critical thermal maximum. *Am. J. Physiol.*, 235:R228–236.
25. Calderon, J., Kiely, S. M., Lefko, S. L., and Unanue, E. R. (1975): The modulation of lymphocyte functions by molecules secreted by macrophages. I. Description and partial biochemical analysis. *J. Exp. Med.*, 142:151–160.
26. Dickson, J. A. (1979): Hyperthermia in the treatment of cancer. *Lancet*, 1:202–205.
27. DiJoseph, C. G., Bayer, M. E., and Kaji, A. (1973): Host cell growth in the presence of the thermosensitive drug resistance factor. *J. Bacteriol.*, 115:399–410.
28. Dinarello, C. A. (1979): Production of endogenous pyrogen. *Fed. Proc.*, 38:52–56.
29. Dinarello, C. A., and Rosenwasser, L. J. (1981): Lymphocyte activating properties of human leukocytic pyrogen. In: *Advances in Immunopharmacology*, edited by J. W. Hadden, P. Mullen, L. Chedid, and F. Spreafice, pp. 419–425. Pergamon Press, Oxford.
30. Dinarello, C. A., and Wolff, S. M. (1978): Pathogenesis of fever in man. *N. Engl. J. Med.*, 298:607–612.
31. Dinarello, C. A., and Wolff, S. M. (1979): Mechanisms in the production of fever in humans. *Semin. Infect. Dis.*, 2:173–192.
32. Dinarello, C. A., Bodel, P., and Atkins, E. (1968): The role of the liver in the production of fever and in pyrogenic tolerance. *Trans. Assoc. Am. Physicians*, 81:334–344.
33. Dinarello, C. A., Goldin, N. P., and Wolff, S. M. (1974): Demonstration and characterization of two distinct human leukocytic pyrogens. *J. Exp. Med.*, 139:1369–1381.
34. Dinarello, C. A., LoPreste, G., and Wolff, S. M. (1980): Human blood lymphocytes produce an endogenous pyrogen-inducing factor. *Clin. Res.*, 28:367A.
35. Dinarello, C. A., Renfer, L., and Wolff, S. M. (1977): Human leukocytic pyrogen: Purification and development of a radioimmunoassay. *Proc. Natl. Acad. Sci. U.S.A.*, 74:4623–4627.
36. Dinarello, C. A., Elin, R. J., Chedid, L., and Wolff, S. M. (1978): The pyrogenicity of synthetic adjuvants muramyl dipetide and two structural analogues. *J. Infect. Dis.*, 138:760–767.
37. Dubois, E. F. (1949): Why are fever temperatures over 106°F rare? *Am. J. Med. Sci.*, 17:361–368.
38. DuPont, H. L., and Spink, W. W. (1969): Infections due to gram-negative organisms: an analysis of 860 patients with bacteremia at the Univ. of Minn. Medical Center 1958–1966. *Medicine*, 48:307–332.

39. Eddington, C. L., Upchurch, H. F, and Kampschmidt, R. (1972): Quantitation of plasma alpha-Z AP globulin before and after stimulation with leukocyte extincts. *Proc. Soc. Exp. Biol. Med.*, 139:565–569.
40. Elin, R. J., and Wolff, S. M. (1974): The role of iron in nonspecific resistance to infection induced by endotoxin. *J. Immunol.*, 112:737–745.
41 Enders, J. F., and Shatter, M. F. (1936): Studies on natural immunity to pneumococcus type III. I. The capacity of strains of pneumococcus type III to grow at 41°C and their virulence for rabbits. *J. Exp. Med.*, 67:1–18.
42. Farrar, J. S., Koopman, W. S., and Fuller-Bonar, J. (1977): Identification and partial purification of two synergistically acting helper mediators in human mixed leukocyte culture supernatants. *J. Immunol.*, 119:47–53.
43. Gibson, J. G., and Kopp, I. (1938): Studies in the physiology of artificial fever. I. Changes in the blood volume and water balance. *J. Clin. Invest.*, 17:219.
44. Gordon, A. H., and Parker, I. D. (1980): A pyrogen from human cells which is active in mice. *Br. J. Exp. Pathol.*, 61:534–539.
45. Grieger, T. A., and Kluger, M. J. (1978): Fever and survival: The role of serum iron. *J. Physiol.*, 279:187–196.
46. Haeseler, F., Bodel, P., and Atkins, E. (1977): Characteristics of pyrogen production by isolated rabbit Kupffer cells *in vitro. J. Reticuloendothel Soc.*, 22:569–581.
47. Hahn, H. H., Char, D. C., Postel, W. B., and Wood, W. B., Jr. (1967): Studies on the pathogenesis of fever. XV. The production of endogenous pyrogen by peritoneal macrophages. *J. Exp. Med.*, 126:385–394.
48. Hanson, D. F., Murphy, P. A., and Windle, B. E. (1980): Failure of rabbit neutrophils to secrete endogenous pyrogen when stimulated with staphylococci. *J. Exp. Med.*, 151:1360–1371.
49. Hoffman-Goetz, L., and Kluger, M. J. (1979): Protein deprivation: its effect on fever and plasma iron during bacterial infection in rabbits. *J. Physiol.*, 295:419–430.
50. Hooper, D. C., Steer, C. J., Dinarello, C. A., and Peacock, A. C. (1981): Haptoglobin and albumin synthesis in isolated rat hepatocytes. Response to potential mediators of the acute-phase reaction. *Biochem. Biophys. Acta*, 653:118–129.
51. Kampschmidt, R., and Pulliam, L. (1975): Stimulation of antimicrobial activity in the rat with leukocytic endogenous mediator. *J. Reticuloendothelial Soc.*, 17:162–169.
52. Kampschmidt, R. F., and Pulliam, L. A. (1978): Effect of human monocyte pyrogen on plasma iron, plasma zinc, and blood neutrophils in rabbits and rats. *Proc. Soc. Exp. Biol. Med.*, 158:32.
53. Kampschmidt, R. F., and Upchurch, H. (1969): Lowering of plasma iron concentration in the rat with leukocytic extracts. *Am. J. Physiol.*, 216:1287–1291.
54. Kampschmidt, R. F., and Upchurch, H. F. (1970): A comparison of the effects of rabbit endogenous pyrogen on the body temperature of the rabbit and lowering of plasma iron in the rat. *Proc. Soc. Exp. Biol. Med.*, 133:128–130.
55. Kampschmidt, R. F., and Upchurch, H. F. (1970): The effect of endogenous pyrogen on the plasma zinc concentration of the rat. *Proc. Soc. Exp. Biol. Med.*, 134:1150–1152.
56. Kampschmidt, R. F., and Upchurch, H. F. (1974): Effect of leukocytic endogenous mediator on plasma fibrinogen and haptoglobin. *Proc. Soc. Exp. Biol. Med.*, 146:904–907.
57. Kampschmidt, R., and Upchurch, H. F. (1977): Possible involvement of leukocytic endogenous mediator in granulopoiesis. *Proc. Soc. Exp. Biol. Med.*, 155:89–93.
58. Kampschmidt, R. F., Long, R. D., and Upchurch, H. F. (1972): Neutrophil releasing activity in rats injected with endogenous pyrogen. *Proc. Soc. Exp. Biol. Med.*, 139:1224–1226.
59. Kampschmidt, R. F., Upchurch, H. F., Eddington, C. L., and Pulliam, L. A. (1973): Multiple biological activities of a partially purified leukocytic endogenous mediator. *Am. J. Physiol.*, 224:530–533.
60. Klastersky, J., and Kass, E. H. (1970): Is suppression of fever or hypothermia useful in experimental and clinical infectious diseases? *J. Infect. Dis.*, 121:81–85.
61. Klempner, M. S., Dinarello, C. A., and Gallin, J. I. (1978): Human leukocytic pyrogen induces release of specific granule contents from human neutrophils. *J. Clin. Invest.*, 61:1330–1336.
62. Klempner, M. S., Dinarello, C. A., Henderson, W. R., and Gallin, J. I. (1979): Stimulation of human neutrophil oxygen metabolism by leukocytic pyrogen. *J. Clin. Invest.*, 64:996–1002.
63. Kluger, M. J., Ringler, D. H., and Anver, M. R. (1975): Fever and survival. *Science*, 188:166–168.

64. Kluger, M. J., and Vaughn, L. K. (1978): Fever and survival in rabbits infected with *Pasteurella multocida*. *J. Physiol.*, 282:243–251.
65. Kochan, I. (1977): Role of iron in the regulation of nutritional immunity. *Adv. Chem.*, 162:55–77.
66. Koren, H. S., Anderson, S. J., and Larrick, J. W. (1979): *In vitro* activation of a human macrophage-like cell line. *Nature (London)*, 279:328–330.
67. Kreger, B. E., Craven, D. E., Carling, P. C., and McCabe, W. R. (1980): Gram-negative bacteremia. IV. Reassessment of etiology, epidemiology and ecology in 612 patients. *Am. J. Med.*, 68:332–343.
68. Lace, J. K., Tan, J. S., and Watanakumakorn, C. (1978): An appraisal of the nitroblue tetrazolium reduction test. *Am. J. Med.*, 58:685–694.
69. Lachman, L. B. (1978): Purification and properties of human lymphocyte activating factor from unstimulated leukocyte cultures. *Fed. Proc.*, 37:1589.
70. Lachman, L. B. (1980): Purification of human interleukin I. *J. Supramol. Struc.*, 13:457–471.
71. Lachman, L. B., and Metzgar, R. S. (1980): Purification and characterization of human lymphocyte activating factor. In: *Biochemical Characterization of Lymphokines*, edited by A. L. deWeck, F. Kristensen, M. Landy, pp. 405–409. Academic Press, New York.
72. Lachman, L. B., Moore, J. O., and Metzgar, R. S. (1978): Preparation and characterization of lymphocyte-activating factor (LAF) from acute monocytic and myelomonocytic leukemia cells. *Cell. Immunol.*, 41:199–206.
73. Ledingham, J. C. G. (1908): The influence of temperature in phagocytosis. *Proc. R. Soc. Lond.*, 80:188–195.
74. Lwoff, A. (1959): Factors influencing the evolution of viral diseases at the cellular level and in the organism. *Bacteriol. Rev.*, 23:109–124.
75. Mackowiak, P. A. (1979): Clinical uses of microorganisms and their products. *Am. J. Med.*, 67:293–306.
76. Mandell, G. L. (1975): Effect of temperature on phagocytosis by human polymorphonuclear neutrophils. *Infect. Immun.*, 12:221–225.
77. Manzella, J. P., and Roberts, N. J., Jr. (1979): Human macrophage and lymphocyte responses to mitogen stimulation after exposure to influenza virus, ascorbic acid and hyperthermia. *J. Immunol.*, 123:1940–1944.
78. McAdam, K. P. W. J., and Dinarello, C. A. (1980): Induction of serum amyloid A synthesis by human leukocytic pyrogen. In: *Bacterial Endotoxins and Host Response*, edited by M. K. Agarwal, pp. 167–178. Elsevier North-Holland, Amsterdam.
79. Merriman, C. R., Pulliam, L. A., and Kampschmidt, R. F. (1975): Effect of leukocytic endogenous mediator on C-reactive protein in rabbits. *Proc. Soc. Exp. Biol. Med.*, 149:782–784.
80. Merriman, C. R., Pulliam, L. A., and Kampschmidt, R. F. (1977): Comparison of leukocytic pyrogen and leukocytic endogenous mediator. *Proc. Soc. Exp. Biol. Med.*, 154:224–227.
81. Mitchell, M. S. (1976): Studies on the immunological effects of BCG and its components: theoretical and therapeutic implications. *Biomedicine*, 24:209–213.
82. Mitchell, R. H., Gander, G. W., and Goodale, F. (1976): The role of phagocytosis in the production of endogenous pyrogen by polymorphonuclear leukocytes. *Adv. Exp. Med. Biol.*, 73:257–266.
83. Mizel, S. B. (1979): Biochemical and biological characterization of lymphocyte-activating factor (LAF) produced by the murine macrophage cell line, P388D. *Ann. N.Y. Acad. Sci.*, 332:539–549.
84. Mizel, S. B., Rosenstreich, D. L., and Oppenheim, J. J. (1978): Phorbol myristic acetate stimulates LAF production by the macrophage cell line, P388D. *Cell. Immunol.*, 40:230–235.
85. Moore, D. M., Murphy, P. A., Chesney, J. P., and Wood, W. B., Jr. (1973): Synthesis of endogenous pyrogen by rabbit leukocytes. *J. Exp. Med.*, 137:1263–1274.
86. Murphy, P. A., Simon, P. L., and Willoughby, W. F. (1980): Endogenous pyrogens made by rabbit peritoneal exudate cells are identical with lymphocyte-activating factors made by rabbit alveolar macrophages. *J. Immunol.*, 124:2498–2501.
87. Nahas, G. G., Tannieres, M. L., and Lennon, J. F. (1971): Direct measurement of leukocyte motility: effect of pH and temperature. *Proc. Soc. Exp. Biol. Med.*, 138:350–352.
88. Nordlund, J. J., Root, R. K., and Wolff, S. M. (1970): Studies on the origin of human leukocytic pyrogen. *J. Exp. Med.*, 131:727–743.

89. Oettgen, H. F., Hoffman, M. K., Clarkson, B. F., and Old, L. J. (1979): Effect of endotoxin and endotoxin-induced mediators on cancer and the immune system. In: *The Role of Non-specific Immunity in the Prevention and Treatment of Cancer*, edited by C. Chagas, pp. 121–145. Pontifical Academy of Science, Vatican City.

90. Parant, M., Riveau, G., Parant, F., Dinarello, C. A., Wolff, S. M., and Chedid, L. (1980): Effect of indomethacin on increased resistance to infection and on febrile responses induced by muramyl dipeptide. *J. Infect. Dis.*, 142:708–715.

91. Pekarek, R. S., Powanda, M. C., and Wannemackes, R. W., Jr. (1972): The effect of leukocytic endogenous mediator (LEM) on serum copper and ceruloplasma in concentration in the rat. *Proc. Soc. Exp. Biol. Med.*, 141:1029–1031.

92. Peterson, P. K., Verhoef, J., Sabath, L. D., and Oruie, P. G. (1976): Extracellular and bacterial factors influencing staphylococcal phagocytosis and killing by human polymorphonuclear leukocytes. *Infect. Immun.*, 14:496–501.

93. Phelps, P., and Stanislaw, D. (1969): Polymorphonuclear leukocyte motility *in vitro*. I. Effect of pH, temperature, ethyl alcohol and caffeine using a modified Boyden chamber technique. *Arthritis Rheum.*, 12:181–188.

94. Puri, J., Shinitzky, M., and Lonai, P. (1980): Concomitant increase in antigen binding and in T cell membrane lipid viscosity induced by the lymphocyte-activating factor, LAF. *J. Immunol.*, 124:1937–1942.

95. Roberts, N. J. (1979): Temperature and host defense. *Microbiol. Rev.*, 43:241–259.

96. Roberts, N. J., Jr., and Sandberg, K. (1979): Hyperthermia and human leukocyte function. II. Enhanced production of and response to leukocyte migration inhibition factor (LIF). *J. Immunol.*, 122:1990–1993.

97. Roberts, N. J., Jr., and Steigbigel, R. T. (1977): Hyperthermia and human leukocyte functions: Effects on response of lymphocytes to mitogen and antigen and bactericidal capacity of monocytes and neutrophils. *Infect. Immun.*, 18:673–679.

98. Root, R. K., Nordlund, J. J., and Wolff, S. M. (1970): Factors affecting the quantitative production and assay of human leukocytic pyrogen. *J. Lab. Clin. Med.*, 75:679–693.

99. Rosenthal, A. S. (1980): Regulation of the immune response—role of the macrophage. *N. Engl. J. Med.*, 303:1153–1156.

100. Rosenwasser, L. J., and Rosenthal, A. S. (1978): Adherent cell function in murine T lymphocyte antigen recognition. I. A macrophage dependent T cell proliferation assay in the mouse. *J. Immunol.*, 120:1991–2001.

101. Rosenwasser, L. J., Dinarello, C. A., and Rosenthal, A. S. (1979): Adherent cell function in murine T-lymphocyte antigen recognition. IV. Enhancement of murine T-cell antigen recognition by human leukocytic pyrogen. *J. Exp. Med.*, 150:709–714.

102. Ruderman, A., Mackowiak, P., and Smith, J. (1978): Enhanced *in vitro* activity of antibiotics at physiologically elevated temperatures. *Clin. Res.*, 26:771A.

103. Sanders, F., Crawford, E. S., DeBakey, M. E. (1957): Effects of hypothermia on experimental intracutaneous pneumococcal infection in rabbits. *Surg. Forum*, 8:92–97.

104. Sebag, J., Reed, W. P., and Williams, R. C., Jr. (1977): Effect of temperature on bacterial killing by serum and by polymorphonuclear leukocytes. *Infect. Immun.*, 16:947–954.

105. Sobocinski, P. Z., McCarthy, J. P., and Critz, W. J. (1980): Stimulation of granulocyte chemiluminescence by endogenous pyrogen: possible relationship to protection against lethal bacterial infection. *Fed. Proc.*, 39:1913.

106. Togawa, A., Oppenheim, J. J., and Mizel, S. B. (1979): Characterization of lymphocyte-activating factor (LAF) produced by human mononuclear cells: biochemical relationship of high and low molecular weight forms of LAF. *J. Immunol.*, 122:2112–2118.

107. Unanue, E. R. (1978): The regulation of lymphocyte functions by the macrophage. *Immunol. Rev.*, 40:227–254.

108. Wagner-Jauregg, J. (1927): The treatment of dementia paralytica by malaria inoculation. In: *Nobel Lectures: Physiology or Medicine, 1992–1941*, pp. 159–169. Elsevier North-Holland, New York.

109. Wallach, D. F. H. (1977): Basic mechanism in tumor thermotherapy. *J. Mol. Med.*, 2:381–403.

110. Weinberg, E. D. (1966): Roles of metallic ions in host-parasite interactions. *Bacteriol. Rev.*, 30:136–146.

111. Wolff, S. M. (1973): Biological effects of bacterial endotoxins in man. *J. Infect. Dis.*, 128:251–256.

112. Wood, D. D. (1979): Purification and properties of human B-cell activating factor. *J. Immunol.*, 123:2395–2400.
113. Wood, D. D. (1979): Mechanism of action of human B cell-activating factor. *J. Immunol.*, 123:2406–2407.

Advances in Host Defense Mechanisms, Vol. 1,
edited by John I. Gallin and Anthony S. Fauci,
Raven Press, New York © 1982.

The Neutrophil as a Secretory Organ
of Host Defense

Daniel G. Wright

*Department of Hematology, Walter Reed Army Institute of Research,
Washington, DC 20012; USUHS School of Medicine, Bethesda, Maryland 20014*

Discoveries made during the 19th century demonstrating the importance of infectious microorganisms in human disease, provoked great interest in the physiologic response of the body to infection. It was at this time that the biology of inflammation was first carefully studied and accurately described. In 1882 Julius Cohnheim presented his lectures on the microscopic vascular events that occur in acutely inflamed tissues, as he observed them in the mesentery and tongue of the frog. His descriptions of capillary dilation, transudation of fluid, sticking of leukocytes to capillary walls, and migration of the leukocytes into extravascular spaces have retained their validity throughout a century of derivative research (37).

It was also at this time that Metchnikoff conducted his celebrated experiments through which he recognized the importance of inflammation and inflammatory leukocytes in protecting the body against infection. "The diapedesis of the white corpuscles, their migration through the vessel wall into the tissues, is one of the principal means of defense possessed by the animal. As soon as the infective agents have penetrated into the body, a whole army of white corpuscles proceed towards the menaced spot, there entering into a struggle with the microorganisms. . . . The leukocytes, having arrived at the spot where the intruders are found, seize them after the manner of Amoebae and within their bodies subject them to intracellular digestion (139)." In describing phagocytosis, Metchnikoff recognized that "cytases," which mediated the intracellular digestion of phagocytized microbes, were most likely derived from cytoplasmic granules that characterized inflammatory phagocytes (neutrophils). He concluded from his studies, however, that these cytases were not released by the cells during their normal function. "The cytases must be grouped with the soluble ferments which are not thrown off by the phagocytes as long as these (cells) remain intact (139)."

This conclusion opposed the hypothesis promoted by some of Metchnikoff's contemporaries (including Paul Ehrlich) that a function of inflammatory leukocytes was to secrete microbicidal substances at sites of infection. In 1887 Ehrlich published a paper titled, "On the significance of the neutrophil granules (49)," in which he described the characteristic granulated morphology of neutrophils that distinguished them from other leukocytes, and he speculated that neutrophils secreted substances that were stored in these granules. Ehrlich summarized this concept in a subsequent lecture on leukocytes given in 1900: "It is likely that the leukocyte granulations are in fact secretory products which the cell dissolves and spreads to the environment as needed. One can recall, in favor of this opinion, ... the results of Hankin and Janowsky, who noted a progressive decrease in the numbers of these granulations in polymorphonuclear leukocytes during emigration, results which are easy to explain if one admits that these granulations are extruded by the protoplasm which contains them. This hypothesis ... will only be proven the day that it is possible to characterize chemically the various types of leukocyte granules (49)."

During the 70 years that followed this lecture, Ehrlich's concept of neutrophils as secretory cells was largely put aside in favor of the Metchnikoffian view that the principal host-defense functions of these cells are phagocytosis and the intracellular killing of microorganisms. In recent years, however, much as Ehrlich predicted, a more detailed understanding of the contents and function of neutrophil granules has revitalized his concept, for it is now increasingly evident that secretory events are intrinsic to the normal host-defense functions of neutrophils in inflammation.

This chapter presents a review of recent experimental information which supports the validity of considering the neutrophil as a secretory cell. This review summarizes current knowledge about the development of granules in neutrophil precursor cells, the contents of these granules, functional distinctions among granule subtypes, and the extracellular release of granule constituents. This review also summarizes information concerning secretory products of neutrophils not derived from granules and discusses the consequences of neutrophil secretion for host defense. It should be noted at the outset that in this review the term "secretion" is applied to several different cellular processes: the extracellular release of substances stored in membrane-bound organelles (granules), the synthesis and direct transport of proteins to the outside of the cell, and the release of plasma-membrane constituents or metabolites at the cell surface.

THE DEVELOPMENT AND CONTENT OF NEUTROPHIL GRANULES

In healthy human beings, neutrophils develop from undifferentiated hematopoietic stem cells only in the bone marrow, and they spend most of their brief life-span there. Commitment of myeloid precursor cells to differentiation into neutrophils is clearly recognizable only with the development of cytoplasmic granules in these cells, which occurs at the promyelocyte stage. Promyelocytes are relatively large cells (approximately 15 μm diameter), which are recognizable because of their large, prominant cytoplasmic granules that have a deep purple-red color in Wright-Giemsa-stained preparations. The striking morphology of these cells was noted by early students of bone marrow histology who used the term azurophil granules for the promyelocyte granulations in recognition of their affinity for the azure dyes of blood stains (10,13,188). As human promyelocytes mature into myelocytes, the granulations lose their azurophilic properties and become neutrophilic, in that they are colored by both acidic and basic dyes. The neutrophilic staining of early myelocytes begins in an area adjacent to the nucleus (the so-called dawn or sunrise of neutrophilia) and then spreads throughout the cytoplasm as myelocytes develop into metamyelocytes and mature neutrophils. The neutrophilic granulations of these more mature cells were called specific granules by early hematologists in that they were specific for neutrophils and distinguished them from other granulocytes (eosinophils and basophils), which were characterized by their own specific granules (12,13,17,225).

It is now recognized, however, that the sequential appearance of azurophilic and specific granulations in neutrophil precursors does not simply represent an evolution in the staining characteristics of the neutrophil granules, but reflects the formation of two distinct types of granules, both of which are present in the mature cell. Electron-microscopic studies of bone marrow cells, using cytochemical techniques that permit staining of granule-associated enzymes, have shown that the azurophil granules, formed during the promyelocyte stage, contain peroxidase and remain with the cell throughout its maturation (Fig. 1). The appearance of neutrophilia in early myelocytes reflects the production of a second type of granule which is peroxidase-negative and ultimately outnumbers the peroxidase-positive granules by more than two to one (1,10,13,181). The terms primary and secondary are now used to classify the peroxidase-positive and peroxidase-negative granules, respectively, in recognition of their sequential development in neutrophil precursor cells (13,224). However, the older terms azurophil granules and specific granules are still commonly used in referring to the primary (peroxidase-positive) and secondary (peroxidase-negative) granules, although these terms are somewhat misleading given their original meaning. In any case, the distinction between primary and secondary granules is important, for, as will be discussed below, the neutrophil mobilizes and uses these organelles in somewhat different ways.

Electron-microscopic studies have shown that both species of granules have a limiting unit membrane that is about 70 to 90 Å in width with a trilaminar structure (1,10,13,224). Although the secondary granules of human neutrophils tend to be smaller and more pleomorphic than the peroxidase-positive, primary granules, the ultrastructural morphology of both the primary and secondary granules is quite heterogeneous, and these distinct granule species can be distinguished reliably in the mature cell only with the aid of cytochemical techniques (13). Primary and secondary granules of rabbit heterophils, on the other hand, can be distinguished reasonably well by their ultrastructural morphology alone. Some investigators have concluded from studies with rabbits that a third type of granule (tertiary) may be distinguished in developing and mature heterophils (147,224). So-called tertiary granules have also been described in electromicrographs of mature human neutrophils (21, 181). However, there is, as yet, no general agreement on the validity or significance of a third type of neutrophil granule.

The contents of neutrophil granules have been studied extensively both by cytochemical techniques and by direct biochemical analysis of isolated granules that have been physically separated from other cellular constituents. Early studies with

MARROW (development, 14 days)

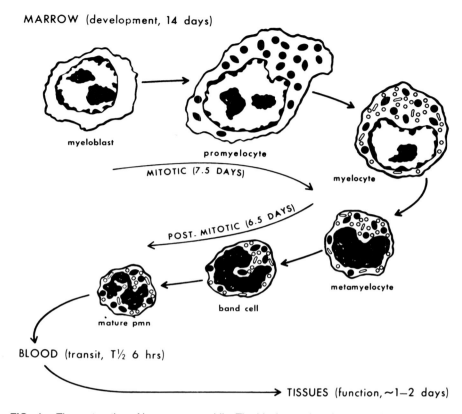

FIG. 1. The maturation of human neutrophils. The black cytoplasmic granule forms represent the peroxidase-positive, primary (or azurophil) granules; the open granule forms represent the peroxidase-negative, secondary (or specific) granules. [From Bainton et al. (13); reproduced by permission of *J. of Exp. Med.*].

crude granule isolates prepared from lysates of rabbit heterophils by differential centrifugation (36) demonstrated that these organelles contained a variety of acid hydrolases such as acid phosphatase and β-glucuronidase, which were characteristic of lysosomes found in other cell types (36,46,98). Moreover, as was characteristic of lysosomes, these acid hydrolases demonstrated latency in that they were fully active only with lysis of the granules and solubilization of the granule contents (36). Lysosomal acid hydrolases (acid phosphatase, arylsulfatase, 5'-nucleotidase, β-glucuronidase, β-galactosidase, and indoxyl esterase) were also identified in rabbit heterophil and/or human neutrophil granules by cytochemical techniques but only in the primary (azurophil) granules of these cells (11,13,223,224). At the same time, it was recognized that other enzymes not characteristic of the lysosomes of other tissues (e.g., lysozyme, alkaline phosphatase, peroxidase, and neutral proteases) were also found in these granules (36,180,231). Nonetheless, the evident analogies between neutrophil granules and lysosomes which had been shown to

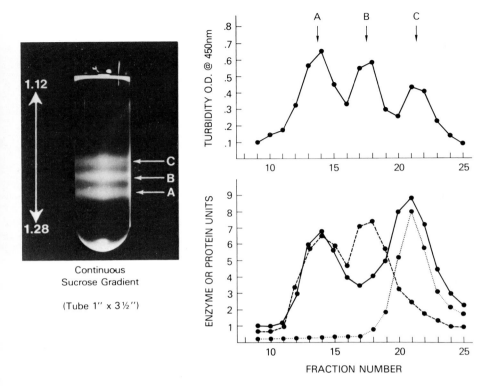

FIG. 2. Analysis of the granule content of human neutrophils by sucrose density gradient techniques. Continuous sucrose gradient is of a range of specific gravities from 1.12 to 1.28; granule separation is from a lysate of 10⁸ neutrophils. In fractionation of the gradient shown at the right, the granule-rich bands A, B, and C were located by optical density measurement of the fractions. Enzyme or protein units represent: *(solid line)* lysozyme: *(dashed line)* β-glucuronidase; *(dotted line)* Vitamin B₁₂-binding protein.

mediate intracellular digestive processes in other cells (36,46,98,212) led to the common use of the term lysosomes when referring to neutrophil granules, a practice that is somewhat misleading (as discussed further below) given the original definition of the lysosome organelle (46).

A significant advance in understanding the content and function of neutrophil granules followed the development of techniques that permitted separation and partial purification of the two distinct types of granules (primary and secondary), which had been shown by cytochemical studies to exist in mature neutrophils. This was accomplished originally by Baggiolini and co-workers with rabbit heterophils (5) and subsequently with human neutrophils (7,8) using zonal centrifugation techniques. However, greater resolution in separating primary and secondary granules, particularly with human neutrophils, has been achieved using isopycnic density gradient centrifugation with continuous sucrose gradients (7,23,112,192,222,239) as illustrated in Fig. 2. Using these techniques, it has been shown that the peroxidase-positive, primary (azurophil) granules from human neutrophils can be resolved into two distinct populations of different densities, s.g. $\simeq 1.22$ and 1.20, respectively (222), [bands A and B in Fig. 2, which are equivalent to bands IIIf and IIIs as described by Spitznagel and co-workers (192)]. The secondary (specific) granules of human neutrophils are resolved by these techniques into a single band of relatively uniform density, s.g. $\simeq 1.18$. Direct biochemical analysis of the isolated granules has confirmed that lysosomal acid hydrolases are contained only in the peroxidase-positive, primary (or azurophil) granules (23,192,222). Moreover, these granules contain all of the granule-associated neutral proteases that have been recovered from neutrophils, with the exception of collagenase (148,190,240). Known constituents of primary (azurophil) and secondary (specific) granules in human neutrophils, demonstrated either with cytochemical or with isolation techniques, are listed in Table 1.

It is apparent from Table 1 that secondary granules, the most numerous type of cytoplasmic granule in neutrophils, are quite distinct from lysosomes with respect to their content. Of note, alkaline phosphatase, which was long considered the classic histochemical marker for secondary granules (13,224), is not found to be associated with secondary granules when these granules are isolated from human neutrophils (23,192,222), and, at present, the most specific biochemical markers for neutrophil secondary granules are lactoferrin and Vitamin B_{12}-binding protein

TABLE 1. *Known constituents of human neutrophil granules[a]*

Primary (azurophil) granules	Secondary (specific) granules
Acid hydrolases	Lysozyme
Acid β-glycerophosphatase	Lactoferrin
β-glucuronidase	
N-acetyl-β-glucosaminidase	Vitamin B_{12}-binding protein
	(cobalophilin)
α-mannosidase	
Arylsulfatase	
β-galactosidase	Collagenase[b]
5′-nucleotidase	
α-fucosidase	Acidic proteins
Acid protease (cathepsin)	
Neutral proteases	
Chymotrypsinlike protease	
Elastase	
Collagenase	
Cationic proteins	
Myeloperoxidase	
Lysozyme	
Acid mucopolysaccharide	

[a]Adapted from Klebanoff and Clark (115).
[b]Secondary granule collagenase is released as a latent enzyme (240).

(cobalophilin) (6,112,125,164,237). Collagenase and lysozyme have been recovered from both the primary and secondary granules, although the collagenases found in the primary and secondary granules appear to be different enzymes (240), and lysozyme is associated with only one of the two primary granule populations separable by density centrifugation (192,222,239). It is likely that additional granule components will be identified with further study, for a number of biologically active granule components have been described which await further characterization. For example, a constituent of the secondary granules of human neutrophils has been shown to activate the complement system in fresh serum (236). Also, secondary granule lysates have been shown to stimulate monocyte migration and their transformation into macrophages *in vitro* (238). However, the relationship of these mediators to previously identified secondary granule components remains unclear. Certain granule components listed in Table 1 will be considered in more detail in the following section, with discussion of their extracellular release.

In addition to differences in the timing of primary and secondary granule formation during neutrophil maturation, and differences in their content, there are also differences in their locus of formation within the cell. Ultrastructural studies of both rabbit and human bone marrow have indicated that granules originate at a complex, central Golgi structure which remains with neutrophil precursors through the myelocyte stage (1,10,13,225). In promyelocytes, numerous ribosomes, both free in the cytoplasm and associated with endoplasmic reticulum membranes, permit the very active synthesis of proteins by these cells. Proteins, such as peroxidase, which are ultimately packaged into granules, have been shown to be formed in the endoplasmic reticulum and their associated membrane cisternae and then apparently transported to stacks of membrane lamellae in the Golgi complex. There, marker proteins are concentrated in membrane buds which develop into cytoplasmic granules. The budding of Golgi membrane that appears to lead to primary granule formation occurs at the inner, concave surface of the membrane lamellae facing the centrally located centrioles. In myelocytes, on the other hand, membrane buds leading to secondary granule formation appear at the outside surface of the Golgi lamellae (10,225).

Whereas budded, progranule vesicles appear to fuse with one another as the granules mature, primary and secondary granules normally remain separate from one another (13). In the abnormal formation of giant granules in Chediak-Higashi disease, however, fusion of primary and secondary granules does appear to occur (167). In other types of cells (e.g., fibroblasts), formation of lysosomal organelles has been shown to involve a complex process with extracellular transport of synthesized protein followed by endocytosis of this protein, which is then concentrated into lysosomes (176). As yet, however, there is no evidence that a comparable process occurs in the formation of granules by neutrophil precursor cells.

DEGRANULATION AND EXTRACELLULAR RELEASE OF GRANULE CONTENTS

The loss of granulations from neutrophils engaged in inflammatory responses did not escape the notice of Ehrlich, Metchnikoff, and contemporary investigators. But, as noted above, the significance of granule loss was a matter of dispute. Early cytochemical studies by Graham in 1920, however, specifically related degranulation to the process of phagocytosis: "Very marked changes in the granules may readily be determined by the study of leukocytes engaged in phagocytosis, as for example . . . in smears of pus . . . When such preparations are stained with a 'peroxidase' reagent, interesting examples of the more or less complete disappearance of the granules from individual cells may be obtained. . . . In general, the granules disappear from the leukocytes progressively as the number of bacterial inclusions in the cell increases (71)." Subsequent studies by Robineaux and Frederick (169) and Hirsch and Cohn (95,96), using phase contrast microscopy, more clearly defined the degranulation of neutrophils which accompanied phagocytosis. The studies of Hirsch (95) using microcinematography were particularly revealing in showing that degranulation occurred almost explosively at the borders of phagocytic vacuoles. This process was most readily observed with chicken and rabbit polymorphonuclear leukocytes because of their relatively large cytoplasmic granules but clearly occurred comparably in phagocytizing human neutrophils. Subsequent ultrastructural studies showed that degranulation resulted from the fusion of granule membranes with the membrane of a phagocytic vacuole, followed by extrusion of granule contents into the vacuole as the granule membranes were incorporated into that of the vacuole (247). These observations defined, at least in part, the mechanism by which Metchnikoff's "digestive ferments" were delivered to the phagocytic vacuole.

Initial biochemical and cell fractionation studies by Cohn and Hirsch using rabbit exudate cells (36,96) indicated that degranulation during phagocytosis was an entirely intracellular phenomenon. These findings were consistent with the concept that neutrophil granules were lysosomes that subserved intracellular digestive processes as in other types of cells (46,212). These studies were also consistent with the original concept of Metchnikoff, who concluded that the neutrophil's "digestive ferments" were normally not "thrown off by the phagocytes." It was recognized at the same time, however, that injury to neutrophils could result in the extracellular release of their lysosomal constituents. There was, in this regard, considerable interest in the effects of the streptococcal exotoxins or streptolysins (97,230,246), and the staphyloccal toxin, leukocidin (228,231), on neutrophils. These toxins were observed to cause degranulation and lysis of the cells *in vitro* with extracellular release of granule contents (97,213,228,230,231,246). This phenomenon appeared to be relevant to the pathogenesis of tissue destruction that characterized infections with these organisms, but it was distinct from the normal intracellular function of neutrophil granules during phagocytosis (97,213,228).

Subsequent studies in various laboratories, however, demonstrated that significant extracellular release of granule constituents by viable, intact neutrophils could also occur during phagocytosis (4,27,40,83,87,88,109,125,136,163,166,215,233,247). The extent of extracellular release during phagocytosis was found to be dependent on the degree of phagocytic challenge (e.g., the number of particles: neutrophils) (88,215,233), the type of particle ingested (85,88,89,93,197,216), and the particular granule component under study (e.g., for a given phagocytic challenge, lysozyme and lactoferrin were noted to be much more accessible for extracellular release by neutrophils than were acid hydrolases or peroxidase) (125,233). Ultrastructural studies demonstrated that extracellular release of granule constituents during phagocytosis occurred when granules fused with phagocytic vacuoles as they were forming at the surface of a cell and were still open to the exterior (9,90,100, 215,247). These observations suggested that under certain conditions of phagocytosis, neutrophils were untidy eaters, and the term "regurgitation while feeding" was coined to describe this phenomenon (216).

In related studies, Henson (87,88) observed that if a surface was "opsonized" by antigen-antibody complexes and complement, neutrophils would attach to and spread against the surface and then undergo degranulation at the plasma membrane adjacent to it, as if the surface had been internalized—a phenomenon called "frustrated phagocytosis." Under these conditions, extracellular release of granule constituents appeared to result from the exteriorization of a normally intracellular event. Extracellular degranulation by neutrophils was also found to be promoted when cells were treated with cytochalasin B. This agent interferes with the microfilamentous, contractile elements of neutrophils (221), and cells treated with it lose their ability to ingest particles (44,45,133,245). Nonetheless, cytochalasin-B-treated neutrophils attach to opsonized particles and undergo extracellular degranulation at the sites of particle attachment (43,44,100,185,216,249).

Each of these experimental observations emphasized that although degranulation is associated with phagocytosis, it is not dependent on phagocytosis. These observations also emphasized that degranulation occurs at the plasma membrane, whether the plasma membrane has been internalized in forming a phagocytic vacuole or whether it remains at the cell surface. Nevertheless, extracellular release of granule constituents under these experimental conditions was generally interpreted as having more relevance to the pathology of inflammation than to the physiology of neutrophil function in host defense. As was implied by such terms as "regurgitation while feeding" and "frustrated phagocytosis" (62,89,216,217), extracellular degranulation was regarded as the consequence of processes by which normal phagocytic responses by neutrophils are stressed or altered. The relevance of extracellular degranulation to the pathology of inflammation was clearly supported by the identification of diverse proteolytic enzymes in neutrophil granules which could digest tissue substrates (34,105,107–109,124,155,158,202,216), and by observations that certain antiinflammatory drugs (e.g., colchicine and corticosteroids) inhibited degranulation and the extracellular release of granule constituents (61,84,103,215,234).

Certain investigators, however were sufficiently impressed by the extracellular release of lysozyme (233) and lactoferrin (125) from resting and phagocytizing neutrophils to suggest that release of these granule components might reflect a secretory response by neutrophils that is relevant to the normal function of these cells in host defense. This latter-day restatement of Ehrlich's original concept of neutrophil granules has now been supported by the identification of various non-phagocytic stimuli that cause neutrophils to release granule constituents extracellularly (Table 2). This concept has also been supported by studies that have recognized significant differences in the accessibility of primary and secondary granules for extracellular degranulation.

During phagocytosis components of both the primary and secondary granules are released extracellularly. However, Leffell and Spitznagel made the important observation that during phagocytosis secondary (specific) granule degranulation is directed primarily toward the outside of the cell, whereas primary (azurophil) granule degranulation is confined primarily to internalized phagocytic vacuoles (125,126). Relative differences in the extracellular release of primary and secondary granule constituents during phagocytosis is explained in part by the observations of Bainton with rabbit heterophils (9), and, subsequently, of Brentwood and Henson with human neutrophils (20) that degranulation of secondary granules occurs before that of primary granules. With sequential granulation of these granule species, secondary granules are more likely to release their contents into phagocytic vacuoles that are forming at the cell surface and still open to the exterior.

However, the particular accessibility of secondary granules for exocytosis has been delineated further by studies of soluble stimuli that cause neutrophil degranulation. The divalent cation ionophore A23187, induces an active secretory response in neutrophils *in vitro* with significant extracellular release of granule constituents, particularly those contained in the secondary granules (66,122,186,239), and, at certain concentrations of this drug, a selective extracellular degranulation of the

TABLE 2. *Stimuli for granule exocytosis by normal human neutrophils*

Stimulus	Primary granule exocytosis	Secondary granule exocytosis
Phagocytosis	+ +	+ + +
Interaction with opsonized non-phagocytosable surface	+ + +	+ + +
Bacterial toxins (e.g., leukocidin)	+ + +	+ + +
Nonspecific adherence to surfaces	±	+ +
Chemoattractants + surface contact	±	+ +
Hydroxyeicotetranoic acid	−	+ +
Calcium ionophore (e.g., A23187)	+	+ + +
PMA	−	+ + +
Lectin (concanavalin A)	−	+ + +
Calcium-dependent, spontaneous exocytosis	−	+

secondary granules occurs (239). This effect of A23187 on neutrophils is analogous to its effect on a variety of secretory cells, [mast cells (35), pancreatic cells (50), and adrenergic neurons (201)], which undergo brisk exocytosis of their storage granules when exposed to this agent. Phorbol myristate acetate (PMA), the cocarcinogenic principal of croton oil, also causes an active exocytosis of neutrophil granules, an effect which appears to be quite selective for the secondary granules (67,226,239). Ultrastructural studies have shown that neutrophils exposed to nanogram concentrations of PMA are rendered entirely devoid of their peroxidase-negative, secondary granules (226), and this observation has been confirmed by studies in which the granule content of neutrophils treated with PMA was analyzed by fractionation techniques (Fig. 3). (239). The lectin, concanavalin A, has also been found to cause a selective exocytosis of neutrophil secondary granules (101). Recently, certain arachidonate metabolites (the hydroxyeicosatetranoic acids, 5-HETE and 12-HETE) (194), and purified leukocytic pyrogen (117) have been shown to have similar effects on neutrophils. Chemotactic factors, such as the synthetic n-formylated peptides and the chemotactic C5 fragment (C5a), also induce neutrophils to undergo granule exocytosis when the cells are adherent to or migrating through micropore filters in vitro (14,15,39,182,237) (Fig. 4). With human neutrophils, granule exocytosis under these conditions predominantly affects the secondary granules (237).

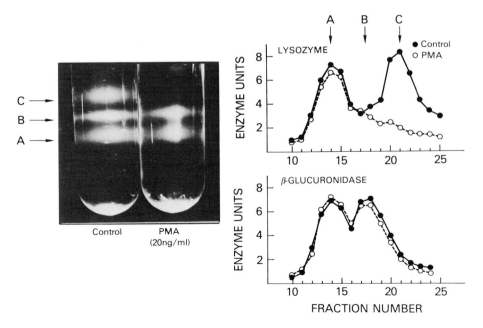

FIG. 3. Granule separations from 10^8 neutrophils incubated 30 min with buffer alone or with PMA, (20 ng/ml). [From Wright and Gallin (237); reproduced by permission of J. Immunol.].

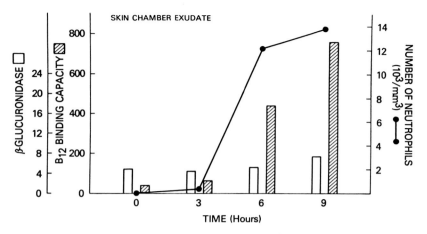

FIG. 4. Changes in β-glucuronidase and Vitamin B_{12}-binding protein in the extracellular fluid of a sterile, experimental inflammatory lesion created on the skin of a normal human subject and their relationship to the influx of exudate neutrophils over time. [From Wright and Gallin (237); reproduced by permission of *J. Immunol.*].

Perhaps the best evidence for the special accessibility of secondary granules for extracellular degranulation comes from the observation that neutrophils spontaneously secrete the contents of these granules. Before it was determined that the neutrophil-associated vitamin B_{12} binding protein is stored in the secondary granules, it was recognized that neutrophils secrete this protein when incubated at 37°C in physiologic media (38). It was also observed that neutrophils secrete lysozyme spontaneously under these same conditions (65,233), a phenomenon that is dependent on extracellular calcium (65) and reflects a selective exocytosis of secondary granules (65,237). The spontaneous secretion of secondary granule contents is significantly enhanced when neutrophils adhere to surfaces such as glass or nylon *in vitro* (237).

Consistent with these *in vitro* observations is the finding that neutrophils undergo secondary granule degranulation and secrete the contents of these granules during exudation *in vivo*. In studies of sterile, experimental inflammatory lesions on the skin of normal human subjects, Wright and Gallin (237) observed that secondary granule constituents (e.g., the vitamin B_{12}-binding protein) appeared in the extracellular fluid as exudate neutrophils arrived at the inflammatory site (Fig. 5). Comparable secretion of primary granule components was not evident, on the other hand. Moreover, when the granule content of the sterile exudate neutrophils was analyzed and compared with that of blood neutrophils, it was found that the exudate cells had lost nearly one-half of their peroxidase-negative, secondary granules. These studies provided direct evidence to support the concept of Ehrlich, stated 80 years earlier (49), that "a progressive decrease in the numbers of granulations in polymorphonuclear leukocytes during emigration" reflects the "extrusion" of granules by these cells. These studies indicated, further, that granule exocytosis (prin-

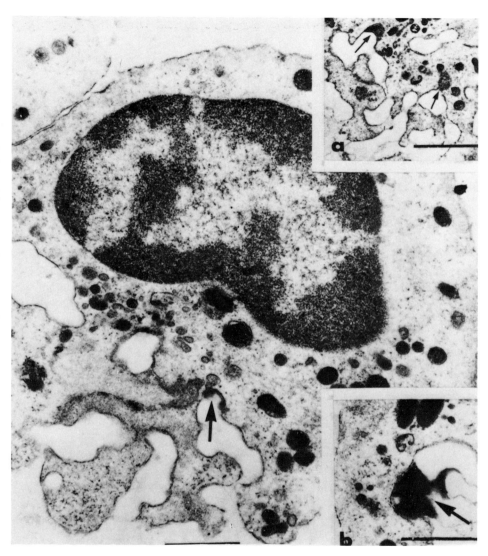

FIG. 5. Human neutrophil exposed to a concentration gradient of a chemoattractant, N-f-Met-Leu-Phe, and adherent to a micropore filter. Examples of granule exocytosis *(arrow and insets)* are seen at the side of cell in contact with the micropore filter and closest to the source of chemoattractant. [From Cramer and Gallin (39); reproduced by permission of *J. Cell Biol.*].

cipally of secondary granules) is intrinsic to the participation of neutrophils in an inflammatory response regardless of whether or not these cells undergo phagocytosis. Indeed, the observation that secondary granule constituents are spontaneously secreted *in vitro* has suggested that neutrophils may release the contents of these granules to a limited extent throughout their life *in vivo*, including the several days that they are stored in the marrow before entering the circulation.

During their functional life, therefore, neutrophils may encounter a variety of stimuli which can induce extracellular degranulation, some of which appear to promote a selective exocytosis of secondary granules, and others the combined exocytosis of both primary and secondary granules. These stimuli are outlined hierarchically in Fig. 6, with a hypothetical schema of primary and secondary granule exocytosis that may occur in different compartments of the neutrophil's life. In this schema it is suggested that neutrophils normally undergo some degree of secondary granule exocytosis during their normal turnover in the body, spontaneously or in association with incidental surface contact. When neutrophils encounter humoral stimuli such as chemotactic factors, become adherent to microvascular endothelium, and emigrate into extravascular spaces, secondary granule exocytosis is significantly increased. Extracellular release of lysosomal constituents from primary granules may also occur, but this would appear to be relatively limited. However, when neutrophils encounter phagocytic stimuli at a site of inflammation (opsonized microorganisms, phagocytosable tissue or cellular debris, or immunoglobulin and complement fixed to a nonphagocytosable substrate), significant se-

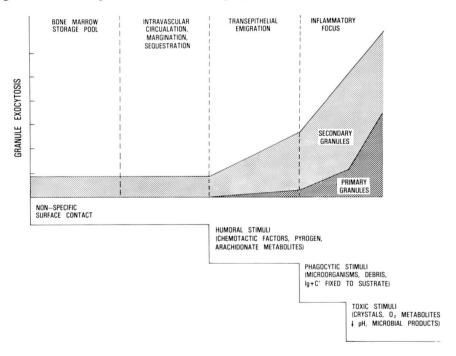

FIG. 6. Diagrammatic representation of the secretion of granule contents by neutrophils during different stages of their functional life *in vivo*.

cretion of primary granule components can occur, which is enhanced further by toxic factors that ultimately lead to neutrophil lysis and death.

GRANULE EXOCYTOSIS: REGULATION AND INTERACTIONS WITH OTHER NEUTROPHIL FUNCTIONS

The cellular events in neutrophils that are necessary and sufficient for fusion of granules with the plasma membrane and for granule exocytosis are not fully understood. Nonetheless, it is evident that calcium fluxes across the plasma membrane or within the cell, the assembly of cytoplasmic microtubules, the state of plasmalemmal microfilaments, glycolysis, and cyclic nucleotide metabolism are critical to granule mobilization and exocytosis. When living neutrophils are examined by phase microscopy, their cytoplasmic granules are seen to be in active Brownian motion. Granule movement is not necessarily random, however, for in preparations of spread cells, granules are observed to oscillate back and forth along fixed paths that radiate out from the center of the cell (16a), and these radial paths of movement are defined by microtubules that extend from the centrioles.

Ordinarily, granules do not appear to come into contact with the plasma membrane without some perturbation at the cell surface. Indeed, the limited, spontaneous exocytosis of secondary granules that has been observed when neutrophils are incubated under physiologic conditions *in vitro* (65,233,237) may reflect the effects of incidental cell-cell or cell-surface contacts that occur unavoidably with neutrophils in culture. In a resting neutrophil, the network of contractile proteins that is distributed throughout the periphery of the cell may act as a barrier that prevents granules from making contact with the plasma membrane, for ultrastructural studies have indicated that granule fusion occurs at regions of the plasma membrane that are relatively devoid of microfilaments made up of these proteins, either as a neutrophil envelopes a particle during phagocytosis (9,90,100,215,247) or spreads against a surface (39,90). Moreover, disruption of microfilaments with cytochalasin B (81,221) significantly facilitates granule fusion events at the cell surface (43,44,65,100,185,216,249).

However, granule contact with the plasma membrane does not appear to be sufficient for fusion and exocytosis, for cytochalasin-B-treated neutrophils still require some exogenous surface stimulation to effect degranulation, such as the occupancy of plasma membrane receptors for chemotactic factors (65,182) or for the immunoglobulin Fc fragment (64,91). There is also evidence that degranulation is an active process dependent on glycolysis for energy (14,84,89,92), although it is not clear to what extent the movement of granules and plasma membrane prior to their contact or the membrane fusion process itself accounts for energy consumption during degranulation.

Nevertheless, it is clear that the requirements for secondary and primary granule degranulation are different. As discussed above, a number of experimental conditions have been described in which a selective exocytosis of secondary granules occurs (66,101,226,237,239), indicating that the changes in neutrophil plasma membrane sufficient for secondary granule fusion are distinct from those necessary for primary granule fusion. Indeed, the observation that secondary and primary granules degranulate sequentially (9,20,86) suggests that primary granule fusion may be promoted by changes in the plasma membrane that follow incorporation of membrane from secondary granules into the plasma membrane. Studies with isolated granules and artificial lipisome membranes by Hawiger and colleagues (82) suggested that granule fusion involves interactions between plasma membrane phospholipid and granule membrane protein. However, freeze-fracture, scanning electron micrographs of intact, degranulating neutrophils (2,144) have indicated that granule fusion occurs at regions of membrane where intramembranous particles (representing floating membrane protein complexes) are absent, suggesting that membrane fusion primarily involves a rearrangement of membrane lipids as proposed by Lucy and others (41,129). In this regard, it is of interest that the lipid content of isolated primary and secondary granule membranes has been shown to be different. Nachman and co-workers (149) found that the membranes of primary and secondary granules from rabbit heterophils have different cholesterol: phospholipid ratios. This finding has been confirmed recently with human neutrophils by Wright and co-workers (241), who found also that the phospholipid of secondary granule membrane is made up of significantly more phosphatidylethanolamine (PE) than is that of primary granules. Increased PE content in secondary granule membrane may contribute to the relative accessibility of these granules for degranulation, since PE has been found to increase membrane instability and to promote membrane fusion events (41).

The critical role of ionic calcium in granule exocytosis has been emphasized by diverse studies of degranulation. Granule exocytosis under most experimental conditions requires extracellular calcium (14,66,92,103,183,186,229). Moreover, facilitated transport of Ca^{2+} across the plasma membrane induced by the ionophore A23187 has been shown to cause a brisk secretion of granule contents (66,122, 186,239). These observations indicate that exogenous stimuli induce granule exocytosis at least in part by opening transport channels for ionic calcium, thereby causing local increases in the intracellular concentration of this cation. Limited granule exocytosis occurs in neutrophils treated with cytochalasin B and C5a (68) or with PMA (67,239), in the absence of extracellular Ca^{2+}, but there is recent evidence to suggest that an intracellular redistribution of calcium stores is a necessary feature of granule mobilization under these conditions (187). The mechanism by which local changes in intracellular calcium may induce or facilitate degranulation is unclear; however, it is evident that calcium affects the contraction of polymerized, plasmalemmal contractile proteins (243a), which may in turn have an active (99,143) or permissive role in bringing granules into contact with the plasma membrane.

Microtubule assembly has also been found to be critical to the process of granule exocytosis. It has been shown convincingly that the inhibition of microtubule formation in neutrophils by colchicine or related drugs is associated with an inhibition of degranulation and granule exocytosis (14,102,132,214,234,250). It has also been shown that stimuli, which induce granule exocytosis, promote microtubule formation (67,101,102,132). Microtubules appear to direct the movement of granules within the neutrophil, as noted above (16a), and to facilitate the delivery of granules to internalized or surface plasma membrane (102,132,218). However, the mechanism by which microtubules influence granule movement remains unclear.

Considerable investigative interest has been directed toward the role of guanyl- and adenylcyclase systems in regulating granule mobilization and exocytosis [reviewed extensively elsewhere (62,104,115,218)], for it is evident that cellular cyclic nucleotide levels may affect granule exocytosis by modulating microtubule assembly (67,218). Agents such as isoproterenol and prostaglandins E and A, which stimulate adenylcyclase and elevate intracellular levels of cyclic AMP, impair both microtubule assembly and granule mobilization. On the other hand, cholinergic agonists, prostaglandin $F_{2\alpha}$, and PMA which elevate intracellular cyclic GMP, promote microtubule assembly and granule exocytosis (62,115,218). Although it is evident from these observations that cyclic nucleotide metabolism modulates neutrophil secretory responses, it is not necessarily evident that cyclic nucleotides act as a critical "second messenger" by which stimuli sensed at the neutrophil surface induce granule translocation and exocytosis.

Although it is now recognized that granule exocytosis and secretion of granule contents (secondary granules in particular) are intrinsic features of neutrophil activation, it is also evident that degranulation at the neutrophil surface changes the character of the plasma membrane and affects the ability of the cell to respond to further stimuli. Granule exocytosis has been shown to cause a significant neutralization of cell-surface charge (56). This change is associated with a marked increase in neutrophil adhesiveness, which may be explained in part by the delivery of secondary granule acidic proteins to the surface of the cell (18). In addition, exocytosis of secondary granules is initially associated with an increase in the number of plasma membrane receptor sites for chemotactic factors, and it has been proposed that delivery of secondary granule membrane to the cell surface may effect a resupply of unoccupied chemotactic factor receptors, which permits a continuation of the neutrophil's migration responses to these stimuli (57,178). However, secondary granule exocytosis leads eventually to greatly decreased chemoattractant receptor numbers and markedly reduced chemotactic responsiveness by neutrophils (57). The hyperadhesiveness and diminished chemotactic factor responsiveness that follows secondary granule exocytosis may represent mechanisms by which exudate neutrophils evolve functionally from wandering cells to cells that are committed to a specific site of inflammation and to the phagocytic and bactericidal tasks to be carried out at this site (178,232).

SECRETORY PRODUCTS OF NEUTROPHILS NOT DERIVED FROM GRANULES

The very active synthesis of protein that takes place during the promyelocyte and myelocyte stages of neutrophil development does not continue in the mature cell, and there is no evidence to suggest that neutrophils can resupply their granules once degranulation has occurred and granule constituents have been released extracellularly or into phagocytic vacuoles. Nonetheless, recent studies have emphasized that neutrophils retain some, albeit limited, capacity for ribonucleic acid (RNA) and protein synthesis (73). Evidence for persistent synthetic capabilities in mature neutrophils comes from studies in which radiolabeled precursor molecules for RNA and protein are taken up by the cell or are detected in secreted products (73). Evidence for active protein synthesis also comes from the identification of discrete mediators that are secreted by stimulated neutrophils but are not recoverable from lysates of resting cells; production of these mediators, moreover, may be prevented by inhibitors of protein synthesis: cycloheximide, puromycin, and actinomycin D. These neutrophil products include leukocytic pyrogen (LP) (3,19,142,152), crystal-induced chemotactic factor (189), and a neutrophil-derived plasminogen activator (72). There is also preliminary evidence to suggest that fibronectin may be synthesized by activated neutrophils (220).

Secretion of granule constituents following exocytosis of granules may be detected within minutes of exposing neutrophils to appropriate stimuli *in vitro* and is usually maximal within about 30 min. Secretion of synthetic products such as pyrogen or plasminogen activator, on the other hand, is fully expressed only after hours of *in vitro* culture (3,72). The stimuli that trigger production of these synthetic products [phagocytosis (3,19,142,152), crystal ingestion (189), concanavalin A (72)] also cause granule mobilization, which may represent a critical step in stimulating synthetic processes.

Phagocytic and humoral stimuli, which promote granule exocytosis, also trigger an oxidative, metabolic burst and production of oxygen metabolites: hydrogen peroxide, superoxide anion, hydroxyl radical, and singlet oxygen (69,92,111,114a, 115,170,171). It is now recognized that the oxidase apparatus responsible for this metabolic response is located at the neutrophil plasma membrane, and that neutrophil activation may result in significant extracellular release of biologically active oxygen metabolites (24,47,69,74,198). The possible extracellular effects of these metabolites has been the object of considerable study, as discussed further below. It has been suggested that peroxidation reactions at the plasma membrane may have a role in degranulation (115); such reactions at the cell surface would not appear to be critical for degranulation, however, since chronic granulomatous disease neutrophils, which are incapable of an oxidative burst, are still able to undergo degranulation (4,205), although the rate of degranulation may be reduced (60).

Metabolic reactions also occur at the cell surface that involve membrane phospholipid and result in the production of various soluble, biologically active mediators. Metabolites of the unsaturated, long-chain fatty acid, arachidonate, have been identified as products of neutrophil activation and include prostaglandins of the E and F series (248), thromboxanes (70), arachidonate (208), and hydroxyeicotetranoic acid (HETE) (193). Production of these metabolites may influence or amplify certain functional responses of neutrophils including degranulation. The HETE in particular has been shown to stimulate granule exocytosis following transport of ionic calcium into the cell, and it has been suggested that this lipid metabolite may act as the neutrophil's own ionophore which promotes degranulation responses to various secretagogues (194). A platelet-activating factor (PAF), structurally similar to the PAF secreted by basophils and monocytes, has been shown to be released by phagocytizing neutrophils, and this molecule appears to be a metabolite of membrane lipid distinct from arachidonate derivitives (30,131).

CONSEQUENCES OF SECRETION FOR HOST DEFENSE

There has been considerable investigative interest in the extracellular release of proteases and lysosomal constituents by neutrophils because of their clear relevance to the pathology of inflammation and to the tissue damage that characterizes inflammatory disease processes [as reviewed elsewhere (61,89,115,212,217,219)]. Particular attention has focused on acid proteases (34,216), neutral elastase (55,107,137), and neutral chymotrypsinlike proteases (108,134) and their ability to destroy tissue substrates. These enzymes are now known to be storage products of the primary granules of neutrophils and, as such, are relatively inaccessible for extracellular release except in the setting of active or altered phagocytosis responses by the cells (see above). Release of these tissue-degrading enzymes may have an important host-defense role in contributing to the "walling-off" and/or spontaneous drainage of an abscess. Yet, abscesses, although a dramatic manifestation of the neutrophil's response to infection, must be regarded as a partial failure of host-defense mechanisms in which pathogenic features of a microorganism, the breakdown of physical barriers, or alterations in normal neutrophil responsiveness have permitted a pathologic accumulation of microorganisms in normally sterile tissues. Indeed, clinical disorders, in which there is a demonstrable abnormality of neutrophil function [e.g., chemotaxis defects or microbicidal defects (116)], are characterized by recurrent abscess formation.

It is now evident, however, that neutrophil secretory responses, particularly those involving secondary granule exocytosis and release of metabolites generated at the plasma membrane, may be as relevant to the physiology of neutrophil function as they are to the pathology of acute inflammation. Secretory products of neutrophils may: a) deliver antimicrobial activity to the extracellular milieu, b) amplify, facilitate, and control various features of the inflammatory response, and c) influence the function of inflammatory monocytes, lymphocytes, and eosinophils and also regulate myelopoiesis (Table 3).

Extracellular Antimicrobial Effects

It is likely that the principal, day-to-day functions of neutrophils are to contribute to integumental barriers and to constantly restore sterility in subcutaneous and submucosal tissues when invaded by small, clinically insignificant numbers of microorganisms that have circumvented these barriers. Neutrophils are short-lived cells which are turned over in the body in enormous numbers daily (10 to 15×10^{10} cells/24 hr in a healthy, adult human being). It has long been recognized that

TABLE 3. *Likely contributions of neutrophil secretory function to host defense*

Enhancement of extracellular antimicrobial systems
Elimination of infected and transformed cells
Amplification and control of acute inflammatory responses
Conditioning of immunocompetent cell function to promote the immunogenicity of potential antigens at sites of inflammation
Release of mediators that regulate myelopoiesis

uninterrupted production, circulation, and turnover of these cells is critical for the maintenance of an uninfected state. It is known, for example, that large numbers of neutrophils are continuously delivered to mucosal surfaces of the body, particularly in the gastrointestinal tract (118,200), where diverse microorganisms reside and proliferate as normal flora. A constant supply of neutrophils to such sites clearly constitutes an important part of the barrier against microbial invasion, for when production and turnover of neutrophils cease, overwhelming sepsis with organisms from this normal flora quickly ensues. Thus, neutrophils do not represent a normally latent system of phagocytes that becomes active only with acute infection or with some other insult to the body.

In host-defense activities of neutrophils, which may contribute to maintenance of an uninfected state, secretion of primary granule constituents would not appear to occur to an extent sufficient to cause tissue damage, although a low level of primary granule exocytosis may occur at sites of neutrophil turnover. On the other hand, a substantial secretion of secondary granule components may occur in the course of normal neutrophil turnover in the absence of phagocytic stimuli, as suggested in the hypothetical schema of Fig. 6, for secondary granule exocytosis appears to be an intrinsic feature of neutrophil adherence, response to chemotactic factors, and emigration into extravascular spaces (237). Therefore, the content of these granules (see Table 1) is of particular interest in considering the secretory activities of neutrophils in host defense.

Lysozyme (or muramidase), the iron-binding protein, lactoferrin, and vitamin B_{12}-binding protein (cobalophilin), structurally related to plasma transcobalamins I and III, are known to be contained in the secondary granules. Each of these proteins has antimicrobial activity.

Lysozyme was originally described in the early 1920s by Fleming, who in searching for naturally occurring antimicrobial substances noted the lytic effect of this enzyme on various gram-positive bacteria (52). About two-thirds of the lysozyme recovered from neutrophils is contained in the secondary granules (5,7,192,222,239), and levels of this enzyme recovered in plasma and urine have been related to the rate of neutrophil turnover in the body (51,78). Lysozyme specifically cleaves the β1-4 linkage between repeating units of N-acetylglucosamine and N-acetylmuramic acid in the polysaccharide structure of bacterial cell walls (196). For those bacterial species in which this linkage is critical to cell wall integrity, lysozyme can exert a direct lytic effect. The mucopolysaccharide substrate for lysozyme may, however, be protected by a lipoprotein coat as in gram-negative bacteria and in some pathogenic gram-positive organisms. Also, secondary cross-linkages between tetrapeptide units that are attached to the N-acetylmuramic acid residues may strengthen the bacterial cell wall structure such that it is resistant to direct lysis by lysozyme (196). Nonetheless, lysozyme resistant organisms may become susceptible to lysis by this enzyme when exposed to an acid environment, proteases, H_2O_2, or specific antibody and complement (58,59,141,161,204,227). The importance of lysozyme in host defense has been disputed, because all bacterial pathogens relevant to human disease are resistant to it. However, this fact may reflect the contribution of lysozyme to the barrier against the microbial world, and, at mucosal surfaces, or other sites where neutrophils appear, secreted lysozyme may combine with other factors to control the colonization of microorganisms that are resistant to this enzyme by itself.

The iron-binding protein, lactoferrin, has been shown to be microbiostatic when not fully saturated with iron; it inhibits the growth of certain gram-negative and gram-positive bacteria and *Candida* species (114,135,157,168) *in vitro*. The inhibitory effect of lactoferrin on microbial growth appears to result from the binding of trace iron necessary for microbial proliferation, for other iron-chelating agents have been shown to have similar effects. Also, the microbiostatic properties of lactoferrin are abolished if the protein is fully saturated with iron (135,157). As with lysozyme, there may be synergism between lactoferrin and other antimicrobial systems (48). Lactoferrin may be detected in the plasma, and lactoferrin levels correlate with total body neutrophil pools and turnover rates (16,79).

Secondary granule exocytosis also results in the extracellular release of a vitamin B_{12}-binding protein or cobalophilin (184,237). This protein is immunologically identical to both transcobalamins (TC) I and III of plasma (106). Although it is now reasonably clear that TC III in plasma represents secreted neutrophil cobalophilin, there is also evidence that TC I, to which most of circulating B_{12} is bound, may also be derived from the neutrophil protein (106). As with lysozyme and lactoferrin, the levels of TC I and TC III in plasma have been shown to be related to the size of total body neutrophil pools and to the rate of neutrophil turnover (106). Neutrophil cobalophilin has been shown to have antibacterial effects (76), although these effects have not been studied as extensively as have those of lysozyme and lactoferrin.

Five case reports have appeared in the literature describing individuals whose neutrophils have a complete absence of secondary granules (22,120,159,191,195), and observations made with these individuals indicate the importance of secondary granule components in neutrophil host-defense functions. All of these patients were found to suffer from recurrent skin infections, and most had recurrent infections of the lung, upper respiratory tract, and/or ears in addition. Variable bactericidal defects *in vitro* were found with the neutrophils from three of these patients (120,191,195), whereas the cells from one patient were normal with respect to intracellular killing of bacteria (22). Recurrent infections, particularly in this last patient, may be related to a deficiency in extracellular antimicrobial activity normally provided by the secretion of secondary granule constituents.

Nonphagocytic stimuli that induce secondary granule exocytosis also coincidentally stimulate an oxidative metabolic response at the neutrophil surface resulting in the extracellular release of H_2O_2 and oxygen derivatives such as superoxide (69,114a,115,127). These oxygen metabolites may provide short-range antimicrobial activity in the extracellular milieu, particularly when combined with exogenous, peroxidases in the environment (114a,115). In addition, oxygen metabolites have been clearly implicated as mediators in the extracellular cytotoxic effects of neutrophils against both normal and transformed cells, particularly when combined with extracellular peroxidase and halide (31,32). Release of these metabolites, therefore, may play an important role in the normal elimination of senescent, viral infected, or otherwise transformed cells in the body.

Pathologic conditions in which there is a large-scale invasion of tissues by microorganisms may provide a sufficient stimulus for the extracellular release of primary granule constituents and the exteriorization of antimicrobial activities that are normally confined to phagocytic vacuoles. This sort of secretory response, however, albeit of probable importance in eliminating infection, is at the expense of normal tissues in the extracellular environment (216).

Amplification and Modulation of the Inflammatory Response

There is now considerable evidence to indicate that secretory responses by neutrophils are critical for the initiation, development, and regulation of acute inflammation. As noted above, chemotactic factors not only promote the directed migration of neutrophils but they also stimulate granule exocytosis (14,237) and trigger oxidative metabolism at the plasma membrane (127). Secondary granule exocytosis and the consequent delivery of acidic proteins to the cell surface has been implicated in the neutralization of neutrophil surface charge and the greatly increased cell adhesiveness that results from exposure of neutrophils to chemotactic factors (18). Increased neutrophil adhesiveness may also be promoted by release of archidonate and the arachidonate derivative, HETE, which have been shown to be products of membrane lipid turnover and metabolism in stimulated neutrophils (154,193,194,208). Changes in adhesiveness appear to be critical to the irreversible adherence of circulating neutrophils to capillary endothelium which initiates the accumulation of these cells at sites of inflammation. Secretory events also appear to be involved in loosening endothelial cell junctions and in splitting the basement membrane, thereby creating gaps in the capillary vessel walls through which neutrophils can emigrate into the tissues. Neutrophils have been shown to loosen the intercellular and surface attachments of endothelial cells and fibroblasts in culture through a combined effect of secreted oxygen metabolites and proteases derived most likely from the primary granules (80,130,137,199). This effect appears to be mediated in part by the digestion of fibronectin by neutrophil elastase (137). Secreted collagenase, stored in both the primary and secondary granules, may facilitate the penetration of neutrophils through the microvascular basement membrane (54,148,156,240).

Secretion also appears to provide a mechanism by which neutrophils initially engaged at an inflammatory site may amplify the inflammatory response and promote the accelerated accumulation of additional neutrophils. This amplification effect may be mediated both by the generation of vasoactive mediators that enhance local blood flow and increase vascular permeability and by the generation of chemotactic factors. Various proteases derived from neutrophil granules have been found to release peptides with bradykininlike activity from a protein substrate in serum (leukokininogen) (29,75,138,145,146). There is also evidence for a plasminogen activator released by activated neutrophils, which acts on plasminogen to produce plasmin, which in turn acts on kininogen to release kinin (140). In addition, granule-derived mediators released by stimulated neutrophils have been found to cause degranulation of tissue mast cells with a consequent release of histamine from these cells (110,113,165,177). Cationic proteins (presumably proteases) stored in neutrophil primary granules also induce the release of vasoactive amines from platelets (77,86). A product of secondary granules has been shown to generate the chemotactic fragment of C5 through activation of the intact complement system in serum (63,235,236), and there appear to be various proteases contained in the primary granules of neutrophils that can generate chemotactic molecules through direct cleavage of complement components (206,210,211,235). Release of mediators derived from plasma membrane lipid metabolism also represents a secretory phenomenon through which stimulated neutrophils may amplify the inflammatory response through generation of chemotactic activity [e.g., HETE (193)] or vasoactive substances [e.g., thromboxanes (70) and prostaglandins (248)].

Although secretory events may serve to amplify the response of neutrophils to inflammatory stimuli, they also appear to provide for a negative feedback regulation of inflammation. Proteases derived from the primary granules have been shown to inactivate chemotactic factors (26,236) and to degrade vasoactive kinins (72,138,145). Moreover, recent studies have shown that extracellular H_2O_2 and myeloperoxidase can also inactivate chemotactic factors (33).

Secretion of granule constituents and oxygen metabolites may also mediate both coagulant and anticoagulant effects at a site of inflammation. As has already been mentioned, release of H_2O_2 by neutrophils can stimulate serotonin release by platelets and platelet aggregation (115,128) both alone or in association with myeloperoxidase and halide. Platelet-release reactions can also be mediated by release of a thromboplastin like substance, which is associated with neutrophil granules, and which can also effect the conversion of fibrinogen to fibrin via thrombin generation (119,151,174). The generation and extracellular release of thromboxane, derived from plasma-membrane lipid metabolism, represents another secretory response of activated neutrophils that may mediate platelet aggregation and serotonin release (70). A platelet-activating factor has also been found to be released by stimulated neutrophils as an apparent by-product of plasma-membrane lipid metabolism (30,131).

On the other hand, extracellular release of primary granule cationic proteins and proteases may be associated with anticoagulant effects either as a direct effect of the protein (173), as a result of proteolytic cleavage of clotting factors (94,155,179,203), or proteolysis of fibrinogen which leads to peptide fragments with anticoagulant activity (162). Moreover, there is substantial evidence to suggest that neutrophils can mediate fibrinolysis either through the release of proteases that digest fibrin directly (153,155,162,175,179) or through the release of a plasminogen activator (72,140,175,243).

Interactions of Secretory Products with Other Cells: Lymphocytes, Monocytes, Eosinophils, and Myeloid Precursor Cells

Neutrophils have been traditionally regarded as cells which respond to inflammatory signals but do not themselves influence the behavior of other inflammatory and/or immunocompetent cells. As has been pointed out previously, however, neutrophils may clearly influence the development and course of an acute inflammatory process by means of secreted mediators. It has also become clear that secretory products of neutrophils may interact with monocytes, lymphocytes, and eosinophils and thereby may condition the immune response of these cells at sites of inflammation. In 1968 Ward described a chemotactic factor derived from the granules of rabbit heterophils that was specific for monocytes (209). The presence of such a factor was recently confirmed in studies with human neutrophils by Wright and co-workers, who isolated a specific chemokinetic (if not chemotactic) factor for monocytes from purified secondary granules and from postsecretory extracellular media (238). Secondary granule protein from human neutrophils was also found to stimulate the transformation of blood monocytes to macrophages *in vitro* as reflected by changes in enzyme markers (238).

Various studies have indicated that neutrophil granule components may also influence the immune responsiveness of lymphocytes. Both human neutrophil elastase and the chymotrypsinlike protease (cathepsin G), which are components of primary granules, have been found to stimulate lymphocyte proliferation *in vitro* as B-cell mitogens (207). A neutral protease has also been recovered from the extracellular media of cultured mouse polymorphonuclear leukocytes, which enhances both thymocyte stimulation by phytohemagglutinin and mitogenic stimulation of mouse splenocytes (123,150,244). Recently, it has been suggested that LP, secreted by neutrophils as a delayed effect of neutrophil stimulation (3,19,142,152), may also have lymphocyte-activating effects (172). These observations suggest that neutrophils may not only influence the emigration of mononuclear phagocytes to sites of inflammation, but they may also promote the immune recognition of potential antigens present at these sites. Neutrophils may, in addition, influence the participation of eosinophils in an inflammatory response through the release of an eosinophil chemotactic factor, which appears to be derived directly from the plasma membrane (42,53,121).

Finally, there is recent evidence from a series of studies by Broxmeyer and co-workers (25) and Pelus and colleagues (160) that lactoferrin, a component of neutrophil secondary granules, acts as a negative feedback regulator of neutrophil precursor cell proliferation and differentiation in the bone marrow. Lactoferrin appears to inhibit myelopoiesis by interfering with the release of colony-stimulating factor (CSF) from marrow mononuclear cells (25). As has been noted above, secondary granule components (including lactoferrin) may be secreted to a limited degree spontaneously by mature neutrophils present in marrow storage pools. Depletion of these cells from storage pools as they enter the circulation may stimulate myelopoiesis by the removal of an inhibitory product of these cells, such as lactoferrin. The probable importance of negative feedback regulation in myelopoiesis is supported by observations made in human and canine cyclic neutropenia (242).

SUMMARY AND CONCLUSIONS

In a reprise of Paul Ehrlich's original concepts that were formulated almost a century ago, it has become appropriate once again to consider the neutrophil as a secretory cell. It is now evident that neutrophils secrete a wide variety of biologically active products, not only during their normal turnover in the body, but also as they accumulate and function at discrete sites of inflammation. Secretory products are derived from the exocytosis of cytoplasmic granules, from the *de novo* synthesis and release of proteins, and from metabolic events that take place at the plasma membrane. Although neutrophil granules have been considered in general to be lysosomes that subserve intracellular digestive functions, more than two-thirds of these granules (the secondary granules) are clearly distinct from lysosomes with respect to their content and appear to have much in common with the storage granules of secretory cells. It is also apparent that the exocytosis of granules (secondary granules in particular) and the release of metabolites that originate at the cell surface are intrinsic features of normal neutrophil function in host defense and are not simply pathologic side effects of acute inflammation. Secretory responses by neutrophils deliver antimicrobial substances to the extracellular milieu, provide mechanisms for the amplification and modulation of inflammatory responses, influence the behavior of other specialized inflammatory cells that are involved with specific immune recognition, and may provide negative feedback signals that regulate the production of neutrophils in the bone marrow. It is no longer possible to view neutrophils as simple-minded cells that can only take and never give orders in host defense. Rather, it is now clear that the secretory activity of neutrophils reflects the experience of these cells at sites of inflammation and can have a profound effect on the development and course of an inflammatory response. Secretion of mediators by neutrophils may also condition the immunogenicity of potential antigens present at the inflammatory site.

ACKNOWLEDGMENTS

The author is indebted to Dr. John I. Gallin for the many rewarding opportunities for collaborative research, discussion, and sharing of ideas which constitute a background for this review article, and to Anda Meierovics, Joyce Powell, and Saundra Goode for their help in preparing the manuscript. The author also wishes to note that the title of this article is adapted from terminology used previously by

Weissmann and co-workers, who have described neutrophils as "secretory organs of inflammation" (217).

REFERENCES

1. Ackerman, G. A. (1971): The human neutrophilic myelocyte. A correlated phase and electron microscopic study. *Z. Zellforsch. M. Krosk. Anat.*, 121:153–170.
2. Amherdt, M., Baggiolini, M., Perrelet, A., and Orci, L. (1978): Freeze-fracture of membrane fusions in phagocytosing polymorphonuclear leukocytes. *Lab. Invest.*, 39:398–404.
3. Atkins, E., and Bodel, P. (1972): Fever. *N. Engl. J. Med.*, 286:27–34.
4. Baehner, R. L., Karnovsky, M. J., and Karnovsky, M. L. (1969): Degranulation of leukocytes in chronic granulomatous disease. *J. Clin. Invest.*, 48:187–192.
5. Baggiolini, M., Hirsch, J. G., and de Duve, C. (1969): Resolution of granules from rabbit heterophil leukocytes into distinct populations by Zonal sedimentation. *J. Cell Biol.*, 40:529–541.
6. Baggiolini, M., De Duve, C., Masson, P. L., and Heremans, J. F. (1970): Association of lactoferrin with specific granules in rabbit heterophil leukocytes. *J. Exp. Med.*, 131:559–570.
7. Baggiolini, M., Bretz, U., and Gusus, B. (1974): Biochemical characterization of azurophil and specific granules from human and rabbit polymorphonuclear leukocytes. *Schweiz. Med. Wschenschr.*, 104:129–132.
8. Baggiolini, M., Dewald, B., Rindler-Ludwig, R., and Bretz, V. (1975): Subcellular localization and heterogeneity of neutral proteases in human polymorphonuclear leukocytes. *Ann. N.Y. Acad. Sci.*, 256:263–265.
9. Bainton, D. F. (1973): Sequential degranulation of the two types of polymorphonuclear leukocyte granules during phagocytosis of microorganisms. *J. Cell Biol.*, 58:249–264.
10. Bainton, D. F., and Farguhar, M. G. (1966): Origin of granules in polymorphonuclear leukocytes. Two types derived from opposite faces of the Golgi complex in developing granulocytes. *J. Cell Biol.*, 28:277–301.
11. Bainton, D. F., and Farquhar, M. G. (1968): Differences in enzyme content of azurophil and specific granules of polymorphonuclear leukocytes. I. Histochemical staining of bone marrow smears. II. Cytochemistry and electro microscopy of bone marrow cells. *J. Cell Biol.*, 39:299–317.
12. Bainton, D. F., and Farquhar, M. G. (1970): Segregation and packaging of granule enzymes in eosinophilic leukocytes. *J. Cell Biol.*, 45:54–73.
13. Bainton, D. F., Ullyot, J. L., and Farquhar, M. G. (1971): The development of neutrophilic polymorphonuclear leukocytes in human bone marrow. Origin and content of azurophil and specific granules. *J. Exp. Med.*, 134:907–934.
14. Becker, E. L., and Showell, H. J. (1974): The ability of chemotactic factors to induce lysosomal enzyme release. II. The mechanism of release. *J. Immunol.*, 112:2055–2062.
15. Becker, E. L., Showell, H. J., Henson, P. M., and Hsu, L. S. (1974): The ability of chemotactic factors to induce lysosomal enzyme release. I. The characteristics of release, the importance of surfaces and the relation of enzyme release to chemotactic responsiveness. *J. Immunol.*, 112:2047–2054.
16. Bennett, R. M., and Kokocinski, T. (1979): Lactoferrin turnover in man. *Clin. Sci.*, 57:453–460.
16a. Bessis, M. (1973): *Living Blood Cells and Their Ultrastructure.* Springer-Verlag, New York, pp. 307–311.
17. Bessis, M., and Thiery, J. (1961): Electron microscopy of human white blood cells and their stem cells. *Int. Rev. Cytol.*, 12:199–241.
18. Bockenstedt, L. K., and Goetzl, E. J. (1980): Constituents of human neutrophils that mediate enhanced adherence to surfaces. Purification and identification as acidic proteins of the specific granules. *J. Clin. Invest.*, 65:1372–1381.
19. Bodel, P. (1970): Studies on the mechanism of endogenous pyrogen production. I. Investigation of new protein synthesis in stimulated human blood leukocytes. *Yale J. Biol. Med.*, 43:145–163.
20. Brentwood, B. J., and Henson, P. M. (1980): The sequential release of granule constituents from human neutrophils. *J. Immunol.*, 124:855–862.
21. Breton-Gorius, J., Coquin, Y., and Guichard, B. S. (1978): Cytochemical distinction between azurophils and catalase-containing granules in leukocytes. *Lab. Invest.*, 38:21–31.

22. Breton-Gorius, J., Mason, D., Buriot, D., Vilde, J-L., and Griscelli, C. (1980): Lactoferrin deficiency as a consequence of a lack of specific granules in neutrophils from a patient with recurrent infections. *Am. J. Pathol.*, 99:413–427.
23. Bretz, V., and Baggiolini, M. (1974): Biochemical and morphological characterization of azurophil and specific granules of human neutrophilic polymorphonuclear leukocytes. *J. Cell Biol.*, 63:251–269.
24. Briggs, R. T., Drath, D. B., Karnovsky, M. L., and Karnovsky, M. J. (1975): Localization of NADH oxidase on the surface of human polymorphonuclear leukocytes by a new cytochemical method. *J. Cell Biol.*, 67:566–586.
25. Broxmeyer, H. E., Smithyman, A., Eger, R. R., Meyers, P. A., and De Sonsa, M. (1978): Identification of lactoferrin as the granulocyte-derived inhibitor of colony stimulating activity production. *J. Exp. Med.*, 148:1052–1067.
26. Brozna, J. P., Senior, R. M., Krentzer, D. L., and Ward, P. A. (1977): Chemotactic factor inactivators of human granulocytes. *J. Clin. Invest.*, 60:1280–1288.
27. Burke, J. S., Uriuhava, T., Macmorine, D. R. L., and Movat, H. Z. (1964): A permeability factor released from phagocytosing PMN-leukocytes and its inhibition by protease inhibitors. *Life Sci.*, 3:1505–1512.
28. Capone, R. J., Weinreb, E. L., and Chapman, G. B. (1964): Electron microscope studies on normal human myeloid elements. *Blood*, 23:300–320.
29. Chang, J., Freer, R., Stella, R., and Greenbaum, L. M. (1972): Studies on leukokinins. II. Studies on the formation, partial amino acid sequence and chemical properties of leukokinins M and PMN. *Biochem. Pharmacol.*, 21:3095–3106.
30. Clark, P. O., Hanahan, D. J., and Pinckard, R. N. (1980): Physical and chemical properties of platelet-activating factor obtained from human neutrophils and monocytes and rabbit neutrophils and basophils. *Biochim. Biophys. Acta*, 628:69–75.
31. Clark, R. A., and Klebanoff, S. J. (1975): Neutrophil-mediated tumor cell cytotoxicity: Role of the peroxidase system. *J. Exp. Med.*, 141:1442–1447.
32. Clark, R. A., and Klebanoff, S. J. (1977): Myeloperoxidase-H_2O_2-halide system: Cytotoxic effect on human blood leukocytes. *Blood*, 50:65–70.
33. Clark, R. A., and Klebanoff, S. J. (1979): Chemotactic factor inactivation by the myeloperoxidase-hydrogen peroxide-halide system. *J. Clin. Invest.*, 64:913–920.
34. Cochrane, C. G., and Aikin, B. S. (1966): Polymorphonuclear leukocytes in immunologic reactions. The destruction of vascular basement membrane *in vivo* and *in vitro*. *J. Exp. Med.*, 124:733–752.
35. Cochrane, D. E., and Douglas, W. W. (1974): Calcium induced extrusion of secretory granules (exocytosis) in mast cells exposed to 48/80 or the ionophores A23187 and X-537A. *Proc. Natl. Acad. Sci. U.S.A.*, 71:408–412.
36. Cohn, Z. A., and Hirsch, J. G. (1960): The isolation and properties of the specific cytoplasmic granules of rabbit polymorphonuclear leukocytes. *J. Exp. Med.*, 112:983–1004.
37. Cohnheim, J. (1882): Lectures on General Pathology, quoted from *The Inflammatory Process*, edited by B. Zweifach, L. Grant, and R. McClusky, Academic Press, New York, 1965.
38. Corcino, J., Krauss, S., Waxman, S., and Herbert, V. (1970): Release of vitamin B_{12}-binding protein by human leukocytes *in vitro*. *J. Clin. Invest.*, 49:2250–2255.
39. Cramer, E. B., and Gallin, J. I. (1979): Localization of submembranous cations to the leading end of human neutrophils during chemotaxis. *J. Cell Biol.*, 82:369–379.
40. Crowder, J. G., Martin, R. R., and White, A. (1969): Release of histamine and lysosomal enzymes by human leukocytes during phagocytosis of staphylcococci. *J. Lab. Clin. Med.*, 74:436–444.
41. Cullis, P. R., and Hope, M. J. (1978): Effects of fusogenic agent on membrane structure of erythrocyte ghosts and the mechanism of membrane fusion. *Nature (London)*, 271:672–674.
42. Czarnetzki, B. M. (1978): Eosinophil chemotactic factor release from neutrophils by *Nippostrongylus brasiliensis* larvae. *Nature (London)*, 271:553–554.
43. Davies, P., Allison, A. C., Fox, R. I., Polyzonis, M., and Haswell, A. D. (1972): The exocytosis of polymorphonuclear-leukocyte lysosomal enzymes induced by cytochalasin B. *Biochem. J.*, 128:78–79.
44. Davies, P., Fox, R. I., Polyzonis, M., Allison, A. C., and Haswell, A. D. (1973): The inhibition of phagocytosis and facilitation of exocytosis in rabbit polymorphonuclear leukocytes by cytochalasin B. *Lab. Invest.*, 28:16–22.

45. Davis, A. T., Estensen, R., and Quie, P. G. (1971): Cytochalasin B. III. Inhibition of human polymorphonuclear leukocyte phagocytosis. *Proc. Soc. Exp. Biol. Med.*, 137:161–164.
46. DeDuve, C., and Wattiaux, R. (1966): Functions of lysosomes. *Annu. Rev. Physiol.*, 28:435–492.
47. Dewald, B., Baggiolini, M., Churnutte, J. T., and Babior, B. M. (1979): Subcellular localization of the superoxide-forming enzyme in human neutrophils. *J. Clin. Invest.*, 63:21–29.
48. Dobrin, R. S., Michael, A. F., Haseman, J., and Holmes, B. (1975): The antibacterial activity of lactoferrin. *Fed. Proc.*, 34:1044.
49. Ehrlich, P. (1887–1900), quoted by Hirsch, J. G., and Hirsch, B. I. (1980): Paul Ehrlich and the discovery of the eosinophil. In *The Eosinophil*, edited by A. Mahmond and K. F. Austen. pp. 3–25. Grune & Stratton, New York.
50. Eimerl, S., Naphtali, S., Heichal, O., and Schinger, Z. (1974): Induction of enzyme secretion in rat pancreatic slices using ionophore A23187 and calcium. *J. Biol. Chem.*, 249:3991–3993.
51. Fink, M. E., and Finch, S. C. (1968): Serum muramidase and granulocyte turnover. *Proc. Soc. Exp. Biol. Med.*, 127:365–367.
52. Fleming, A., and Allison, V. D. (1922): Observations on a bacteriolytic substance ("lysozyme") found in secretions and tissues. *Br. J. Exp. Pathol.*, 3:252–260.
53. Frickhofen, N., and Konig, W. (1979): Subcellular localization of the eosinophil chemotactic factor (ECF) and its inactivator in human polymorphonuclear leukocytes (PMN). *Immunology*, 37:111–122.
54. Gadek, J. E., Fells, G. A., Wright, D. G., and Crystal, R. G. (1980): Human neutrophil elastase functions as a type III collagen "collagenase." *Biochem. Biophys. Res. Commun.*, 95:1815–1822.
55. Gladston, M., Janoff, A., and Davis, A. L. (1973): Familial variation of leukocyte lysosomal protease and serum αl-anti-trypsin as determinants in chronic obstructive pulmonary disease. *Am. Rev. Resp. Dis.*, 107:718–727.
56. Gallin, J. I. (1980): Degranulating stimuli decrease the negative surface charge and increase the adhesiveness of human neutrophils. *J. Clin. Invest.*, 65:298–306.
57. Gallin, J. I., Wright, D. G., and Schiffmann, E. (1978): Role of secretory events in modulating human neutrophil chemotaxis. *J. Clin. Invest.*, 62:1364–1374.
58. Gemsa, D., Davis, S. D., and Wedgwood, R. J. (1966): Lysozyme and serum bactericidal action. *Nature (London)*, 210:950–951.
59. Glynn, A. A. (1969): The complement lysozyme sequence in immune bacteriolysis. *Immunology*, 16:463–471.
60. Gold, S. B., Hanes, D. M., Stites, D. P., and Fudenberg, H. H. (1974): Abnormal kinetics of degranulation in chronic granulomatous disease. *N. Engl. J. Med.*, 291:332–337.
61. Goldstein, I. M. (1976): Pharmacologic modulation of lysosomal enzyme release from polymorphonuclear leukocytes. *J. Invest. Dermatol.*, 67:622–624.
62. Goldstein, I. M. (1976): Polymorphonuclear leukocyte lysosomes and immune tissue injury. *Prog. Allergy*, 20:301–340.
63. Goldstein, I. M., and Weissman, G. (1974): Generation of C5-derived lysosomal enzyme-releasing activity (C5a) by lysates of leukocyte lysosomes. *J. Immunol.*, 113:1583–1588.
64. Goldstein, I. M., and Weissmann, G. (1979): Non-phagocytic stimulation of human polymorphonuclear leukocytes: Role of the plasma membrane. *Semin. Hematol.*, 16:175–187.
65. Goldstein, I., Hoffstein, S., Gallin, J., and Weissmann, G. (1973): Mechanisms of lysosomal enzyme release from human leukocytes: Microtubule assembly and membrane fusion induced by a component of complement. *Proc. Nat. Acad. Sci. U.S.A.*, 70:2916–2920.
66. Goldstein, I. M., Horn, J. K., Kaplan, H. B., and Weissmann, G. (1974): Lysosomal enzyme release from human polymorphonuclear leukocytes. *Biochem. Biophys. Res. Commun.*, 60:807–812.
67. Goldstein, I. M., Hoffstein, S. T., and Weissmann, G. (1975): Mechanisms of lysosomal enzyme release from human polymorphonuclear leukocytes. Effects of phorbol myristate acetate. *J. Cell Biol.*, 66:647–652.
68. Goldstein, I. M., Hoffstein, S. T., and Weissmann, G. (1975): Influence of divalent cations upon complement-mediated release from human polymorphonuclear leukocytes. *J. Immunol.*, 115:665–670.
69. Goldstein, I. M., Cerqueira, M., Lund, S., and Kaplan, H. B. (1977): Evidence that the super-oxide-generating system of human leukocytes is associated with the cell surface. *J. Clin. Invest.*, 59:249–254.

70. Goldstein, I. M., Malmsten, C. L., Kindahl, H., Kaplan, H. B., Radmark, O., Samuelsson, B., and Weissmann, G. (1978): Thromboxane generation by human peripheral blood polymorphonuclear leukocytes. *J. Exp. Med.*, 148:787–792.

71. Graham, G. S. (1920): The neutrophilic granules of the circulating blood in health and disease. A preliminary report. *N.Y. State J. Med.*, 20:46–55.

72. Granelli-Piperno, A., Vassalli, J -D., and Reich, E. (1977): Secretion of plasminogen activator by human polymorphonuclear leukocytes. Modulation by glucocorticoids and other effectors. *J. Exp. Med.*, 146:1693–1706.

73. Granelli-Piperno, A., Vassalli, J -D., and Reich, E. (1979): RNA and protein synthesis in human peripheral blood polymorphonuclear leukocytes. *J. Exp. Med.*, 149:284–289.

74. Green, T. R., Schaefer, R. E., and Makler, M. T. (1980): Orientation of the NADPH dependent superoxide generating osidoreductase on the outer membrane of human PMN's. *Biochem. Biophys. Res. Commun.*, 94:262–269.

75. Greenbaum, L. M. (1972): Leukocyte kininogenases and leukokinins from normal and malignant cells. *Am. J. Pathol.*, 68:613–623.

76. Gullberg, R. (1974): Possible antimicrobial function of the large molecular size vitamin B_{12}-binding protein. *Scand. J. Gastroenterol.*, 9(Suppl. 29):19–21.

77. Hallgren, R., and Venge, P. (1976): Cationic proteins of human granulocytes. Effects on human platelet aggregation and serotonin release. *Inflammation*, 1:359–370.

78. Hansen, N. E., Karle, H., Anderson, V., and Olgaard, K. (1972): Lysozyme turnover in man, *J. Clin. Invest.*, 51:1146–1155.

79. Hansen, N. E., Malmquist, J., and Thorell, J. (1975): Plasma myeloperoxidase and lactoferrin measured by radioimmunoassay: Relations to neutrophil kinetics. *Acta. Med. Scand.*, 198:437–443.

80. Harlan, J. M., Killen, P. D., Harker, L. A., and Striker, G. E. (1980): Endothelial denudation mediated by neutrophil derived neutral proteases. *Clin. Res.*, 28:547a.

81. Hartwig, J. H., and Stossel, T. P. (1978): Cytochalasin B dissolves actin gels by breaking actin filaments. *J. Cell Biol.*, 79:271a.

82. Hawiger, J., Collins, R. D., Horn, R. G., and Koenig, M. G. (1969): Interaction of artificial phospholipid membranes with isolated polymorphonuclear leukocytic granules. *Nature (London)*, 222:276–278.

83. Hawkins, D. (1972): Neutrophilic leukocytes in immunologic reactions: Evidence for the selective release of lysosomal constituents. *J. Immunol.*, 108:310–317.

84. Hawkins, C. (1974): Neutrophilic leukocytes in immunologic reactions *in vitro*. III. Pharmacologic modulation of lysosomal constituent release. *Clin. Immunol. Immunopathol.*, 2:141–152.

85. Hawkins, D., and Peeters, S. (1971): The response of polymorphonuclear leukocytes to immune complexes *in vitro*. *Lab. Invest.*, 24:483–491.

86. Henson, P. M. (1970): Mechanisms of release of constituents from rabbit platelets by antigen-antibody complexes and complement. II. Interaction of platelets with neutrophils. *J. Immunol.*, 105:490–501.

87. Henson, P. M. (1971): Interaction of cells with immune complexes: Adherence, release of constituents, and tissue injury. *J. Exp. Med.*, 134:114–135.

88. Henson, P. M. (1971): The immunologic release of constituents from neutrophil leukocytes. II. Mechanisms of release during phagocytosis and adherence to nonphagocytosable surfaces. *J. Immunol.*, 107:1547–1557.

89. Henson, P. M. (1972): Pathologic mechanisms in neutrophil-mediated injury. *Am. J. Pathol.*, 68:593–606.

90. Henson, P. M. (1973): Mechanisms of release of granule enzymes from human neutrophils phagocytosing aggregated immunoglobulin. An electron microscopic study. *Arthritis Rheum.*, 16:208–216.

91. Henson, P. M., and Oades, Z. G. (1973): Enhancement of immunologically induced granule exocytosis from neutrophils by cytochalasin B. *J. Immunol.*, 110:290–293.

92. Henson, P. M., and Oades, Z. G. (1975): Stimulation of human neutrophils by soluble and insoluble immunoglobulin aggregates. Secretion of granule constituents and increased oxidation of glucose. *J. Clin. Invest.*, 56:1053–1061.

93. Henson, P. M., Johnson, H. B., and Spiegelberg, H. L. (1972): The release of granule enzymes from human neutrophils stimulated by aggregated immunoglobulins of different classes and subclasses. *J. Immunol.*, 109:1182–1192.

94. Herion, J. C., Bucher, J. R., Penniall, R., Walker, R. I., Baker, M., and Roberts, H. R. (1979): Isolation and characterization of granulocyte lysosomal proteins and study of their effects on the clotting system. *Am. J. Hematol.*, 7:265–279.

95. Hirsch, J. G. (1962): Cinemicrophotographic observations on granule lysis in polymorphonuclear leukocytes during phagocytosis. *J. Exp. Med.*, 116:827–834.

96. Hirsch, J. G., and Cohn, Z. A. (1960): Degranulation of polymorphonuclear leukocytes following phagocytosis of microorganisms. *J. Exp. Med.*, 112:1005–1014.

97. Hirsch, J. G., Bernheimer, A. W., and Weissmann, G. (1963): Motion picture study of the toxic action of streptolysins on leukocytes. *J. Exp. Med.*, 118:223–227.

98. Hirschorn, R., and Weissmann, G. (1965): Isolation and properties of human leukocyte lysosomes *in vitro*. *Proc. Soc. Exp. Biol. Med.*, 119:36–39.

99. Hoffstein, S., and Weissmann, G. (1978): Microfilaments and microtubules in calcium ionophore-induced secretion of lysosomal enzymes from human polymorphonuclear leukocytes. *J. Cell Biol.*, 78:769–781.

100. Hoffstein, S., Zurier, R. B., and Weissmann, G. (1974): Mechanisms of lysosomal enzyme release from human leukocytes. III. Quantitative morphologic evidence for an effect of cyclic nucleotides and colchicine on degranulation. *Clin. Immunol. Immunopathol.*, 3:201–217.

101. Hoffstein, S., Soberman, R., Goldstein, I., and Weissmann, G. (1976): Conconavalin A induces microtubule assembly and specific granule discharge in human polymorphonuclear leukocytes. *J. Cell Biol.*, 68:781–787.

102. Hoffstein, S., Goldstein, I. M., and Weissmann, G. (1977): Role of microtubule assembly in lysosomal enzyme secretion from human polymorphonuclear leukocytes. A re-evaluation. *J. Cell Biol.*, 73:242–256.

103. Ignarro, L. J. (1974): Regulation of lysosomal enzyme secretion: Role in inflammation. *Agents Actions*, 4:241:258.

104. Ignarro, L. J. (1975): Hormonal control of lysosomal enzyme release from human neutrophils by cyclic nucleotides and autonomic neurohormones. In: *Cyclic Nucleotides in Disease*, edited by H. Weiss, pp. 187–210. University Park Press, Baltimore.

105. Ignarro, L. J., Oronsky, A. L., and Perper, R. J. (1973): Breakdown of noncollagenous chondro-mucoprotein matrix by leukocyte lysosome granule lysates from guinea pig, rabbit and human. *Clin. Immunol. Immunopathol.*, 2:36–51.

106. Jacob, E., Baker, S. J., and Herbert, V. (1980): Vitamin B_{12}-binding proteins. *Physiol. Rev.*, 60:918–960.

107. Janoff, A. (1972): Human granulocyte elastase. Further delineation of its role in connective tissue damage. *Am. J. Pathol.*, 68:579–591.

108. Janoff, A. (1975): At least three human neutrophil lysosomal proteases are capable of degrading joint connective tissues. *Ann. N.Y. Acad. Sci.*, 256:402–408.

109. Janoff, A., and Zeligs, J. D. (1968): Vascular injury and lysis of basement membrane *in vitro* by neutral protease of human leukocytes. *Science*, 161:702–704.

110. Janoff, A., Shaefer, S., Scherer, J., and Bean, M. A. (1965): Mediators of inflammation in leukocyte lysosomes. II. Mechanism of action of lysosomal cationic protein upon vascular permeability in the rat. *J. Exp. Med.*, 722:841–851.

111. Johnston, R. B., Jr., and Lehmeyer, J. E. (1976): Elaboration of toxic oxygen by-products by neutrophils in a model of immune complex disease. *J. Clin. Invest.*, 57:836–841.

112. Kane, S. P., and Peters, T. J. (1975): Analytical subcellular fractionation of human granulocytes with reference to the localization of vitamin B_{12}-binding proteins. *Clin. Sci. Mol. Med.*, 49:171–182.

113. Kelly, M. T., Martin, R. R., and White, A. (1971): Mediators of histamine release from human platelets, lymphocytes, and granulocytes. *J. Clin. Invest.*, 50:1040–1049.

114. Kirkpatrick, C. H., Green, I., Rich, R. R., and Schade, A. L. (1971): Inhibition of growth of *Candida albicans* by iron unsaturated lactoferrin: Relation to host-defense mechanisms in chronic mucocutaneous candidiasis. *J. Infect. Dis.*, 124:539–544.

114a. Klebanoff, S. J. (1980): Oxygen metabolism and the toxic properties of phagocytes. *Ann. Intern. Med.*, 93:480–489.

115. Klebanoff, S. J., and Clark, R. A. (1978): *The Neutrophil: Function and Clinical Disorders*, pp. 217–281. North-Holland, Amsterdam.

116. Klebanoff, S. J., and Clark, R. A. (1978): *The Neutrophil: Function and Clinical Disorders*, pp. 489–783. North-Holland, Amsterdam.

117. Klempner, M. S., Dinarello, C. A., and Gallin, J. I. (1978): Human leukocytic pyrogen induces release of specific granule contents from human neutrophils. *J. Clin. Invest.*, 61:1330–1336.
118. Klinkhamer, J. M. (1963): Human oral leukocytes. *Periodontics*, 1:109–117.
119. Kociba, G. J., and Griesemer, R. A. (1972): Disseminated intravascular coagulation induced with leukocyte procoagulant. *Am. J. Pathol.*, 69:407–416.
120. Komiyama, A., Morosawa, H., Nakahata, T., Miyagawa, Y., and Akabane, T. (1979): Abnormal neutrophil maturation in a neutrophil defect with morphologic abnormality and impaired function. *J. Pediatr.*, 94:19–25.
121. Konig, W., Frickhofen, N., and Tesch, H. (1978): Generation and secretion of eosinophilotactic activity from human polymorphonuclear neutrophils by various mechanisms of cell activation. *Immunology*, 36:733–742.
122. Koza, E. P., Wright, T. E., and Becker, E. L. (1975): Lysosomal enzyme secretion and volume contraction induced by cytochalasin B, chemotactic factor and A23187. *Proc. Soc. Exp. Biol. Med.*, 149:476–479.
123. Lamster, I. B., Sonis, S. T., Mirando, D. M., and Wilson, R. E. (1979): Influence of supernatants from polymorphonuclear leukocytes on blastogenesis of syngeneic and allogeneic murine splenocytes. *Clin. Exp. Immunol.*, 36:285–291.
124. Lazarus, G. S., Daniels, J. R., Brown, R. S., Bladen, H. A., and Fullmer, H. M. (1968): Degradation of collagen by a human granulocyte collagenolytic system. *J. Clin. Invest.*, 47:2622–2629.
125. Leffell, M. S., and Spitznagel, J. K. (1974): Intracellular and extracellular degranulation of human polymorphonuclear azurophil and specific granules induced by immune complexes. *Infect. Immun.*, 10:1241–1249.
126. Leffell, M. S., and Spitznagel, J. K. (1975): Fate of human lactoferrin and myeloperoxidase in phagocytizing human neutrophils: Effects of immunoglobulin G subclasses and immune complexes coated on latex beads. *Infect. Immun.*, 12:813–820.
127. Lehmeyer, J. E., Synderman, R., and Johnston, R. B. (1979): Stimulation of neutrophil oxidative metabolism by chemotactic peptides: Influence of calcium ion concentration and cytochalasin B and comparison with stimulation by phorbol myristate acetate. *Blood*, 54:35–45.
128. Levine, P. H., Weinger, R. S., Simon, J., Scoon, K. L., and Krinsky, N. I. (1976): Leukocyte-platelet interaction. Release of hydrogen peroxide by granulocytes as a modulator of platelet reactions. *J. Clin. Invest.*, 57:955–963.
129. Lucy, J. A. (1970): The fusion of biological membranes. *Nature (London)*, 227:814–817.
130. Lungren, G., Zukoski, C. F., and Moller, G. (1968): Differential effects of human granulocytes and lymphocytes on human fibroblasts *in vitro*. Clin. Exp. Immunol., 3:817–836.
131. Lynch, J. M., Lotner, G. Z., Betz, S. J., and Henson, P. M. (1979): The release of a platelet-activating factor by stimulated rabbit neutrophils. *J. Immunol.*, 123:1219–1226.
132. Malawista, S. E. (1975): Microtubules and the mobilization of lysosomes in phagocytizing human leukocytes. *Ann. N.Y. Acad. Sci.*, 253:738–749.
133. Malawista, S. E., Gee, J. B. L., and Bensch, K. G. (1971): Cytochalasin B reversibly inhibits phagocytosis: Functional, metabolic, and ultrastructural effects in human blood leukocytes and rabbit alveolar macrophages. *Yale J. Biol. Med.*, 44:286–300.
134. Malemud, C. J., and Janoff, A. (1975): Human polymorphonuclear leukocyte elastase and cathepsin G mediate the degradation of lapine articular cartilage proteoglycan. *Ann. N.Y. Acad. Sci.*, 256:254–262.
135. Masson, P. L., Heremans, J. F., and Schonne, E. (1969): Lactoferrin, an iron-binding protein in neutrophilic leukocytes. *J. Exp. Med.*, 130:643–658.
136. May, C. D., Levine, B. B., and Weissmann, G. (1970): Effects of compounds which inhibit antigenic release of histamine and phagocytic release of lysosomal enzyme on glucose utilization by leukocytes in humans. *Proc. Soc. Exp. Biol. Med.*, 133:758–763.
137. McDonald, J. A., Baum, B. J., Rosenberg, D. M., Kelman, J. A., Brin, S. C., and Crystal, R. G. (1979): Destruction of a major extracellular adhesive glycoprotein (fibronectin) of human fibroblasts by neutral proteases from polymorphonuclear leukocyte granules. *Lab. Invest.*, 40:350–357.
138. Melmon, K. L., and Cline, M. J. (1967): Interaction of plasma kinins and granulocytes. *Nature (London)*, 213:90–92.
139. Metchnikoff, E. (1905): *Immunity in Infective Diseases*, pp. 540; 551. Cambridge University Press, Cambridge, England.

140. Miller, R. L., Webster, M. E., and Melmon, K. L. (1975): Interaction of leukocytes and endotoxin with the plasmin and kinin systems. *Eur. J. Pharmacol.*, 33:53–60.

141. Miller, T. E. (1969): Killing and lysis of gram-negative bacteria through the synergistic effect of hydrogen peroxide, ascorbic acid, and lysozyme. *J. Bactiol.*, 98:949–955.

142. Moore, D. M., Murphy, P. A., Chesney, P. J., and Wood, W. B. Jr. (1973): Synthesis of endogenous pyrogen by rabbit leukocytes. *J. Exp. Med.*, 137:1263–1274.

143. Moore, P. L., Bank, N. L., Brissie, N. T., and Spicer, S. S. (1976): Association of microfilament bundles with lysosomes in polymorphonuclear leukocytes. *J. Cell Biol.*, 71:659–666.

144. Moore, P. L., Bank, H. L., Brissie, N. T., and Spicer, S. S. (1978): Phagocytosis of bacteria by polymorphonuclear leukocytes: A freeze-fracture, scanning electron microscope, and thin section investigation of membrane structure. *J. Cell Biol.*, 76:158–174.

145. Movat, H. Z., Steinberg, S. G., Habal, F. M., and Ranadive, N. S. (1973): Demonstration of a kinin-generating enzyme in the lysosomes of human polymorphonuclear leukocytes. *Lab. Invest.*, 29:669–684.

146. Movat, H. Z., Habal, F. M., and Macmorine, D. R. L. (1976): Generation of a vasoactive peptide by a neutral protease of human neutrophil leukocytes. *Agents Actions*, 6:183–190.

147. Murata, F., and Spicer, S. S. (1973): Morphologic and cytochemical studies of rabbit heterophilic leukocytes. Evidence for tertiary granules. *Lab. Invest.*, 29:65–72.

148. Murphy, G., Reynolds, J. J., Bretz, V., and Baggiolini, M. (1977): Collagenase is a component of the specific granules of human neutrophil leukocytes. *Biochem. J.*, 162:195–197.

149. Nachman, R., Hirsch, J. G., and Baggiolini, M. (1972): Studies on isolated membranes of azurophil and specific granules from rabbit polymorphonuclear leukocytes. *J. Cell Biol.*, 54:133–140.

150. Nakamura, S., Yoshinaga, M., and Hayashi, H. (1976): Interaction between lymphocytes and inflammatory exudate cells. II. A proteolytic enzyme released by PMN as a possible mediator for enhancement of thymocyte response. *J. Immunol.*, 117:1–6.

151. Niemetz, J. (1972): Coagulant activity of leukocytes. Tissue factor activity. *J. Clin. Invest.*, 51:307–313.

152. Nordlund, J. J., Root, R. K., and Wolff, S. M. (1970): Studies on the origin of human leukocytic pyrogen. *J. Exp. Med.*, 131:727–743.

153. Odeberg, H., Olsson, I., and Venge, P. (1975): Cationic proteins of human granulocytes. IV. Esterase activity. *Lab. Invest.*, 32:86–90.

154. O'Flaherty, J. T., Showell, H. S., Becker, E. L., and Ward, P. A. (1979): Arachidonic acid aggregates neutrophils. *Inflammation*, 3:431–436.

155. Ohlsson, K., and Olsson, I. (1973): The neutral proteases of human granulocytes. Isolation and partial characterization of two granulocyte collagenases. *Eur. J. Biochem.*, 36:473–481.

156. Ohlsson, K., Olsson, I., and Spitznagel, J. K. (1977): Localization of chymotrypsin-like cationic protein, collagenase, and elastase in azurophil granules of human neutrophilic polymorphonuclear leukocytes. *Hoppe Syler Z. Physiol. Chem.*, 358:361–366.

157. Oram, J. D., and Reiter, B. (1968): Inhibition of bacteria by lactoferrin and other iron-chelating agents. *Biochim. Biophys. Acta.*, 170:351–365.

158. Oronsky, A. L., Ignarro, L., and Perper, R. (1973): Release of cartilage mucopolysaccharide-degrading neutral protease from human leukocytes. *J. Exp. Med.*, 138:461–472.

159. Parmley, R. T., Ogawa, M., Darby, C. P., Jr., and Spicer, S. S. (1975): Congenital neutropenia: Neutrophil proliferation with abnormal maturation. *Blood*, 46:723–734.

160. Pelus, L. M., Broxmeyer, H. E., Kurland, J. I., and Moore, M. A. S. (1979): Regulation of macrophage and granulocyte proliferation. Specificities of prostaglandin E and lactoferrin. *J. Exp. Med.*, 150:277–292.

161. Peterson, R. G., and Hartsell, S. E. (1955): The lysozyme spectrum of the gram-negative bacteria. *J. Infect. Dis.*, 96:75–81.

162. Plow, E. F., and Edgington, T. S. (1975): Alternative pathway for fibrinolysis I. Cleavage of fibrinogen by leukocyte proteases at physiologic pH. *J. Clin. Invest.*, 56:30–38.

163. Pruzansky, J. J., and Patterson, R. (1967): Subcellular distribution of histamine in human leukocytes. *Proc. Soc. Exp. Biol. Med.*, 124:56–59.

164. Pryzwansky, K. B., Rausch, P. G., Spitznagel, J. K., and Herion, J. C. (1979): Immunocytochemical distinction between primary and secondary granule formation in developing human neutrophils: Correlations with Romanowsky stains. *Blood*, 53:179–185.

165. Ranadive, N. S., and Cochrane, C. G. (1968): Isolation and characterization of permeability factors from rabbit neutrophils. *J. Exp. Med.*, 128:605–622.

166. Ranadive, N. S., Sajnani, A. N., Alimurka, K., and Movat, H. Z. (1973): Release of basic proteins and lysosomal enzymes from neutrophil leukocytes of the rabbit. *Int. Arch. Allergy Appl. Immunol.*, 45:880–898.

167. Rausch, P. G., Pryzwansky, K. B., and Spitznagel, J. K. (1978): Immunocytochemical identification of azurophilic and specific granule markers in the giant granules of Chediak-Higashi neutrophils. *N. Engl. J. Med.*, 298:693–698.

168. Reiter, B., Brock, J. H., and Steel, E. D. (1975): Inhibition of *E. coli.* by bovine colostrum and post-colostral milk. II. The bacteriostatic effect of lactoferrin on a serum susceptible and serum resistant strain of *E. coli. Immunology*, 28:83–95.

169. Robineaux, J., and Frederick, J. (1955): Contribution à l'étude des granulations neutrophiles des polynucléaires par la microcinematographie en contraste de phase. *C.R. Soc. Biol. (Paris)*, 149:486–489.

170. Roos, D., Goldstein, I. M., Kaplan, H. B., and Weissmann, G. (1976): Dissociation of phagocytosis, metabolic stimulation, and lysosomal enzyme release in human leukocytes. *Agents Actions*, 6:256–259.

171. Root, R. K., Metcalf, J., Oshino, N., and Chance, B. (1975): H_2O_2 release from human granulocytes during phagocytosis. I. Documentation, quantitation, and some regulating factors. *J. Clin. Invest.*, 55:945–955.

172. Rosenwasser, L. J., Dinarello, C. A., and Rosenthal (1979): Adherent cell function in murine T-lymphocyte antigen recognition. IV. Enhancement of murine T-cell antigen recognition by human leukocytic pyrogen. *J. Exp. Med.*, 150:709–714.

173. Saba, H. I., Roberts, H. R., and Herion, J. C. (1967): The anti-coagulant activity of lysosomal cationic proteins from polymorphonuclear leukocytes. *J. Clin. Invest.*, 46:580–589.

174. Saba, H. I., Herion, J. C., Walker, R.'I., and Roberts, H. R. (1973): The procoagulant activity of granulocytes. *Proc. Soc. Exp. Biol. Med.*, 142:614–620.

175. Saba, H. I., Herion, J. C., Walker, R. I., and Roberts, H. R. (1975): Effect of lysosomal cationic proteins from polymorphonuclear leukocytes upon fibrinogen and fibrinolysis system. *Thromb. Res.*, 7:543–554.

176. Sando, G. N., and Neufeld, E. F. (1977): Recognition and receptor mediated uptake of a lysosomal enzyme, alpha-l-iduronidase, by cultured human fibroblasts. *Cell*, 12:619–627.

177. Scherer, J., and Janoff, A. (1968): Mediators of inflammation in leukocyte lysosomes. VII. Observations on mast cell disrupting agents in different species. *Lab. Invest.*, 18:196–202.

178. Schiffmann, E., and Gallin, J. I. (1979): Biochemistry of phagocyte chemotaxis. In: *Current Topics in Cellular Regulation*, Vol. 15, pp. 203–261. Academic Press, New York.

179. Schmidt, W., Egbring, R., and Havermann, K. (1975): Effect of elastase-like and chymotrypsin-like neutral proteases from human granulocytes on isolated clotting factors. *Thromb. Res.*, 6:315–326.

180. Schultz, J., Corlin, R., Oddi, F., Kaminker, K., and Jones, W. (1965): Myeloperoxidase of the leukocyte of normal human blood. III. Isolation of the peroxidase granule. *Arch. Biochem. Biophys*, 111:73–79.

181. Scott, R. E., and Horn, R. G. (1970): Ultrastructural aspects of neutrophil granulocyte development in humans. *Lab. Invest.*, 23:202–215.

182. Showell, H. J., Freer, R. J., Zigmond, S. H., Schiffmann, E., Aswanikumar, S., Corcoran, B., and Becker, E. L. (1976): The structure-activity relations of synthetic peptides as chemotactic factors and inducers of lysosomal enzyme secretion for neutrophils. *J. Exp. Med.*, 143:1154–1169.

183. Showell, H. J., Naccache, P. H., Sha'afi, R. I., and Becker, E. L. (1977): The effects of extracellular K^+, Na^+, and Ca^{++} on lysosomal enzyme secretion from polymorphonuclear leukocytes. *J. Immunol.*, 119:804–811.

184. Simon, J. D., Houck, W. E., and Albala, M. M. (1976): Release of unsaturated vitamin B_{12}-binding capacity from human granulocytes by the calcium ionophore A23187. *Biochem. Biophys. Res. Commun.*, 73:444–450.

185. Skosey, J. L., Damagaard, E., Chow, D., and Sorensen, L. B. (1974): Modification of zymosan-induced release of lysosomal enzymes from human polymorphonuclear leukocytes by cytochalasin B. *J. Cell Biol.*, 62:625–634.

186. Smith, R. J., and Ignarro, L. J. (1975): Bioregulation of lysosomal enzyme secretion from human neutrophils: Roles of guanosine 3', 5'-monophosphate and calcium in stimulus-secretion coupling. *Proc. Natl. Acad. Sci. U.S.A.*, 72:108–112.

187. Smith, R. J., and Iden, S. S. (1979): Phorbol myristate acetate-induced rlease of granule enzymes from human neutrophils: Inhibition by the calcium antagonist, B-(N,N-diethylamino)-octyl 3,4,5-trimethoxybenzoate hydrochloride. *Biochem. Biophys. Res. Commun.*, 91:263–271.
188. Spicer, S. S., and Hardin, J. H. (1969): Ultrastructure, cytochemistry, and function of neutrophil leukocyte granules. A review. *Lab. Invest.*, 20:488–497.
189. Spilberg, I., Gallacher, A., Mehta, J. M., and Mandell, B.: Urate crystal-induced chemotactic factor. Isolation and partial characterization. *J. Clin. Invest.*, 58:815–819.
190. Spitznagel, J. K. (1975): Advances in the study of cytoplasmic granules of human neutrophilic polymorphonuclear leukocytes. In: *The Phagocytic Cell in Host Resistance*, edited by J. Bellanti and D. Dayton, pp. 77–85. Raven Press, New York.
191. Spitznagel, J. K., Cooper, M. R., McCall, A. E., DeChatelet, L. R., and Welsh, I. R. H. (1972): Selective deficiency of granules associated with lysozyme and lactoferrin in human polymorphs (PMN) with reduced microbicidal capacity. *J. Clin. Invest.*, 51:93a.
192. Spitznagel, J. K., Dalldorf, F. G., Leffell, M. S., Folds, J. D., Welsh, R. H., Cooney, M. H., and Martin, L. E. (1974): Character of azurophil and specific granules purified from human polymorphonuclear leukocytes. *Lab. Invest.*, 30:774–785.
193. Stenson, W. F., and Parker, C. W. (1979): Metabolism of archidonic acid in ionophore stimulated neutrophils. Esterification of a hydroxylated metabolite into phospholipids. *J. Clin. Invest.*, 64:1457–1465.
194. Stenson, W. F., and Parker, C. W. (1980): Monohydroxyeicosatetranoic acids (HETEs) induce degranulation of human neutrophils. *J. Immunol.*, 124:2100–2104.
195. Strauss, R. G., Boue, K. E., Jones, J. E., Mauer, A. M., and Fulginiti, V. A. (1974): An anomaly of neutrophil morphology with impaired function. *N. Engl. J. Med.*, 290:478–484.
196. Strominger, J. L., and Tipper, D. J. (1974): Structure of bacterial cell walls: The lysozyme substrate. In: *Lysozyme*, edited by E. Osserman, W. Canfield, and C. Bechok, pp. 169–184. Academic Press, New York.
197. Taichman, N. S., Pruzanski, W., and Ranadive, N. S. (1972): Release of intracellular constituents from rabbit polymorphonuclear leukocytes exposed to soluble and insoluble immune complexes. *Int. Arch. Allergy Appl. Immunol.*, 43:182–195.
198. Takanaka, K., and O'Brien, P. J. (1975): Mechanisms of H_2O_2 formation by leukocytes. Evidence for a plasma membrane location. *Arch. Biochem. Biophys.*, 169:428–435.
199. Taubman, S. B., and Cogen, R. B. (1975): Cell detaching activity mediated by an enzyme(s) obtained from human leukocyte granules. *Lab. Invest.*, 32:555–560.
200. Teir, H., Rytomaa, T., Cedarburg, A., and Kiviniemi, K. (1963): Studies on the elimination of granulocytes in the intestinal tract of the rat. *Acta Pathol. Microbiol. Scand.*, 59:311–324.
201. Thoa, N. B., Costa, J. L., Moss, J., and Kopin, I. J. (1974): Mechanism of release of norepinephrine from peripheral adrenergic neurons by calcium ionophores X-537a and A23187. *Life Sci. (I)*, 14:1705–1719.
202. Thomas, L. (1964): Possible role of leukocyte granules in the Shwartzman and Arthus reactions. *Proc. Soc. Exp. Biol. Med.*, 115:235–240.
203. Thompson, A. R., Takaki, A., Enfield, D. L., and Wright, D. G. (1980): Calcium dependent activation cleavages of ^{125}I-human factor IX by a human granulocyte (PMN) constituent. *Clin. Res.*, 28:326A.
204. Thorne, K. J. I., Oliver, R. C., and Barrett, A. J. (1976): Lysis and killing of bacteria by lysosomal proteinases. *Infect. Immun.*, 14:555–563.
205. Ulevitch, R. J., Henson, P., Holmes, B., and Good, R. A. (1974): An in vitro study of exocytosis of neutrophil granule enzymes in chronic granulomatous disease neutrophils. *J. Immunol.*, 112:1383–1386.
206. Venge, P., and Olsson, I. (1975): Cationic proteins of human granulocytes. VI. Effects on the complement system and mediation of chemotactic activity. *J. Immunol.*, 115:1505–1508.
207. Vischer, T. L., Bretz, V., and Baggiolini, M. (1976): In vitro stimulation of lymphocytes by neutral proteinases from human polymorphonuclear leukocyte granules. *J. Exp. Med.*, 133:100–112.
208. Waite, M., DeChatelet, L. R., King, L. and Shirley, P. S. (1979): Phagocytosis-induced release of arachidonic acid from human neutrophils. *Biochem. Biophys. Res. Commun.*, 90:984–992.
209. Ward, P. A. (1968): Chemotaxis of mononuclear cells. *J. Exp. Med.*, 128:1201–1221.
210. Ward, P. A., and Hill, J. H. (1970): C5 chemotactic fragment produced by an enzyme in lysosomal granules of neutrophils. *J. Immunol.*, 104:535–543.

211. Ward, P. A., and Zvaifler, N. J. (1973): Quantitative phagocytosis by neutrophils. II. Release of the C5-cleaving enzyme and inhibition of phagocytosis by rheumatoid factor. *J. Immunol.*, 111:1777–1782.

212. Weissmann, G., and Dukor, P. (1970): The role of lysosomes in immune responses. *Adv. Immunol.*, 12–283–331.

213. Weissmann, G., Becher, B., and Thomas, L. (1964): Studies on lysosomes. V. The effects of streptolysins and other hemolytic agents on isolated leukocyte granules. *J. Cell Biol.*, 22:115–126.

214. Weissmann, G., Dukor, P., and Zurier, R. B. (1971): Effect of cylic AMP on release of lysosomal enzymes from phagocytes. *Nature (New Biol.)*, 231:131–135.

215. Weissmann, G., Zurier, R. B., Spieler, P. J., and Goldstein, I. M. (1971): Mechanisms of lysosomal enzyme release from leukocytes exposed to immune complexes and other particles. *J. Exp. Med.*, 134:149–165.

216. Weissmann, G., Zurier, R. B., and Hoffstein, S. (1972): Leukocytic proteases and the immunologic release of lysosomal enzymes. *Am. J. Pathol.*, 68:539–559.

217. Weissmann, G., Zurier, R. B., and Hoffstein, S. (1973): Leukocytes as secretory organs of inflammation. *Agents Actions*, 3:370–379.

218. Weissmann, G., Goldstein, I., Hoffstein, S., Chauvet, G., and Robineaux, R. (1975): Yin/Yang modulation of lysosomal enzyme release from polymorphonuclear leukocytes by cyclic nucleotides. *Ann. N.Y. Acad. Sci.*, 256:222–232.

219. Weissmann, G., Smolen, J. E., and Korchak, H. M. (1980): Release of inflammatory mediators from stimulated neutrophils. *N. Engl. J. Med.*, 202:27–34.

220. Weissmann, G., Pearlstein, E., Perez, H. D., Falkow, S., Goldstein, I. M., and Hoffstein, S. T. (1980): Neutrophils synthesize and deposit fibronectin on surfaces to which they attach. *Clin. Res.*, 28:552A.

221. Wessells, N. K., Spooner, B. S., Ash, J. F., Bradley, M. O., Ludena, M. S., Taylor, E. L., Wrenn, J. T., and Yamada, K. M. (1971): Microfilaments in cellular and developmental processes. *Science*, 171:135–143.

222. West, B. C., Rosenthal, A. S., Gelb, N. A., and Kimball, H. R. (1974): Separation and characterization of human neutrophil granules. *Am. J. Pathol.*, 77:41–62.

223. Wetzel, B. K., Horn, R. G., and Spicer, S. S. (1963): Cytochemical localization of nonspecific phosphatase activity in rabbit myeloid elements. *J. Histochem. Cytochem.*, 11:812–814.

224. Wetzel, B. K., Spicer, S. S., and Horn, R. G. (1967): Fine structural localization of acid and alkaline phosphatases in cells of rabbit blood and bone marrow. *J. Histochem. Cytochem.*, 15:311–334.

225. Wetzel, B. K., Horn, R. G., and Spicer, S. S. (1967): Fine structural studies on the development of heterophil, eosinophil, and basophil granulocytes in rabbits. *Lab. Invest.*, 16:349–382.

226. White, J. G., and Estensen, R. D. (1974): Selective labilization of specific granules in polymorphonuclear leukocytes by phorbol myristate acetate. *Am. J. Pathol.*, 75:45–54.

227. Wilson, L. A., and Spitznagel, J. K. (1968): Molecular and structural damage to *E. coli* produced by antibody, complement, and lysozyme systems. *J. Bacteriol.*, 96:1339–1348.

228. Woodin, A. M. (1973): The leukocidin-treated leukocyte. In: *Lysosomes in Biology and Pathology*, edited by J. T. Dingle, pp. 395–422. North-Holland, Amsterdam.

229. Woodin, A. M., and Wieneke, A. A. (1963): The accumulation of calcium by the polymorphonuclear leukocyte treated with staphylococcal leukocidin and its significance in the extrusion of protein. *Biochem. J.*, 87:487–495.

230. Woodin, A. M., and Wieneke, A. A. (1966): The secretion of protein by the polymorphonuclear leukocyte treated with streptolysin O. *Exp. Cell Res.*, 43:319–331.

231. Woodin, A. M., French, J. E., and Marchesi, V. T. (1963): Morphological changes associated with the extrusion of protein induced in the polymorphonuclear leukocyte by staphylococcal leukocidin. *Biochem. J.*, 87:567–571.

232. Wright, D. G. (1981): The activation and deactivation of neutrophils. In: *Physiology and Biochemistry of Acute Infections*, edited by M. C. Powanda, and P. G. Canonico. North-Holland, Amsterdam (in press).

233. Wright, D. G., and Malawista, S. E. (1972): The mobilization and extracellular release of granular enzymes from human leukocytes during phagoctyosis. *J. Cell Biol.*, 53:788–797.

234. Wright, D. G., and Malawista, S. E. (1973): Mobilization and extracellular release of granular enzymes from human leukocytes during phagocytosis: Inhibition by colchicine and corticosteroid but not by salicylates. *Arthritis Rheum.*, 16:749–758.
235. Wright, D. G., and Gallin, J. I. (1975): Modulation of the inflammatory response by-products released from human polymorphonuclear leukocytes during phagocytosis. Generation and inactivation of the chemocactic factor C5a. *Inflammation*, 1:23–39.
236. Wright, D. G., and Gallin, J. I. (1977): A functional differentiation of human neutrophil granules: Generation of C5a by a specific (secondary) granule product and inactivation of C5a by azurophil (primary) granule products. *J. Immunol.*, 119:1068–1076.
237. Wright, D. G., and Gallin, J. I. (1979): Secretory responses of human neutrophils: Exocytosis of specific (secondary) granules by human neutrophils during adherence *in vitro* and during exudation *in vivo*. *J. Immunol.*, 123:285–294.
238. Wright, D. G., and Greenwald, D. (1979): Increased motility and maturation of human blood monocytes stimulated by products released from neutrophil secondary granules. *Blood*, 54 (Suppl. 1):95a.
239. Wright, D. G., Bralove, D. A., and Gallin, J. I. (1977): The differential mobilization of human neutrophil granules. Effects of phorbol myristate acetate and ionophore A23187. *Am. J. Pathol.*, 87:273–281.
240. Wright, D. G., Kelman, J. A., Gallin, J. I., and Crystal, R. G. (1978): Extracellular release by human neutrophils (PMN) of a latent collagenase stored in the specific (secondary) granules. *Clin. Res.*, 26:387A.
241. Wright, D. G., Meierovics, A. I., Richards, R. L., and Alving, C. R. (1981): Studies of cytoplasmic granules in human neutrophils (PMN): Differences in the membrane phospholipid content of azurophil and specific granules. *Fed. Proc.*, 40:375.
242. Wright, D. G., Dale, D. C., Fauci, A. S., and Wolff, S. M. (1981): Human cyclic neutropenia: Clinical review and long-term follow-up of patients. *Medicine*, 60:1–13.
243. Wunschmann-Henderson, B., Horwitz, D., and Astrup, T. (1972): Release of plasminogen activator from viable leukocytes of man, baboon, dog, and rabbit. *Proc. Soc. Exp. Biol. Med.*, 141:634–638.
243a. Yin, H. L., and Stossel, T. P. (1979): Control of cytoplasmic actin gel-sol transformation by gelsolin, a calcium-dependent regulatory protein. *Nature (London)*, 281:583–586.
244. Yoshinaga, M., Nishime, K., Nakamura, S., and Goto, F. (1980): A PMN-derived factor that enhances DNA-synthesis in PHA or antigen-stimulated lymphocytes. *J. Immunol.*, 124:94–99.
245. Zigmond, S. H., and Hirsch, J. G. (1972): Effects of cytochalasin B on polymorphonuclear leukocyte locomotion, phagocytosis and glycolysis. *Exp. Cell Res.*, 73:383–393.
246. Zucker-Franklin, D. (1965): Electron microscope study of the degranulation of polymorphonuclear leukocytes following treatment with streptolysin. *Am. J. Pathol.*, 47:419–433.
247. Zucker-Franklin, D., and Hirsch, J. G. (1964): Electron microscope studies on the degranulation of rabbit peritoneal leukocytes during phagocytosis. *J. Exp. Med.*, 120:569–576.
248. Zurier, R. B. (1976): Prostaglandin release from human polymorphonuclear leukocytes. *Adv. Prostaglandin Thromboxane Res.*, 2:815–818.
249. Zurier, R. B., Hoffstein, S., and Weissmann, G. (1973): Cytochalasin B: Effect on lysosomal enzyme release from human leukocytes. *Proc. Natl. Acad. Sci. U.S.A.*, 70:844–848.
250. Zurier, R. B., Hoffstein, S., and Weissmann, G. (1973): Mechanisms of lysosomal enzyme release from human leukocytes. I. Effect of cyclic nucleotides and colchicine. *J. Cell Biol.*, 58:27–41.

Advances in Host Defense Mechanisms, Vol. 1,
edited by John I. Gallin and Anthony S. Fauci,
Raven Press, New York © 1982.

Oxygen-Dependent Cytotoxic Mechanisms of Phagocytes

Seymour J. Klebanoff

*Department of Medicine, University of Washington School of Medicine,
Seattle, Washington 98195*

In 1933, Baldridge and Gerard (38) described "the extra respiration of phagocytosis" which occurred when dog leukocytes were incubated with *Sarcina lutea*. The increase in oxygen consumption "began at once, reached a maximum value twice that at the start in about 15 minutes and was over in 90–150 minutes." Thus began a new era in the physiology of phagocytes, the oxidative phase in which attention was drawn to the mechanism of the respiratory burst and to its function.

All phagocytic leukocytes [neutrophils, eosinophils, mononuclear phagocytes (monocytes, macrophages)] have in common a mechanism or mechanisms by which perturbation of the plasma membrane results in a burst of oxygen consumption. This plasma membrane disturbance is generally a prelude to phagocytosis but need not be so. The leukocyte may be exposed to an antigen-antibody complex on a nonphagocytosable surface and respond to it as it would to an appropriately opsonized particle. In addition, there are a number of soluble agents which can react with cell-surface components to initiate the respiratory burst.

The mechanism of the respiratory burst has been reviewed elsewhere (24,30,109,253) and will not be considered in detail here. Its presence suggests that there is an enzyme in phagocytes which is dormant when the cell is at rest but which is activated by exposure of the phagocyte to a stimulus, such as an opsonized particle, with a resultant increase in oxygen consumption. The early finding that cyanide did not inhibit the respiratory burst of the polymorphonuclear leukocyte (PMN) (45,95,405) distinguished this activity from the mitochondrial respiratory chain, which is cyanide-sensitive, and drew attention to flavoprotein oxidases, which are unaffected by cyanide. Although the precise nature of the oxidase(s) has yet to be definitively established, the most widely held view is that it is a reduced pyridine nucleotide oxidase which, in some species at least, is associated with the plasma membrane (24,30,94,109,154,253). There is some controversy as to whether the primary nucleotide oxidized is NADPH or NADH and the structure of the enzyme and its organization within the membrane is only beginning to be understood. Some solubilization of the human enzyme has been recently achieved (146,147,442). The NAD(P)H oxidase(s) of PMNs appears to be a flavoprotein, requiring flavin adenine dinucleotide (FAD) for optimum activity (27,146,223). There is growing support for a transmembrane electron transport system [possibly involving the oxidation and reduction of a cytochrome of the b type (57,58,186,409–412,414,421)], which links the oxidation of intracellular reduced pyridine nucleotides to the reduction of oxygen in the extracellular fluid or, following membrane invagination, in the intraphagosomal space. The NAD(P)H oxidase activity also has been detected in preparations of mononuclear phagocytes (390,422) and eosinophils (31,111,444).

Early studies had indicated that the extra oxygen consumed by neutrophils was not needed for the generation of the metabolic energy required for the ingestion process; phagocytosis was unaffected by hypoxia or by inhibitors of oxidative phosphorylation such as dinitrophenol (12,45,95,405,406). Phagocytosis by eosinophils also occurred in the absence of oxygen (91), whereas mononuclear phagocytes varied in the need for oxidative metabolism. Thus, guinea pig (354), rabbit (355), and human (93) alveolar macrophages appeared to require oxidative metabolism for optimum phagocytic activity, whereas guinea pig (354) and mouse (445) peritoneal macrophages and human monocytes (90) and monocyte-derived macrophages (89) did not.

Oxygen is required for the optimum microbicidal activity of phagocytes. Thus, hypoxia inhibits (but does not abolish) the antimicrobial activity of neutrophils (198,255,279,281,295,315,416) and the tumoricidal activity of macrophages (338, 342). Studies of the effect of hypoxia on the microbicidal activity of macrophages, however, have yielded conflicting results with some studies showing a decrease in killing (89,327) and others (335,445) no effect. An important role for the respiratory burst in the microbicidal activity of phagocytes was further emphasized by the major defect in the respiratory burst of neutrophils from patients with chronic granulomatous disease (CGD) (197). These cells ingest but do not kill certain microorganisms (199,369). A comparable killing defect was found in CGD monocytes (108,379) and eosinophils (278) suggesting that the antimicrobial systems of these cells also are dependent, in part, on the respiratory burst.

Thus, attention was drawn to oxygen as a potential source of the toxic agents required to kill ingested organisms and extracellular targets. The agents of greatest interest are the products of oxygen reduction and excitation, namely the superoxide anion (O_2^-), hydrogen peroxide (H_2O_2) hydroxyl radicals ($\cdot OH$) and singlet oxygen ($^1O_2$). This review will deal with the role of these agents in the cytocidal activity of phagocytes.

SUPEROXIDE ANION

Production

Oxygen in its ground state contains two unpaired valence electrons. Each occupies a separate orbital which can be filled by the addition of a second electron. When oxygen accepts a single electron, it is converted to O_2^- or its protonated form, the perhydroxyl radical (HO_2) as follows:

$$O_2 \xrightarrow{ e } \begin{matrix} HO_2^{\cdot} \\ \updownarrow \\ H^+ + O_2^{\bar{}} \end{matrix} \quad \begin{matrix} \text{perhydroxyl radical} \\ \\ \text{superoxide anion} \end{matrix} \qquad (a)$$

The pKa for the dissociation of the perhydroxyl radical is 4.8 (47,51), so that the radical exists almost entirely as the superoxide anion at neutral pH. Assay systems for the detection of $O_2^{\bar{}}$ have been reviewed (62,143–145).

A new chapter in the continuing saga of the respiratory burst began in 1973 with the report by Babior and co-workers (29) that phagocytosis by neutrophils is associated with the formation of $O_2^{\bar{}}$. Superoxide production was based on the reduction of cytochrome C by intact neutrophils (a reaction which can be induced by $O_2^{\bar{}}$) and its inhibition by superoxide dismutase. The confirmation of this finding by a number of investigators using a variety of assays, and the finding that stimulated eosinophils (111,263,444) and mononuclear phagocytes (119,216,436,465) also generate $O_2^{\bar{}}$, has led to the generally held view that $O_2^{\bar{}}$ is the initial product of the respiratory burst. A number of oxidases reduce oxygen, in part or totally, to $O_2^{\bar{}}$; the oxidase responsible for the respiratory burst of phagocytes appears to be one of these, catalyzing the reaction

$$NAD(P)H + 2O_2 \rightarrow 2O_2^{\bar{}} + NAD(P)^+ + H^+ \qquad (b)$$

The conclusion that $O_2^{\bar{}}$ is the primary product of the respiratory burst has been questioned by Segal and Meshulam (413) based on the lack of inhibition of neutrophil oxygen consumption by cytochrome C or superoxide dismutase. Oxygen is reformed from $O_2^{\bar{}}$ by these agents and this recycling of oxygen should theoretically decrease the total amount of oxygen consumed by neutrophils. It has been proposed, however, that the absence of a reduction in oxygen consumption by cytochrome C or superoxide dismutase may be due to the high cell concentrations employed in the experiments of Segal and Meshulam (25) or to the development of an oxygen-diffusion barrier at the active site of the membrane oxidase (159).

Toxic Properties

Interest in the toxicity of $O_2^{\bar{}}$ in biological systems stemmed from the finding that superoxide dismutase, an enzyme which scavenges $O_2^{\bar{}}$, is widely distributed in nature, raising the possibility that the primary function of this enzyme is to protect cells from the toxic effect of $O_2^{\bar{}}$ (143–145). In general, organisms which require oxygen for growth (aerobes), and thus have the potential for $O_2^{\bar{}}$ production, contain relatively large amounts of superoxide dismutase, strict anaerobes contain little or none, and organisms which tolerate but do not require oxygen (aerotolerant anaerobes) contain intermediate amounts (310). Some anaerobes contain superoxide dismutase (166,194,440), which may be responsible in part for the variability in the susceptibility of anaerobes to oxygen toxicity.

Certain $O_2^{\bar{}}$-generating systems are toxic to cells, particularly those deficient in superoxide dismutase, and in some instances the addition of superoxide dismutase is protective, implicating O_2^- in the toxicity (163–165,167,181,182,234,349.) The O_2^- also inhibits the gelation of collagen solutions (161) and has been reported to generate a chemotactic factor *in vivo* or when added to plasma *in vitro* (361). It should be emphasized that inhibition by superoxide dismutase does not necessarily indicate a direct effect of O_2^-; an agent dependent on O_2^- for its formation may be responsible. Indeed it is now a widely held view that O_2^- itself has relatively weak direct toxic activity (30,124,145,215,249). Superoxide is both a one-electron reductant and a one-electron oxidant, which can react with a number of compounds (276,404). However, with many biologically important compounds [e.g., amino acids (51)], the reaction rate is exceedingly slow as compared to that observed with other reactants (e.g., ·OH), and there is little evidence to suggest that these direct actions of O_2^- are cytotoxic. Fee and Valentine (124) stated: "It is the opinion of the authors that no chemical reactions have yet been found which would explain how superoxide could act as a 'deleterious' or 'cytotoxic' species. So far superoxide itself does not have the necessary reactivity." Thus it is probable that O_2^- exerts its toxicity largely through the products which it forms, namely H_2O_2, ·OH, and possibly $^1O_2$ as indicated below.

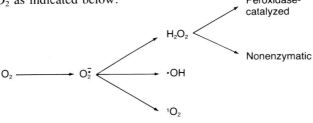

Superoxide can cross the erythrocyte cell membrane (293) either through anion channels (294) or by penetration of the lipid bilayer (392), and this permeability may allow the passage of O_2^- to a site where its more reactive products can exert their toxic effect. The *Escherichia coli* cell envelope, however, appears to be impermeable to O_2^- (183).

HYDROGEN PEROXIDE

Production

The formation of H_2O_2 by PMNs during phagocytosis was first proposed by Iyer and co-workers (205) based on the oxidation of formate – ^{14}C to $^{14}CO_2$, a reaction which is catalyzed by catalase in the presence of H_2O_2, and H_2O_2 formation by stimulated PMNs has since been confirmed by a number of investigators using a variety of techniques (for review see 253). The generation of H_2O_2 by eosinophils (31,111,263) and mononuclear phagocytes (250,337,339,380,389) also have been repeatedly demonstrated. H_2O_2 is formed when oxygen accepts two electrons. It is a weak acid which can dissociate to form the corresponding anion (HO_2^-). The pKa of this dissociation, however, is high (pKa $-$ 11.7), and ionization of the second proton of H_2O_2 does not appear to occur in aqueous solutions (pKa $>$ 14) (124). Thus, H_2O_2 exists almost entirely in the fully protonated form at neutral or acid pH. Hydrogen peroxide can be formed from oxygen either directly by divalent reduction without an apparent O_2^- intermediate [as by glucose oxidase (298,347,428)], or at least in part via the intermediate formation of O_2^- [as by xanthine oxidase (142)]. The NAD(P)H oxidase of leukocytes falls into the second category in which H_2O_2 formation is preceded, in part or totally, by the univalent reduction of oxygen.

Hydrogen peroxide is formed from two superoxide (or perhydroxyl) radicals by a dismutation reaction in which one radical is oxidized and the other reduced as follows:

$$HO_2^. + O_2^- + H^+ \rightarrow O_2 + H_2O_2 \qquad (c)$$

This dismutation can occur spontaneously or be catalyzed by the enzyme, superoxide dismutase. Spontaneous dismutation occurs most rapidly at pH 4.8 [rate constant $8.5 \times 10^7\,M^{-1}sec^-$ (47)], where the perhydroxyl and superoxide radicals are present in equal concentrations (reaction c). When the pH is decreased below 4.8, the perhydroxl radical predominates, and the rate of dismutation decreases to a plateau (rate constant $7.6 \times 10^5\,M^{-1}sec^{-1}$) at pH 2.0. When the pH increases above 4.8, the superoxide anion predominates, and the rate of dismutation falls sharply; indeed it is probable that at very high pH or in aprotic solvents where O_2^- is the sole species, spontaneous dismutation does not occur (50). The rate constant at neutral pH is $4.5 \times 10^5\,M^{-1}sec^{-1}$ (47). The dismutation of O_2^- is catalyzed by superoxide dismutase over a wide pH range [rate constant $1.9 \times 10^9\,M^{-1}sec^{-1}$, with little variation from pH 5.0 to 9.5 (370)]; however, the catalysis is most significant at neutral or alkaline pH, where the rate of spontaneous dismutation falls. A number of distinct superoxide dismutases exist which differ in their metal component (copper-zinc, manganese or iron), their primary structure, and their distribution in tissues and microorganisms (143–145).

The pH within the phagosome is acidic, with values in neutrophils in one study (211) of approximately 6.5 at 3 min and 4.0 at 7 to 15 min following phagocytosis. Thus, the vacuolar pH appears to be in the region where spontaneous dismutation is very rapid. Presumably, the pH also falls to a comparable level in the pockets formed between adherent phagocytes and extracellular targets. Two distinct superoxide dismutases have been detected in neutrophils, one cyanide-sensitive and present in the cytosol and the other cyanide-insensitive and present in the particulate fraction (217,375,398). These are the properties expected of the copper-zinc and the manganese enzymes, respectively. The release of these leukocytic enzymes into the phagosome (or extracellarly) has not been demonstrated; superoxide dismutase, however, may be introduced into the phagosome as a component of the ingested organism.

Toxic Properties

The demonstration that H_2O_2 is a product of the respiratory burst immediately focused attention on the role of this agent in the cytotoxic activity of phagocytes. Hydrogen peroxide is an oxidant which, in high concentrations, is a well-known germicidal agent. Furthermore, this germicidal activity of H_2O_2 is increased many fold by peroxidase and a halide, a catalysis which is of special interest, because peroxidases are present in high concentration in certain phagocytes. The peroxidase-catalyzed and nonenzymatic toxic activities of H_2O_2 in phagocytes are considered below.

Peroxidase-Catalyzed Toxicity

Peroxidases are, in general, hemeproteins which catalyze the oxidation of a number of substances (termed hydrogen or electron donors) by H_2O_2. A number of distinct peroxidases exist in mammalian tissues which differ in primary structure, heme prosthetic group, and in the rate at which they oxidize different electron donors. Among the electron donors oxidized are certain halides (or pseudohalides such as thiocyanate ions) and the products formed have very potent cytocidal activity. This was first demonstrated with the milk peroxidase lactoperoxidase (LPO), which is the same enzyme as that found in saliva (329). Lactoperoxidase inhibited the growth of a variety of organisms when combined with H_2O_2 and thiocyanate ions (207,257,262,373). The LPO and thiocyanate ions were effective in concentrations present in milk or saliva; enzymes (e.g., xanthine oxidase of milk), microorganisms (177), or stimulated phagocytes may theoretically serve as sources of H_2O_2 in these secretions. The toxic product of the LPO-H_2O_2-thiocyanate system has been identified as the hypothiocyanite ion or its protonated form hypothiocyanous acid (23,200). Thiocyanate ions could be replaced by iodide or bromide ions in the antimicrobial system of milk and saliva although in concentrations greater than those present in these biological fluids (116,477).

It has been known since the development of cytochemical stains for peroxidase over 60 years ago and their application to blood smears, that eosinophils, neutrophils, and, to a lesser degree, monocytes contain an abundance of peroxidase-positive granules. More recently, peroxidase also has been detected in basophil (1,49) as well as in mast-cell (190) granules. The presence of a peroxidase-catalyzed antimicrobial system in milk and saliva raised the possibility of a comparable system in those phagocytes which contain peroxidase-positive granules.

Neutrophils

The neutrophil peroxidase was first isolated by Agner (2), who called it verdoperoxidase due to its intense green color. The name was subsequently changed to myeloperoxidase (MPO), the name now generally used. The physical and chemical properties of MPO have recently been reviewed (408,478). Myeloperoxidase, although a different enzyme than LPO, could replace it as the peroxidase component of the peroxidase-H_2O_2-thiocyanate antimicrobial system (257,262); furthermore, when MPO was used, chloride as well as iodide or bromide could meet the halide requirement [for a review see (249)].

The MPO-H_2O_2-halide antimicrobial system is toxic to a wide variety of organisms: bacteria (241,242,316), fungi (113–115, 201,245,277,283), viruses (48), mycoplasma (206), chlamydia (476), protozoa such as *Leishmania donovani* (74) and *Trypanosoma dionisii* (451), and multicellular organisms such as the schistosomula of *Schistosoma mansoni* (221). The peroxidase system is also toxic to certain mammalian cells, e.g., spermatozoa (260,424), erythrocytes (251), leukocytes (79), platelets (81), and tumor cells (86) and can inactivate certain soluble mediators, e.g., the chemotactic factors C5a and formyl-methionyl-leucyl-phenylalanine (82) and $\alpha 1$ proteinase inhibitor ($\alpha 1$ antitrypsin) (72,87,300). Methionine is oxidized to the sulfoxide derivative by the MPO system (452), and the inactivation of the soluble mediators is due to the oxidation of essential methionine residues (77,212,213).

The peroxidase-H_2O_2-halide system, although generally toxic to intact cells, can, when the conditions are mild, stimulate certain cells to secrete biological mediators. Thus, incubation of platelets with the MPO-H_2O_2-halide system can, under certain conditions, release the granule component serotonin to a considerably greater degree than the cytoplasmic marker, adenine, suggesting a nonlytic response analogous to the platelet-release reaction (81). Similarly, mast cells are stimulated to secrete histamine without the concomitant release of the cytoplasmic marker lactic dehydrogenase by the peroxidase-H_2O_2-halide system under mild conditions (191). Both the eosinophil and neutrophil peroxidases are effective in this regard, and electron microscopic studies confirm a degranulation rather than a lytic process. Under these conditions, perturbation of the cell membrane is adequate to trigger a physiological response without being sufficient to induce lasting damage.

The mechanism of action of the peroxidase system is complex. Peroxidase and H_2O_2 form an enzyme-substrate complex which oxidizes the halide to a toxic agent or agents which can attack the cell in a variety of ways. It is probable that both halogenation and oxidation reactions contribute to the toxicity (for reviews see 246,249,253,478). When chloride is the halide, the primary product appears to be hypochlorous acid or its ionized form the hypochlorite ion (4,179).

$$H_2O_2 + Cl^- + H^+ \xrightarrow{\hspace{1cm}} H_2O + HOCl \qquad\qquad (d)$$
$$\text{MPO} \qquad\qquad \updownarrow$$
$$H^+ + OCl^-$$

The pKa of the dissociation of HOCL is 7.5, so that the two forms are at approximately equal concentrations at physiological pH; when the pH is lowered, as would be anticipated in the phagosome, HOCl predominates. The HOCl can react with chloride to form chlorine as follows

$$HOCl + Cl^- \rightarrow Cl_2 + OH^- \qquad\qquad (e)$$

so that a mixture of OCl^-, $HOCl$, and Cl_2 would be anticipated, with the relative proportions of each dependent on the pH and the concentration of components (478). The possible role of singlet oxygen in the toxic activity of the peroxidase system is considered in the section on the hydrogen peroxide-hypochlorite system, p 136. The products of the $MPO-H_2O_2$-chloride system are very reactive agents which can chlorinate and/or oxidize a large variety of compounds (5,37,253,418,434, 446,447,449,478,479) and presumably do so on the surface of the ingested organisms. Chlorine derivatives are widely used as disinfectants, and the body has thus devised a means for their generation within the phagosome as needed for microbicidal activity.

By analogy, the oxidation of bromide by the MPO system would be expected to generate hypobromous acid (HOBr) with consequences similar to those resulting from the generation of HOCL. The pKa for the dissociation of HOBr is 8.7 so that the $HOBr - OBr^-$ couple is more predominantly in the undissociated form than is the $HOCl - OCl^-$ couple at the pHs present in the phagosome. The oxidation of iodide by the peroxidase system also results in the halogenation and oxidation of surface components of the target cell; it is not clear whether hypoiodous acid is an intermediate in these reactions. The effectiveness of iodide in very low concentrations may be due in part to its cyclic oxidation by MPO and H_2O_2 and reduction by bacterial components with reutilization by the peroxidase system (448).

There is considerable evidence to support an important role for the $MPO-H_2O_2$-halide system in the antimicrobial activity of neutrophils (for reviews see 246,247,249,253). Myeloperoxidase is present in very high concentrations in the azurophil (primary) granules of neutrophils, and, following phagocytosis, these granules fuse with the phagosome, the connecting membrane ruptures, and the granule contents, including MPO, are discharged into the phagosome (Fig. 1). The H_2O_2 required for the antimicrobial system is generated by the leukocytic respiratory burst (see above) and has been localized in the phagosome by cytochemical techniques (65). An additional source of H_2O_2 is microbial metabolism. Certain bacteria (e.g., pneumococci, streptococci, lactobacilli) lack heme and thus use flavoproteins for terminal oxidations, which generally reduce oxygen to H_2O_2. These organisms also lack the

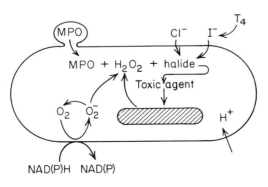

FIG. 1. The myeloperoxidase-H_2O_2-halide antimicrobial system. [Reproduced from Klebanoff and Clark (253), with permission of North-Holland Publishing Company.]

heme enzyme catalase, and the H_2O_2 thus accumulates in the medium. The H_2O_2 so formed can be autoinhibitory, particularly when the leukocytic H_2O_2-generating system is defective as in CGD. Of the halides, chloride would appear to be of most significance since it is present in phagocytes at concentrations considerably greater than those required in the cell-free system. Iodide and bromide are more effective than chloride on a molar basis; however, their concentrations in biological fluids are considerably lower than that of chloride and their contribution to the halide pool within the phagosome is unknown. When iodide is the halide used, iodination of the ingested organism occurs (241,244) indicating that MPO, H_2O_2, and iodide interact within the phagosome. Iodide can be replaced in the isolated system by thyroxine (T_4) and triiodothyronine (T_3) (241), due to their deiodination by the peroxidase system; the thyroid hormones are deiodinated by intact neutrophils following phagocytosis (254,472) and thus may be an additional source of iodide for the intact cell. Thiocyanate ions have a dual effect on the MPO-mediated antimicrobial system; under some conditions it can serve as a required cofactor and contribute to the antimicrobial activity (257,262), whereas when iodide, bromide, or chloride is used as the halide cofactor, thiocyanate can inhibit antimicrobial activity (241,242,253). It is probable that the halide pool is not the limiting factor in the intact leukocyte; chloride is present in excess, and to this halide can be added the small amounts of iodide (absorbed as such or released from the thyroid hormones), bromide, and possibly thiocyanate ions present in biological fluids. Although the pH optimum of the MPO-H_2O_2-chloride system varies with the H_2O_2 and chloride concentrations (478,480), the system functions well at the acid pH believed to be present in the phagosome, as do the iodide- and bromide-dependent systems.

Studies of leukocytes from patients with a genetic defect in microbicial activity further support a role for the peroxidase system in the microbicidal activity of neutrophils. The neutrophils of patients with *CGD* lack a respiratory burst (197); these cells also do not kill certain organisms normally (199,369), and, as a result, the organisms multiply and disseminate, and severe infection results. This finding emphasizes the importance of the respiratory burst and its oxygen products in the normal microbicidal activity of neutrophils. The contribution of H_2O_2 deficiency to the microbicidal defect in CGD is emphasized by the partial reversal of the defect by the introduction of H_2O_2 into the cell (214,381). The H_2O_2-generating enzyme, glucose oxidase, can be used for this purpose; this enzyme forms H_2O_2 without a superoxide intermediate (298,347,428) and thus superoxide (and its products) remains deficient under these conditions. Organisms that generate H_2O_2 and lack catalase, e.g., pneumococci, streptococci, lactobacilli, are readily killed by CGD leukocytes (261,297) and are rarely found in the lesions in this condition. They presumably can provide the H_2O_2 required for their own destruction.

The other inborn error of neutrophil function of particular pertinence to this review is hereditary MPO deficiency, a condition in which neutrophils (and monocytes) lack MPO. These cells have a microbicidal defect, although it is not as severe as in CGD (281,284). Fungicidal activity is low, and bactericidal activity is characterized by a lag period following which, the organisms are killed. In contrast to CGD, the respiratory burst of MPO-deficient cells is intact; indeed it appears to be greater than normal (255,258,382,384) possibly due to a requirement for MPO for the termination of the respiratory burst (208). When MPO is absent, the products of the respiratory burst, produced in increased amounts, combine with the oxygen-independent antimicrobial systems (e.g., acid pH, lysozyme, lactoferrin, cationic proteins) to eventually kill the ingested organisms. As a result, patients with hereditary MPO-deficiency are generally in good health.

Although the primary function of neutrophils is the phagocytosis and destruction of intracellular organisms, leakage or secretion of the toxic systems can occur with the destruction of adjacent cells or soluble mediators. This extracellular toxicity can be mediated by the peroxidase system. Evidence for such a mechanism would be: a) the demonstration of a halide requirement for optimum activity; b) the inhibition of toxicity by peroxidase inhibitors (e.g., azide, cyanide) and by catalase; c) decreased toxicity when CGD leukocytes are used, which is overcome by the addition of H_2O_2 or a H_2O_2-generating system; and d) decreased toxicity when MPO-deficient leukocytes are used, which is overcome by the addition of MPO. Evidence of this sort has implicated the MPO-H_2O_2-halide system in the destruction of tumor cells and other targets by neutrophils stimulated by phagocytosis (78), concanavalin A (83), or phorbal myristate acetate (PMA) (85,219,423). In one study (80), the antibody-dependent tumor-cell cytotoxic activity of neutrophils was not dependent on peroxidase; toxicity was unaffected by azide or by the substitution of MPO-deficient for normal leukocytes. Toxicity to the tumor cells, however, was decreased (but not abolished) when granulocytes from patients with CGD were used, suggesting a requirement for oxidative metabolism for optimum activity. In another study (172), the respiratory burst of neutrophils was triggered by exposure to antibody-coated tumor cells and a requirement for oxidative metabolism for tumor-cell damage was suggested by the inhibitory effect of hypoxia and agents that block the respiratory burst; the peroxidase inhibitors azide or cyanide, however, were ineffective. In both of the above studies (80,172) cytotoxicity was unaffected by catalase or superoxide dismutase possibly due to the inability of these proteins to penetrate to the space between adherent effector and target cells. Capsoni and co-workers (71) also observed a decrease in antibody-dependent tumor cytotoxicity when CGD leukocytes were used and the absence of inhibition of normal leukocytes by azide; however, in their studies superoxide dismutase was inhibitory, implicating O_2^- in the toxicity. In a study of toxicity to antibody-coated human erythrocytes (227), CGD neutrophils were found to be normally cytotoxic when target cell monolayers were used, whereas cytotoxicity was depressed when the target cells were in suspension unless phagocytosis was inhibited by colchicine. It was proposed that an oxidative mechanism was responsible for toxicity to ingested sensitized targets but not for toxicity to extracellular targets. Intact neutrophils activated by phagocytosis also were toxic to platelets as indicated by the release of the granule marker serotonin and the cytoplasmic component adenine (84). This lytic effect was dependent on a halide, was inhibited by catalase, and was not observed when CGD or MPO-deficient leukocytes were used, with the latter effect reversed by the addition of a H_2O_2-generating system or MPO, respectively. The hemeprotein inhibitors azide and cyanide, however, did not inhibit the release of serotonin and adenine from platelets but, rather, increased it. This was believed to be due to the inhibition of platelet catalase (in addition to the neutrophil peroxidase) which allowed H_2O_2 to exert a nonenzymatic toxic effect (84). Finally, intact neutrophils stimulated by PMA can inactivate the chemotactic factors C5a and formyl-methionyl-leucyl-phenylalanine through the release of the components of the peroxidase system (77).

Eosinophils

Human eosinophils are characterized by large cytoplasmic granules containing a crystalloid body, and peroxidase can be detected by cytochemical techniques in the matrix of these granules surrounding the central crystalline core (35). The eosinophil peroxidase (EPO) differs from the neutrophil peroxidase both genetically and in its structure and properties. Patients with hereditary MPO deficiency lack peroxidase activity in neutrophils but contain normal amounts of peroxidase in eosinophils (168,401), indicating that the two enzymes are coded by different genes. Purified guinea pig EPO and MPO differ immunologically and in their absorption spectra, electrophoretic mobility, molecular weight, chromatographic behavior, subunit structure, and heme prosthetic group (112). Eosinophil peroxidase and MPO differ in the rate at which they oxidize different substances by H_2O_2 (123,323,324) and in their response to inhibitors (323). Both enzymes are inhibited by high H_2O_2 concentrations (19,323), and this inhibition is decreased by certain phenolic estrogens (248).

As in neutrophils, phagocytosis by eosinophils is associated with granule fusion and lysis with the discharge of the granule contents, including peroxidase (99), into the phagosome. The EPO can be released into the extracellular fluid when granule rupture occurs prior to the completion of the act of engulfment (18), when the eosinophils lyse in the interstitial space (388), or when eosinophils come into contact with opsonized particles too large to be ingested. Thus, eosinophils adherent to the antibody and/or complement-coated schistosomula of *S. mansoni* release their granule contents, and peroxidase can be detected on the worm surface (312,313).

Like MPO, EPO combines with H_2O_2 and a halide to form a cytotoxic system effective against bacteria (220,324), fungi (277), tumor cells (219), mast cells (191), and the schistosomula of *S. mansoni* (221). The EPO is considerably less effective with chloride (relative to iodide or bromide) than is MPO; however, we have been able to use chloride as the halide, particularly at low pH and relatively high EPO concentrations.

Eosinophil peroxidase is a strongly basic protein. As a result, it binds firmly to negatively charged surfaces with retention of peroxidatic activity. Among the surfaces to which it can bind in this way is that of the target cell. Thus, if *Staphylococcus aureus* is incubated with EPO for a short period and then washed extensively to remove all unbound peroxidase, a portion of the enzyme remains firmly bound to the surface of the organism (371). If H_2O_2 and a halide are added to staphylococci with surface-bound peroxidase, the organisms are very rapidly killed under conditions in which control staphylococci without bound EPO are unaffected. The halides are effective at lower concentrations, and the cytotoxic system is considerably less sensitive to protein inhibition when EPO is bound to the surface of the target cell than when the enzyme is free. Lactoperoxidase (365,432) and MPO (417) also bind to microorganisms with retention of bactericidal activity; these enzymes, however, do not appear to bind to microorganisms as avidly as does EPO.

Mononuclear Phagocytes

Mononuclear phagocytes are a continuum of cells beginning with the bone marrow precursors and continuing through the blood monocyte to the mature tissue macrophage. Macrophages acquire distinct structural and functional characteristics depending on their location and state of activation. Bone marrow promonocytes, like the neutrophil and eosinophil precursors, contain peroxidase-positive granules as do the circulating monocytes of most species [an exception is the rabbit, which lacks peroxidase-positive granules in both promonocytes and monocytes (344)]. Peroxidase-positive granules, however, are fewer in number in monocytes than in neutrophils or eosinophils.

The monocyte peroxidase appears to be identical to that of the neutrophil. Peroxidase is absent from both cell types in patients with hereditary MPO deficiency (168) suggesting that the same gene is responsible for their synthesis, and purified monocyte and neutrophil peroxidase have comparable structural and functional characteristics (63). The monocyte peroxidase appears to be responsible in part for the toxic activity of these cells (250,256,380). The evidence is as follows.

a. Peroxidase is released from the cytoplasmic granules of monocytes into the phagosome containing the ingested organism (105). Hydrogen peroxide is generated by monocytes during phagocytosis (32,372,396), and the iodination associated with phagocytosis (32,54,280) (a reaction which, in the neutrophil, is dependent on MPO and H_2O_2 (252)] suggests the interaction of peroxidase, H_2O_2, and a halide in monocytes.

b. The peroxidase inhibitors azide, cyanide, and sulfadiazine inhibit the fungicidal activity of human monocytes (280).

c. Monocytes from patients with CGD have a bactericidal (108,379) and fungicidal (278) defect, suggesting a requirement for the products of the respiratory burst for optimum microbicidal activity.

d. Monocytes of patients with hereditary MPO deficiency have a fungicidal defect. Thus the monocytes of 3 patients killed 9.5, 4.0, and 4.0% of ingested *Candida albicans* in 2½ hr under conditions in which normal monocytes killed 63.4% of ingested organisms (280).

These data taken together suggest a role for MPO in the microbicidal activity of blood monocytes. Monocytes retain their peroxidase-positive granules for a period following passage into the tissues (101,102,104–106,422,456), and this enzyme is released into the phagosome of tissue monocytes (105). Since many of the mono-nuclear phagocytes present in inflammatory lesions have recently emigrated from the blood stream (17,348,426), their peroxidase may contribute to the microbicidal and cytotoxic activity of these cells. It is of interest in this regard that, in one study (391), the toxicity of mouse peritoneal macrophages on tumor cells in the presence of lymphokines from specifically sensitized spleen cells correlated closely with the proportion of peroxidase-positive macrophages in the cell population.

During the process of maturation in tissues, macrophages, in general, lose their granule peroxidase. This loss of peroxidase has been demonstrated experimentally both *in vivo* (456) and *in vitro* (36,64,455). Although resident macrophages do not contain granule peroxidase, some mature macrophages contain cytochemically iden-tifiable peroxidase in the endoplasmic reticulum, perinuclear cisternae, and Golgi lamellae (for review see 34,46,103). Furthermore, monocytes or macrophages which do not ordinarily contain peroxidase in the endoplasmic reticulum may develop peroxidase activity in this location following adherence of the cells to a surface *in vitro* (34,55,56). The peroxidase appears following several hours of adherence, remains for a period, and then disappears despite continued adherence. The nature of this peroxidase is unknown. It appears in the endoplasmic reticulum of adherent monocytes from patients with hereditary MPO deficiency (34,64) suggesting that it is not MPO. The peroxidase present in the endoplasmic reticulum is not packaged into granules nor is it released into the phagosome (105). Thus, this peroxidase does not appear to be used to kill ingested organisms.

Mature macrophages also can acquire peroxidase by endocytosis; that is, by the uptake of fluid-phase peroxidase by pinocytosis (52,99,433) or particulate perox-idase by phagocytosis (21,187,388). In an inflammatory locus this peroxidase can originate in adjacent neutrophils, eosinophils or monocytes and may contribute to the microbicidal activity of the macrophage. Thus, EPO bound to the surface of staphylococci was carried into mononuclear phagocytes during the phagocytic proc-ess and the EPO-coated organisms were killed more rapidly by rabbit monocytes or alveolar macrophages than were uncoated organisms (371). This potentiation of bactericidal activity by bound EPO was prevented by the addition of azide to the reaction mixture.

Catalase generally inhibits the peroxidase-mediated antimicrobial system by the degradation of H_2O_2. However, when the pH is low, i.e., 4.5, iodide is the halide used and the H_2O_2 is maintained at a low steady-state concentration by a H_2O_2-generating system such as glucose oxidase, then catalase can substitute for per-oxidase as the catalyst for the peroxidase-H_2O_2-halide microbicidal system (243,256). Rabbit alveolar macrophages contain catalase in high concentration (149), and granule preparations from these cells have bactericidal activity at acid pH in the presence of iodide and low levels of H_2O_2 (358). Catalase is released in part into the phagosome of rabbit alveolar macrophages (437), raising the possibility that catalase can serve a microbicidal function in these cells. However, procedures that decrease the catalase content of rabbit alveolar macrophages (148,256) or inhibit catalase (53) were not found to decrease the bactericidal activity of these cells, suggesting either that catalase is present in considerable excess or is not involved in microbicidal activity. Other mononuclear phagocytes, e.g., mouse peritoneal macrophages, contain very little catalase (422), and presumably do not use this enzyme for microbicidal activity.

Mast Cells

Mast-cell granules, which contain a small amount of peroxidase (190), are toxic to bacteria (193) and tumor cells (192) when supplemented with H_2O_2 and a halide. The EPO-H_2O_2-halide system at low H_2O_2 concentrations (191) and H_2O_2 alone at relatively high concentrations (192,351,352) can initiate mast-cell secretion, and intact mast cells incubated with secretory levels of H_2O_2 are toxic to tumor cells in the presence of a halide (192). Hydrogen peroxide serves here both to initiate mast cell secretion and as a component of the peroxidase-mediated cytotoxic system. The toxicity of mast cell granules is considerably increased by binding EPO to the granule surface. Because of its positive charge, EPO binds to the negatively charged granule matrix to form a complex which retains peroxidatic activity (193); indeed, the complex has considerably greater bactericidal (193) and tumoricidal (192) activity than does the free enzyme when standardized to the same guaiacol units of peroxidase activity.

Nonenzymatic Toxicity

Hydrogen peroxide is an oxidant and at relatively high concentrations (as compared to those required for peroxidase-catalyzed toxicity) is toxic to microorganisms and mammalian cells. This toxicity may be potentiated by certain low-molecular-weight compounds. Thus, the toxicity of H_2O_2 is potentiated by combination with iodide (241,256) or with ascorbic acid and a trace metal such as Cu^{2+} or Co^{2+} (110,118,122,224,247). Gram-negative organisms exposed to ascorbic acid and H_2O_2 are more susceptible to the lytic action of lysozyme (326). The toxicity of H_2O_2 also can be potentiated by ultraviolet irradiation (42) or by trace metals (41) possibly by $\cdot OH$ formation. Thus, H_2O_2 reacts with iron (Fenton's reagent) to form $\cdot OH$ (171,460) (see also the section on the Haber-Weiss reaction, p 125).

$$Fe^{2+} + H_2O_2 \rightarrow Fe^{3+} + OH^- + \cdot OH \qquad (f)$$

It is possible that H_2O_2 exerts its toxicity in part through this reaction. Base-catalyzed disproportionation of H_2O_2 has been reported to yield singlet oxygen (425) as follows.

$$H_2O_2 + OH^- \rightleftharpoons HOO^- + H_2O \qquad (g)$$
$$H_2O_2 + HOO^- \rightarrow H_2O + OH^- + {}^1O_2 \qquad (h)$$
$$\overline{2H_2O_2 \rightarrow 2H_2O + {}^1O_2} \qquad (i)$$

The generation of singlet oxygen and its role in the toxicity of phagocytes is considered in the section on singlet oxygen (page 134). It is not clear whether the generation of $^1O_2$ by H_2O_2 disproportionation is possible under the conditions of pH, etc., present in phagocytes.

The H_2O_2 generated by phagocytes can be toxic to a number of targets in the absence of peroxidase under certain experimental conditions. Thus, H_2O_2 has been implicated in the killing of the newborn larvae of *Trichinella spiralis* by human neutrophils and eosinophils in the presence of immune serum (39,40), and stimulated neutrophils may be self-destructive through the formation of H_2O_2 (33,453). Hydrogen peroxide has been identified as the toxic substance in the killing of tumor cells by activated macrophages stimulated by PMA, and the absence of peroxidase in the effector cells and the lack of inhibition by the peroxidase inhibitors azide and cyanide excluded peroxidase as a catalyst of the toxicity (337,340,342). Although lysis of tumor cells by activated macrophages in the presence of antitumor cell antibody was shown to involve an oxidative mechanism, H_2O_2 was not definitively established as the toxic substance, since lysis was not inhibited by catalase (338). Lymphocyte transformation is inhibited by H_2O_2 generated by *Corynebacterium parvum* or thioglycollate-induced mouse peritoneal macrophages (320) or by the xanthine oxidase system (395). Inhibition by catalase also has implicated H_2O_2 in the cytocidal activity of human pulmonary macrophages against human skin fibroblasts; toxicity to human-tumor cell lines, however, was unaffected by catalase (285). Finally, the inhibition of growth of intracellular trypomastigotes of *Trypanosoma cruzi* by mouse peritoneal macrophages correlates well with the formation of H_2O_2 by these cells (341). These findings have implicated H_2O_2 as a toxic substance in phagocytes, which may be active in the absence of peroxidase under some conditions.

HYDROXYL RADICALS

It is now generally accepted that a strong oxidant, resembling hydroxyl radicals in its properties, is generated by certain biochemical systems, and there is increasing interest in the formation of this substance within phagocytes and its role in the cytotoxic activity of these cells.

Production

Haber-Weiss Reaction

In 1934, Haber and Weiss (171) proposed the following sequence of reactions to account for the large amount of H_2O_2 decomposed on the interaction of H_2O_2 with iron salts.

$$Fe^{2+} + H_2O_2 \rightarrow Fe^{3+} + OH^- + \cdot OH \qquad (f)$$
$$\cdot OH + H_2O_2 \rightarrow H_2O + HO_2 \qquad (j)$$
$$HO_2 + H_2O_2 \rightarrow O_2^- + H_2O + \cdot OH \qquad (k)$$
$$\cdot OH + Fe^{2+} \rightarrow Fe^{3+} + OH^- \qquad (l)$$

This sequence is a chain reaction initiated by the decomposition of H_2O_2 by iron salts to form $\cdot OH$ [reaction (f)] and maintained by reactions (j) and (k), in which $\cdot OH$ is initially used [reaction (j)] and then formed [reaction (k)] and reused [reaction (j)] to maintain the chain reaction until either the H_2O_2 is depleted or the chain is broken by reaction (l). Reaction (k) expressed as follows:

$$O_2^- + H_2O_2 \rightarrow O_2 + OH^- + \cdot OH \tag{m}$$

is commonly referred to as the Haber-Weiss reaction.

The Haber-Weiss reaction has been invoked as a possible mechanism for the formation of $\cdot OH$ by biological systems. In a study of the mechanism of ethylene formation from methional by the xanthine oxidase system, Beauchamp and Fridovich (44) observed that this reaction was inhibited by superoxide dismutase, catalase, and the $\cdot OH$ scavengers ethanol and benzoate. Furthermore, ethylene formation was associated with a brief lag phase which was overcome by the addition of H_2O_2. They proposed that ethylene formation was initiated by $\cdot OH$ generated by the interaction of O_2^- and H_2O_2 by the Haber-Weiss reaction. Subsequently, many investigators have used the inhibition of a reaction by superoxide dismutase, catalase, and $\cdot OH$ radicals as evidence for $\cdot OH$ formation by the Haber-Weiss reaction and its use in the reaction.

There is now a large body of evidence which indicates that the direct reductive cleavage of H_2O_2 by O_2^- as depicted in reaction (m) does not occur at an appreciable rate in aqueous solution (100,107,126,150,173,271,306,308,317,378,429,463). Weinstein and Bielski (463) report a rate constant of 0.50 $M^{-1}sec^{-1}$ for $HO_2^- + H_2O_2$ and 0.13 $M^{-1}sec^{-1}$ for $O_2^- + H_2O_2$; the rate of direct interaction is thus very slow as compared to competing reactions such as the spontaneous dismutation of O_2^- (see the section on H_2O_2 production, page 115). It is now the widely held view that a trace metal acts as an oxidation-reduction catalyst of the interaction of O_2^- and H_2O_2 (100,170,175,176,308) with the metal being alternately reduced by O_2^- and oxidized by H_2O_2 as follows

$$O_2^- + M^{n+} \rightarrow O_2 + M^{(n-1)+} \tag{n}$$
$$\underline{M^{(n-1)+} + H_2O_2 \rightarrow M^{n+} + OH^- + \cdot OH} \tag{o}$$
$$O_2^- + H_2O_2 \rightarrow O_2 + OH^- + \cdot OH \tag{m}$$

with the overall reaction being that originally proposed by Haber and Weiss (171). Of a number of metals tested, iron has been the only one found to catalyze the Haber-Weiss reaction (175,308,386). Furthermore, the catalytic activity of iron was increased considerably by the chelator ethylenediamine tetraacetic acid (EDTA) (68,73,170,175,176,308,386). The EDTA could not be replaced in this reaction by the iron chelators diethylenetriamine pentaacetic acid (DTPA) (175,176,386), bathophenanthroline sulfonate (176,386), or desferrioxamine (170,386); indeed, in most studies these chelators inhibited $\cdot OH$ formation by the iron-EDTA complex. The demonstration of a requirement for iron chelation by EDTA for optimum catalysis of the Haber-Weiss reaction raises the question of possible natural chelators of this reaction. Halliwell (175) could not replace iron-EDTA with MPO or ferritin; McCord and Day (308), however, report that iron chelated with the plasma protein transferrin was "at least as effective as iron chelated by EDTA." Lactoferrin is of particular interest in this regard in view of its high concentration in neutrophils. Ambruso and Johnston (13) have reported that fully saturated milk or neutrophil lactoferrin stimulated $\cdot$OH formation by intact PMNs, a PMN particulate preparation and the xanthine oxidase system; partially iron-saturated lactoferrin, however, was ineffective (13,386). Thus, to summarize, iron is the only metal which has been found to catalyze the Haber-Weiss reaction, chelation with EDTA greatly potentiates its action, and certain other chelators are ineffective or inhibitory. The biological chelator, if any, of the iron-catalyzed Haber-Weiss reaction is unknown.

Although these studies support the generation of $\cdot$OH by a modified Haber-Weiss reaction, its formation has been questioned by some investigators. Thus, Bors and co-workers (61), using the bleaching of *p*-nitrosodimethylaniline as a sensitive measure of $\cdot$OH could not detect the formation of $\cdot$OH by a number of biochemical systems (autoxidation of 6-hydroxydopamine, the hydroxylating system NADH-phenazine methosulfate, the oxidation of xanthine, or acetaldehyde by xanthine oxidase), which had been previously reported to generate $\cdot$OH. They concluded that no freely diffusable $\cdot$OH was formed by these systems and proposed an $\cdot$OH-analogous substance present in a complexed state. An H_2O_2-Fe^{2+} complex, the intermediary oxidant of a Fenton-type reaction,

$$Fe^{2+} + H_2O_2 \rightarrow [H_2O_2 - Fe^{2+}] \rightarrow Fe^{3+} + OH^- + \cdot OH \qquad (p)$$

has been proposed as a possibility (61). When the Fe^{3+} formed in the Fenton reaction is reduced by O_2^-, the metal-catalyzed Haber-Weiss reaction is constituted. However, reduction of Fe^{3+} can occur in other ways, and the generation of $\cdot$OH or the $\cdot$OH analogous substance under these conditions may be either unaffected or stimulated by superoxide dismutase as has been observed in some systems (121,133,174). The reaction sequence would be as follows

$$Fe^{2+} + H_2O_2 \rightarrow Fe^{3+} + OH^- + \cdot OH \qquad (f)$$
$$\underline{Fe^{3+} \rightarrow Fe^{2+}} \qquad (q)$$
$$H_2O_2 \rightarrow OH + \cdot OH \qquad (r)$$

A reaction analogous to the Haber-Weiss reaction is the reductive cleavage of organic hydroperoxides by O_2^- as follows

$$O_2^- + ROOH \rightarrow O_2 + RO\cdot + OH^- \qquad (s)$$

(360,366,450), and this reaction has been proposed as a mechanism for the generation of toxic substances other than $\cdot$OH by the leukocyte oxidase (443). Bors and colleagues (60), however, could not detect the formation of alkoxy radicals by the interaction of O_2^- generated by pulse radiolysis and either *t*-butyl hydroperoxides or linoleic acid hydroperoxide.

Phagocytes

Hydroxyl radical formation by phagocytes has been sought using a variety of techniques (62). These include the formation of ethylene from methional or 2-keto-4-thiomethylbutyric acid (KMB), the formation of methane from dimethylsulfoxide (DMSO), the formation of $^{14}CO_2$ from ^{14}C-benzoic acid, and the demonstration of an ·OH spin-trap adduct by electron spin resonance (ESR) spectroscopy. If an ·OH product is found, inhibition of its formation by superoxide dismutase, catalase, and ·OH scavengers has been sought as evidence for the involvement of ·OH generated by the metal-catalyzed Haber-Weiss reaction.

Ethylene Formation from Thioethers

The report by Beauchamp and Fridovich (44) that ethylene formation from methional by the xanthine oxidase system is initiated by ·OH, prompted a study of the formation of ethylene from methional or the related thioether KMB by phagocytes. Appropriately stimulated neutrophils (120,259,374,441,467), eosinophils (259), and mononuclear phagocytes (120,464) form ethylene from methional or KMB. In general, ethylene formation in these studies was inhibited (but not abolished) by superoxide dismutase, catalase, and hydroxyl radical scavengers implicating, at least in part, ·OH generated by the metal-catalyzed Haber-Weiss reaction. In one study, however, ethylene formation by stimulated neutrophils was not significantly reduced by catalase or by the ·OH scavengers ethanol and mannitol (441).

Ethylene formation from methional is initiated by the abstraction of an electron from the sulfur atom of the thioether to form the radical cation, which decays under nucleophilic attack by OH^- to form ethylene, methyldisulfide, and formic acid (474,475) as follows:

$$CH_3 - \overset{..}{S} - CH_2 - CH_2 - CHO + \cdot OH \rightarrow CH_3 - \overset{+}{\overset{.}{S}} - CH_2 - CH_2 - CHO$$
$$+ OH^- \rightarrow CH_2 = CH_2 + \tfrac{1}{2} CH_3 - S - S - CH_3 + HCOOH \qquad (t)$$

Degradation of KMB is comparable except that the final products are ethylene, methyldisulfide, and carbon dioxide (475). Although ·OH are powerful one electron oxidants capable of this reaction [the second order rate constant for reaction with methional is 8.2×10^9 $M^{-1}sec^{-1}$ (59)], it should be emphasized that a number of oxidants other than ·OH can initiate the formation of ethylene (59,259,367,403). Superoxide reacts sluggishly with methional to yield ethylene (59), and organic free radicals can initiate this reaction with the relative reactivity ·OH > RO· > ROO· > RCO−O· > R· (367). The formation of reactive organic radicals as a product of the interaction between O_2^- and organic hydroperoxides (see Haber-Weiss reaction p 127) may account for the weak inhibitory effect of catalase on ethylene formation in some systems (443).

In neutrophils, ethylene formation from either methional or KMB is dependent largely on MPO; it is inhibited by the peroxidase inhibitors azide and cyanide and is less than 10% of normal when MPO-deficient neutrophils are used (259). This is in sharp contrast to the phagocytosis-induced respiratory burst [oxygen consumption (255,382), superoxide production (382), H_2O_2 production (258,382), glucose C-1 oxidation (258,382)], which is greater in MPO-deficient than in normal neutrophils. The addition of purified MPO to MPO-deficient leukocytes increases ethylene formation to a level greater than that of similarly treated normal neutrophils (259). Presumably under these conditions, ethylene formation reflects the increased respiratory burst of MPO-deficient leukocytes. This suggests that ethylene formation by neutrophils is initiated largely by an oxidant (or oxidants) which is dependent on MPO for its formation, and indeed a cell-free, MPO-dependent system has been described which can form ethylene from methional or KMB (259). The nature of the reactive oxidant formed by MPO either in the cell-free system or the intact cell is unknown. The formation of ·OH by MPO is theoretically possible but has not been demonstrated. Since chloride or bromide are required for optimum ethylene formation by the cell-free MPO system (259), oxidation of the thioethers by hypohalites or other halide-derived oxidants is possible. Ethylene is formed from KMB by dye-sensitized photooxidation (259); stimulation of this reaction by D_2O and its inhibition by $^1O_2$ quenchers is compatible with a $^1O_2$ mechanism. There is, however, no evidence that $^1O_2$ is involved in ethylene formation by intact phagocytes.

In summary, although ethylene is formed from methional or KMB by phagocytes, there is some question as to whether ·OH is the primary oxidant responsible at least in phagocytes which contain peroxidase. Certainly in these cells, ethylene formation is not due primarily to ·OH generated by the Haber-Weiss reaction, unless that reaction is catalyzed by MPO. The ethylene formed by phagocytes which lack MPO (e.g., macrophages) and a small portion of the ethylene formed by PMNs (<10%) may, however, depend on ·OH generated nonenzymatically by the metal-catalyzed Haber-Weiss reaction.

Methane formation from DMSO

Dimethylsulfoxide is a potent scavenger of ·OH; the rate constant for the interaction is $4.8 \times 10^9 \text{ M}^{-1}\text{sec}^{-1}$ (151,376). Among the products formed is the methyl radical, which gives rise to methane by hydrogen abstraction as follows.

$$(CH_3)_2SO + \cdot OH \rightarrow \cdot CH_3 + CH_3SO_2H \qquad (u)$$
$$\cdot CH_3 + RH \rightarrow CH_4 + R\cdot \qquad (v)$$

The methane formed can be readily detected by gas chromatography. Repine and co-workers (374) demonstrated the formation of methane from DMSO by human neutrophils, monocytes, or alveolar macrophages stimulated by PMA, or opsonized zymosan. Methane formation was inhibited by superoxide dismutase, catalase, and ·OH scavengers suggesting that it was due, at least in part, to ·OH formed by the metal-catalyzed Haber-Weiss reaction. It is not known whether methane formation from DMSO by PMNs, like ethylene formation from methional or KMB, is dependent on MPO; studies with MPO-deficient leukocytes would be of interest in this regard. Recently Klein and co-workers (264) have reported that formaldehyde also is formed by the interaction of DMSO and ·OH, and that some ·OH-generating systems yield considerably greater amounts of formaldehyde than methane. These authors propose formaldehyde formation from DMSO as a more sensitive measure of the presence of ·OH in biological systems.

CO_2 Release from Benzoic Acid

The decarboxylation of carboxyl-labeled ^{14}C-benzoic acid with the release of $^{14}CO_2$ has been used as a measure of ·OH formation by the xanthine oxidase system and by neutrophils stimulated by the phagocytosis of opsonized zymosan (394). Benzoic acid oxidation by phagocytes was inhibited by superoxide dismutase, catalase, azide, and mannitol and was not observed when cells from a patient with CGD were used. Studies with MPO-deficient leukocytes were not performed.

ESR Spectroscopy

Highly reactive short-lived free radicals can react with certain compounds (spin traps) to form relatively long-lived radicals (spin adducts), which can be detected by ESR spectroscopy (131,209). Spin traps are generally nitrones or nitroso compounds. Nitroso compounds are not used for the detection of ·OH, because the spin adducts are too short-lived; adducts formed with nitrones, however, are sufficiently long-lived for detection. One of the nitrones used for this purpose is 5,5 dimethyl-pyrroline-N-oxide (DMPO) (Fig. 2), which forms an ·OH adduct with a characteristic ESR spectrum (178,210) (Fig. 3).

When human PMNs ingest particles in the presence of DMPO, the characteristic ESR spectrum of the ·OH adduct is seen (Fig. 3) (158,384). (DMPO/OH)· adduct formation is not observed when PMNs from patients with CGD are used and, in sharp contrast to ethylene formation, is not decreased when MPO-deficient leukocytes are used (384). Indeed, like the respiratory burst, adduct formation by MPO-deficient leukocytes is greater than normal, an effect that is reversed by the addition of MPO (384). (DMPO/OH)· adduct formation is also increased by the addition of the peroxidase inhibitors azide and cyanide to normal neutrophils stimulated by phagocytosis (158). Adduct formation by PMNs is inhibited by superoxide dismutase and mannitol but is unaffected by catalase (158,384), suggesting that its formation has little or no requirement for free H_2O_2. Hydroxyl radical formation by a mechanism that does not require H_2O_2, or the formation of the DMPO adduct

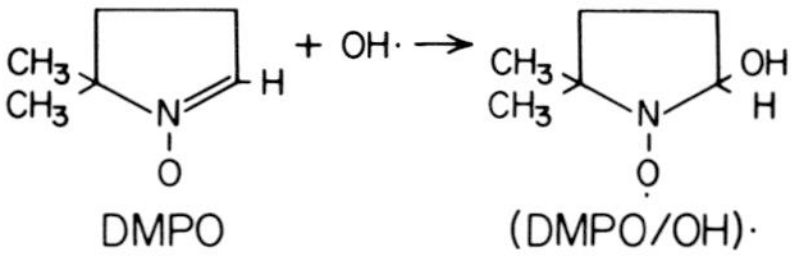

FIG. 2. The formation of the (DMPO/OH) · adduct. [Reproduced from Rosen and Klebanoff (384), with permission of the *Journal of Clinical Investigation*.]

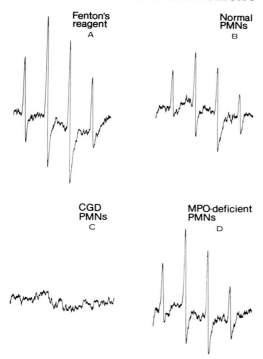

FIG. 3. ESR spectra of (DMPO/OH)· adduct formation by Fenton's reagent (Fe^{2+} + H_2O_2) **(A)** and by phagocytosing normal **(B)**, CGD **(C)** or MPO-deficient **(D)** PMNs. [Reproduced from Rosen and Klebanoff (384), with permission of the *Journal of Clinical Investigation.*]

with O_2^- (or HO_2^-) with subsequent reduction to form the (DMPO/OH)· adduct may occur (384). The latter mechanism would not account for the inhibition by the ·OH scavenger mannitol. An adduct is formed when DMPO reacts with O_2^-, (DMPO/OOH)·, which has an ESR spectrum distinct from that of the OH· adduct (178,129); however, decomposition of (DMPO/OOH)· to (DMPO/OH)· has been reported (129).The rate constants for the reaction of DMPO with HO_2^- and O_2^- are 6.6 × 10^3 and 10 $M^{-1}sec^{-1}$, respectively, values considerably lower than that for reaction with ·OH (3.4 × 10^9 $M^{-1}sec^{-1}$ (130). It is of interest that the (DMPO/OOH)· spectrum was detected when human PMNs were stimulated with PMA (158), whereas when stimulation was by phagocytosis of zymosan or latex, only the (DMPO/OH)· spectrum was seen (158,384). The O_2^- adduct also was detected when azide and, to a lesser degree, cyanide was added to latex particle-stimulated PMNs (158). In contrast to these studies with human neutrophils, in a study in which mixed rat leukocytes, opsonized *E. coli* and three spin-trapping agents, phenyl-tert-butyl nitrone (PBN), 2 methyl-2-nitrosopropane (MNP) and DMPO were used, an ESR signal was detected only with MNP, and this signal appeared to be identical to that formed on reaction of the spin trap with O_2^- (305). The use of spin traps for the detection of ·OH is further complicated by the possibility that the spin trap DMPO can form an adduct with $^1O_2$ which, on hydration, would yield the ·OH adduct (137).

Toxicity

The hydroxyl radical is a powerful one-electron oxidant capable of the abstraction of electrons from a large variety of compounds with the formation of a radical

$$·OH + R^- \rightarrow OH^- + R· \qquad\qquad (w)$$

which may then degrade to other products. It would be anticipated, therefore, that its formation in close proximity to an ingested organism or an extracellular target would contribute to the toxicity of phagocytes. Evidence in favor of a contribution by ·OH has come from studies with model systems and intact phagocytes (for reviews see 26,253).

Model Systems

Hydroxyl radicals have been implicated as the toxic agents in the injury to microorganisms induced by radiation (328,402), exposure of riboflavin and methionine to light (165), or the autoxidation of dialuric acid (458). Hydroxyl radicals may also be damaging to leukocytes (314,399,400), pancreatic islet cells (92,132), and neurons (92). This toxicity may be mediated in some systems by the degradation of DNA (69,97,286,292,457). An additional action of ·OH that may be pertinent to its role in the inflammatory response is the depolymerization of hyaluronic acid (162,170,176,307). Xanthine oxidase has been used extensively as a model of the ·OH-generating cytotoxic system of phagocytes. These studies are described in more detail below.

Xanthine oxidase, in the course of the oxidation of its substrate, xanthine, hypoxanthine, or acetaldehyde, reduces oxygen to O_2^- and H_2O_2 (142), and the interaction of these two products to form ·OH (44) and $^1O_2$ (232) has been proposed. The bactericidal activity of the xanthine oxidase system was demonstrated over 35 years ago (157,289). In these early studies inhibition by catalase implicated H_2O_2 in the toxicity. Since the discovery of the enzymatic activity of superoxide dismutase (309), this enzyme has been used, along with catalase, in the search for the toxic substance formed by the xanthine oxidase system. In some instances, e.g., the effect of the xanthine oxidase system on *E. coli* (28) or *Neisseria gonorrhoeae* (202), toxic activity was inhibited by catalase and not superoxide dismutase, implicating H_2O_2. In other instances, e.g., with *Staphylococcus epidermidis* (28), *Staphylococcus aureus* (385,386), or *Toxoplasma gondii* (331) as the test organism, both catalase and superoxide dismutase were inhibitory, raising the possibility of ·OH involvement. The ·OH scavenger mannitol did not inhibit the toxicity to *S. epidermidis* (28) but did inhibit the toxicity to *S. aureus* (385,386) or *T.gondii* (331) under the conditions used in these studies.

We have compared the staphylocidal activity of the acetaldehyde-xanthine oxidase system in the presence and absence of MPO and chloride as a model for the oxygen-dependent antimicrobial systems of phagocytes (385,386). The xanthine oxidase system was toxic to *S. aureus* in the absence of MPO and chloride at relatively high acetaldehyde concentrations (385). This toxicity was inhibited by superoxide dismutase, catalase, the hydroxyl radical scavengers mannitol and benzoate, and the singlet oxygen quenchers azide, histidine, and 1,4-diazabicyclo[2,2,2] octane (DABCO), findings compatible with the Haber-Weiss reaction in which O_2^- and H_2O_2 interact to form the toxic substance ·OH and $^1O_2$ as follows.

$$O_2^- + H_2O_2 \xrightarrow[\text{metal}]{} {}^1O_2 + OH^- + \cdot OH \qquad (x)$$

Further evidence for $^1O_2$ formation by this system was the conversion of 2,5-diphenylfuran to *cis*-dibenzoylethylene, a reaction which can occur by a $^1O_2$ mechanism. Iron chelated by EDTA was required for the bactericidal activity of the acetaldehyde-xanthine oxidase system (386) supporting the requirement for trace-metal catalysis of the Haber-Weiss reaction. The staphylocidal activity of the acetaldehyde-xanthine oxidase system was considerably increased by the addition of MPO and chloride (385). In contrast to the unsupplemented xanthine oxidase system, the bactericidal activity of the MPO- and chloride-supplemented system was inhibited by catalase but not by superoxide dismutase or mannitol, suggesting that under these conditions, H_2O_2 is the required product.

Phagocytes

Johnston and co-workers (217) proposed the involvement of ·OH in the microbicidal activity of neutrophils, based on the inhibition of bactericidal activity by superoxide dismutase and catalase bound to latex beads and by some ·OH scavengers. [The inhibitory effect of superoxide dismutase bound to latex beads on PMN bactericidal activity has recently been questioned (305).] Other studies also have indicated an inhibition of the bactericidal activity of phagocytes by catalase (255,296,315) and by superoxide dismutase (396,400). In one study (296) superoxide dismutase did not decrease the staphylocidal activity of neutrophils *in vivo* and *in vitro* under conditions in which catalase did. Both H_2O_2 and O_2^- have been implicated in the killing of *T. gondii* by macrophages (331–334), in the toxic effect of neutrophils stimulated by activated complement on cultured endothelial cells (393), and in the lysis of erythrocytes by monocytes stimulated by PMA (466). In the latter study a number of hydroxyl radical or singlet oxygen scavengers did not affect cytolysis. It has been proposed that the bactericidal defect induced in neutrophils by galactose is due, in part, to the ·OH scavenging activity of this compound (290).

In summary, the accumulated evidence strongly suggests, but does not definitively establish, the formation of ·OH by phagocytes and its involvement in microbicidal activity.

SINGLET OXYGEN

Properties

Electrons generally occur in pairs stabilized by spins in the opposite directions. Ground-state oxygen ($^3\Sigma_g^+ O_2$), however, has two unpaired valence electrons in separate orbitals with spins in the same direction. It is thus in the triplet state and has the properties of a diradical. Singlet oxygen ($^1O_2$) is formed when one of the unpaired electrons is lifted to an orbital of higher energy with an inversion of spin (for reviews see 8,135,226,229,461,470). There are two forms of singlet oxygen, delta and sigma. In delta singlet oxygen ($^1\Delta g O_2$) the newly paired electrons with opposite spins occupy the same orbital, whereas in sigma singlet oxygen ($^1\Sigma_g^+ O_2$), the two electrons with opposite spins occupy separate orbitals as indicated diagrammatically below:

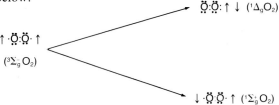

Sigma $^1O_2$ has a higher energy above-ground state (37 kcal) than does delta $^1O_2$ (22 kcal) but a considerably shorter lifetime. The intrinsic mean lifetime (i.e., in the gas phase at zero pressure) is 7.1 sec for $^1\Sigma_g^+ O_2$ and 45 min for $^1\Delta g O_2$ (226). In solution, however, the lifetime of $^1O_2$ is considerably shorter. In water the lifetime of $^1\Sigma_g^+ O_2$ does not exceed 10^{-11} sec, and values reported for $^1\Delta g O_2$ range from 2 to 4 μsec (156,287,318). The lifetime of $^1\Delta g O_2$ in solution, however, is strikingly solvent-dependent ranging from 2 μsec in water to 1,000 μsec in freon (230) (Table 1). Furthermore, its lifetime in a number of solvents is increased by a factor of 10 or more when the solvent is deuterated (319). Thus, values for the lifetime of $^1\Delta g O_2$ in D_2O of 20 μsec (319), 30 μsec (156), 32 μsec (299), and 53 μsec (288) have been reported. The corresponding increase in a chemical reaction on the substitution of D_2O for H_2O has been used as evidence for $^1O_2$ involvement (222,230,319,346). The lifetime of $^1\Delta g O_2$ is little affected by a change in temperature, with a 50% decrease resulting from an increase in temperature from $-50°$ to $+25°C$ (291). Because of its relatively long lifetime, $^1\Delta g O_2$ is the predominant form of $^1O_2$ in solution; indeed, it is probably the sole reactive form in biological systems.

Singlet oxygen reverts to the ground state with the emission of light. The emission spectrum, however, is complex due to the two forms of $^1O_2$ and the possibility of both single molecule transitions and simultaneous transitions resulting from the collision of pairs of $^1O_2$ molecules (Table 2). The emission spectrum is further complicated by its decay both to the ground (0-0) state (Table 2) and to different vibrational levels. Since $^1\Delta g O_2$ is the predominant form of singlet oxygen in solution, the emission spectrum largely reflects its decay with major peaks at 1,270

TABLE 1. *Lifetime of delta singlet oxygen in various solvents[a]*

Solvent	Lifetime (μsec)
H_2O	2
CH_3OH	7
C_2H_5OH	12
C_6H_{12}	17
C_6H_6	24
$CH_3\overset{\text{O}}{\overset{\|}{C}}CH_3$	26
CH_3CN	30
$CHCl_3$	60
CS_2	200
C_6F_6	600
CCl_4	700
Freon 11	1000

[a]Adapted from Kearns (230) with permission.

TABLE 2. *Emission spectra of singlet oxygen decay to the ground state[a]*

Transitions	Wavelength (nm)
Single molecule transitions	
$^1\Delta_g O_2$	1268.7
$^1\Sigma_g^+ O_2$	762.1
Simultaneous transitions	
$(^1\Delta_g O_2)\ (^1\Delta_g O_2)$	634.3
$(^1\Delta_g O_2)\ (^1\Sigma_g^+ O_2)$	476.1
$(^1\Sigma_g^+ O_2)\ (^1\Sigma_g^+ O_2)$	381.0

[a]Adapted from Kasha and Brabham (225).

nm for the single molecule transition and 634 and 703 nm for the simultaneous transition to the 0-0 and 0-1 vibrational levels, respectively.

The chemical reactivity of $^1O_2$ in aqueous solution is due largely, if not entirely, to the delta form due to its relatively long lifetime and its electronic configuration. Singlet oxygen is a strong electrophile which reacts with compounds in areas of high electron density to form characteristic, often oxygenated, products (for review see 461). This reactivity of $^1O_2$ produced by the H_2O_2-OCl$^-$ system (see H_2O_2-OCl$^-$ system, page 136) could be used to oxygenate a number of mono- and diolefins (134,139). The products formed were identical to those produced by some dye-sensitized photooxidation reactions (134,139), lending support to the proposal originally made by Kautsky (228) that $^1O_2$ can be an active intermediate formed in photosensitized oxidations. Simultaneous with these studies was the report that $^1O_2$ produced by microwave discharge initiated comparable chemical reactions (98).

Production

Singlet oxygen can be produced in a variety of ways. These include electrical or microwave discharge, dye-sensitized photooxidations, and a number of chemical reactions (230,330,350,470). Only the latter will be considered here, with special emphasis on those reactions that may occur in phagocytes.

Hydrogen Peroxide-Hypochlorite System

A major advance in the field of $^1O_2$ chemistry was the discovery that the weak red chemiluminescence produced by the reaction between H_2O_2 and hypochlorite was due to the production of $^1O_2$ (239) as follows.

$$H_2O_2 + OCl^- \rightarrow {}^1O_2 + H_2O + Cl^- \qquad (y)$$

This luminescence is readily apparent to the dark-adapted eye when hypochlorite (Chlorox) and H_2O_2 are rapidly mixed (419). The reaction rate is optimum at a pH of about 10 and falls sharply as the pH is raised or lowered (222). The $^1O_2$ formed is derived from H_2O_2 rather than hypochlorite (70), and the chloroperoxy ion ($OOCl^-$) is believed to be an intermediate (226). Hypochlorite can be replaced in this reaction by chlorine (66,67,415) or bromine (311).

The initial product formed by the MPO-H_2O_2-chloride antimicrobial system is HOCl (or OCl^-) (3,4,179), and HOCl and chloride may interact to form chlorine (see Neutrophils, page 117). Comparable products would be anticipated from the MPO-H_2O_2-bromide system, and the interaction of these products of the peroxidase system with excess H_2O_2 to form $^1O_2$ might be expected. Evidence compatible with $^1O_2$ formation by the peroxidase system has appeared. Thus, the MPO-H_2O_2-halide system emits light (6,7,382) and catalyzes the conversion of 2,5 diphenylfuran to its singlet oxygen product *cis*-dibenzoylethylene. The latter reaction is inhibited by the $^1O_2$-quenchers β-carotene, bilirubin, histidine, and DABCO and is stimulated by D_2O (383). Both light emission and diphenylfuran conversion by this system had an acid pH optimum (approximately 4.5), and the effectiveness of the halides varied in the order $Br^- > Cl^- > I^-$. Chemiluminescence, product analysis, $^1O_2$-quenchers, and the deuterium effect also have provided evidence for $^1O_2$ formation by the LPO-H_2O_2-bromide system (362,363). The chemiluminescence appears to be due to secondary excitation of components of the reaction mixture rather than to primary $^1O_2$ decay (362,383).

The evidence presented for the formation of $^1O_2$ by the peroxidase-H_2O_2-halide system has been brought into question (180,188,454). The methods used for the detection of $^1O_2$ by the peroxidase system, i.e., furan oxidation with product analysis, inhibition by $^1O_2$-quenchers, stimulation by D_2O, lack specificity, and evidence implicating HOCl (or HOBr) and/or Cl_2 (or Br_2) as the reactive substances, without the intermediate formation of $^1O_2$, has been presented. In this regard, it should be noted that the generation of $^1O_2$ by the interaction of H_2O_2 and hypochlorite occurs best at alkaline pH (222), whereas the peroxidase-H_2O_2-halide system has an acid pH optimum (383).

Superoxide Anion

There have been a number of reports of the formation of $^1O_2$ from O_2^-. The mechanisms proposed include spontaneous dismutation, the Haber-Weiss reaction, reaction with ·OH, and reaction with diacyl peroxides.

Spontaneous Dismutation

It has been proposed that spontaneous dismutation of O_2^- results in the formation of O_2 in the excited state (235–238,303,430) in contrast to superoxide dismutase-catalyzed dismutation which produces ground-state oxygen. The protonated form of the superoxide anion (HO_2) was reported to be required for $^1O_2$ formation (430), suggesting either of the following reactions.

$$HO_2 + O_2^- + H^+ \rightarrow {}^1O_2 + H_2O_2 \tag{z}$$
$$HO_2 + HO_2 \rightarrow {}^1O_2 + H_2O_2 \tag{aa}$$

On the basis of the marked water quenching of O_2^--sensitized luminescence, Khan (235) initially proposed that $^1\Sigma_g^+ O_2$ was preferentially formed; however, a subsequent theoretical analysis indicated that $^1O_2$ generation was critically dependent on the number of water molecules present (237,238). According to this analysis, $^1O_2$ is formed only when the number of water molecules associated with O_2^- in a cluster is ≥ 5; over a narrow water concentration range $^1\Delta g O_2$ is the product, beyond which $^1\Sigma_g^+ O_2$ predominates.

Although the formation of $^1O_2$ by dismutation of O_2^- is thermodynamically possible (269,270), a number of studies have cast doubt on the spontaneous dismutation of O_2^- as an efficient mechanism for the formation of $^1O_2$ (100,141,169,345,364). This may be due in part to the quenching of $^1O_2$ by O_2^- (169,237,238,387) as follows.

$$^1O_2 + O_2^- \rightarrow O_2^- + {}^3O_2 + 22 \text{ kcal} \tag{ab}$$

Superoxide quenching of $^1O_2$ in aqueous solutions of biological interest however, would not be appreciable because of the relatively low concentration of O_2^- expected (169). Foote and colleagues (141) have concluded from their data that $^1O_2$ is produced in amounts of no greater than 0.2% of the oxygen formed by the dismutation of O_2^- under conditions in which the quenching of $^1O_2$ by O_2^- did not occur.

Haber-Weiss Reaction

Lipid peroxidation by the xanthine oxidase system was reported by Pederson and Aust (359), to require iron and EDTA and to be inhibited by superoxide dismutase and by the $^1O_2$-quencher 1,3-diphenylisobenzofuran, with the latter being converted to its $^1O_2$ product, o-dibenzoylbenzene. They proposed that $^1O_2$, formed from $O_2^{\bar{\ }}$ generated by the xanthine oxidase system, reacts with lipid to form fatty acid hydroperoxides. Kellogg and Fridovich (232) confirmed these findings and provided evidence which implicated the Haber-Weiss reaction in the formation of $^1O_2$. Lipid peroxidation was inhibited by superoxide dismutase, catalase and $^1O_2$ scavengers, but not by scavengers of $\cdot OH$. The xanthine oxidase system also converted 2,5 dimethylfuran (232) and 2,5 diphenylfuran (385) to their $^1O_2$ products. Dimethylfuran conversion was inhibited by superoxide dismutase and catalase, but not by the $\cdot OH$-scavenger, mannitol (232), and diphenylfuran conversion was inhibited by superoxide dismutase, catalase, the $^1O_2$-quenchers azide, DABCO and histidine, and, to a considerably lesser degree, by the $\cdot OH$-scavengers mannitol and benzoate (385). Furthermore, the conversion of 1,3 diphenylisobenzofuran to its $^1O_2$ product by a potassium superoxide-H_2O_2 mixture was inhibited by the $^1O_2$-quenchers β carotene and DABCO (267). These studies are compatible with the formation of $^1O_2$ by the metal-catalyzed Haber-Weiss reaction as follows:

$$O_2^{\bar{\ }} + H_2O_2 \xrightarrow[\text{metal}]{} {}^1O_2 + OH^- + \cdot OH \tag{x}$$

a reaction which is possible on thermodynamic grounds (269). By analogy $^1O_2$ may also be formed by reaction of $O_2^{\bar{\ }}$ with organic peroxides (see the Haber-Weiss reaction, page 127) as follows:

$$O_2^{\bar{\ }} + ROOH \rightarrow {}^1O_2 + RO\cdot + OH^- \tag{ac}$$

Reaction with Hydroxyl Radicals

On the basis of studies of the chemiluminescence of the xanthine oxidase and aldehyde oxidase systems Arneson (20) proposed that $^1O_2$ can be generated by the interaction of $O_2^{\bar{\ }}$ and $\cdot OH$ as follows:

$$O_2^{\bar{\ }} + \cdot OH \rightarrow {}^1O_2 + OH^- \tag{ad}$$

This interaction is possible on thermodynamic grounds (269,270); however, it is unlikely in biological systems, since $\cdot OH$ will be scavenged by its nearest neighbors because of its high reactivity, and thus be unavailable for reaction with $O_2^{\bar{\ }}$ (100).

Reaction with Diacyl Peroxides

The reaction of $O_2^{\bar{\ }}$ with diacyl peroxides has been reported to yield $^1O_2$ (107) as follows:

$$2O_2^{\bar{\ }} + R\overset{\overset{O}{\parallel}}{C}OO\overset{\overset{O}{\parallel}}{C}R \rightarrow 2{}^1O_2 + 2RCO_2^{\bar{\ }} \tag{ae}$$

Other Mechanisms for $^1O_2$ Formation

Other mechanisms for $^1O_2$ production, which may be relevant to the phagocyte, include the base-catalyzed disproportionation of H_2O_2 (see section on nonenzymatic toxicity, page 124) (425) and the peroxidative decomposition of lipids (22,336,438,439,459,473). However, the pH within the phagosome would not appear to favor $^1O_2$ formation by disproportionation of H_2O_2, and the evidence suggesting that $^1O_2$ is formed as a by-product of lipid peroxidation has come mainly from studies with liver-microsome preparations, and its applicability to leukocytes is unknown.

Generation by Leukocytes

A number of attempts have been made to detect $^1O_2$ formation by leukocytes; the results have been inconclusive due to the difficulties inherent in the detection of $^1O_2$ in complex aqueous solutions (137,273). In general, two methods have been used: a) the detection of the chemiluminescence of $^1O_2$ decay and b) product analysis, i.e., the detection of the product of a $^1O_2$-dependent chemical reaction.

Detection by Chemiluminescence

Interest in $^1O_2$ involvement in phagocytic cell function began with the finding by Allen and co-workers (10) that phagocytosis by human PMNs is associated with the emission of light. Subsequent studies indicated that chemiluminescence is a general property of stimulated phagocytes; light is emitted by eosinophils (263) and mononuclear phagocytes (9,43,185,218,325,343) as well as by neutrophils. Under comparable conditions, the maximum light emission by PMNs and eosinophils was similar, although the interval between phagocytic stimulus and peak activity, and the duration of the chemiluminescence were longer with eosinophils than with neutrophils (263). In general, mononuclear leukocytes do not emit as much light as do neutrophils under comparable conditions and require, in some instances, amplification of the light by the addition of luminol for the demonstration of the luminescent response (9,185,468). Light also is emitted by stimulated mast cells and basophils (189). Chemiluminescence by stimulated phagocytes was not observed in the absence of particle ingestion (or other forms of leukocyte stimulation) or when leukocytes from patients with CGD were used (217,382,435). Thus, attention was directed to the phagocytosis-induced respiratory burst as the source of the emitted light and raised the possibility of $^1O_2$ involvement (10).

Chemiluminescence by phagocytes appears to be due to two general mechanisms, one involving peroxidase and the other, the superoxide anion. The evidence for peroxidase involvement is as follows.

a. PMNs that lack MPO, i.e., from patients with hereditary MPO deficiency have a decreased chemiluminescent response during the early postphagocytic period (382).

b. The peroxidase-inhibitor, azide, inhibits the phagocytosis-induced chemilu-minescent response of PMNs (382,397) and eosinophils (263) while having little or no effect on the response of guinea pig peritoneal or alveolar macrophages to stimulation by formyl-methionyl peptides (185). Azide is a scavenger of $^1O_2$ (125,140,184,231) and ·OH (117) as well as a hemeprotein inhibitor; however, the chemiluminescence of MPO-deficient PMNs is unaffected by azide (382), sug-gesting that its effect on normal cells is due to an inhibition of peroxidase.

c. The MPO-H_2O_2-halide system emits light (6,7,382) with an emission spectrum the same as that of phagocytosing PMNs (15). As with the intact cell, the chem-iluminescence of this isolated system is inhibited by azide (382).

The following evidence suggests the involvement of O_2^- in the chemiluminescent response of intact phagocytes.

1. Light emission by neutrophils (11,217,382,396,462), eosinophils (263), and mononuclear phagocytes (9,43,185,218,343) is inhibited by superoxide dismutase. This inhibition is independent of peroxidase, since it is observed when MPO-deficient leukocytes are used (382). A direct quenching effect of superoxide dis-mutase on $^1O_2$ has been proposed (128,356,357,377,469); however, this action of superoxide dismutase has been questioned by a number of investigators (153,195,303,321,407), suggesting that superoxide dismutase inhibits chemilu-minescence by its primary effect on O_2^-.

2. Potassium superoxide or O_2^--generating systems such as the xanthine oxi-dase system emit light, and this light emission is inhibited by superoxide dismutase (20,127,128,152,153,160,382,431). In contrast to the isolated MPO system or intact PMNs, light emission by the xanthine oxidase system is not inhibited by azide (382).

Chemiluminescence indicates the formation of electronically excited states but, without spectral analysis, does not indicate the nature of the excited species. Anal-ysis of the light emitted by stimulated PMNs did not reveal the specific spectrum of singlet oxygen decay but, rather, broad peak activity with a maximum at about 570 nm (15,75). This suggests that the light emitted by phagocytes is not due directly to $^1O_2$ decay. Energy transfer from $^1O_2$ to a variety of acceptors can occur with the formation of excited products, and indeed in complex aqueous solutions it is probable that much of the light emitted as a result of $^1O_2$ formation is due to these secondary excitations. Thus, for example, reaction of $^1O_2$ with olefins form dioxetanes, which are often unstable, decomposing to form excited carbonyl prod-ucts which decay with light emission (275,304,471, Fig. 4). Furthermore, some

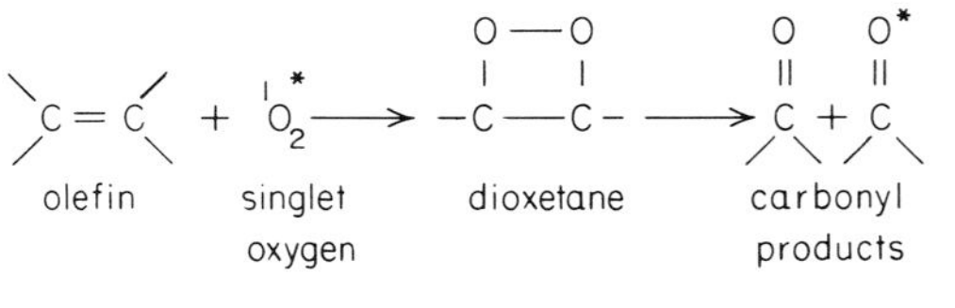

FIG. 4. Formation of dioxetanes and excited carbonyl products by singlet oxygen. *Excited state. [Reproduced from Klebanoff and Clark (253), with permission of North-Holland Publish-ing Company.

biologically important compounds, e.g., tryptophan, serum albumin, arachidonic acid, produce a shift in the emission spectrum of the $^1O_2$-generating system NaOCl + H_2O_2, suggesting secondary excitations (16).

Chemiluminescence also can be a consequence of secondary excitations initiated by oxygen products other than $^1O_2$. Thus, the weak blue-green chemiluminescence produced by O_2^--generating systems is dependent on the presence of carbonate ions in the reaction mixture (196,368,430), and the mechanism proposed is the oxidation of carbonate by ·OH formed by the Haber-Weiss reaction to yield the carbonate radical which dimerizes to form an excited species (196). The substitution of D_2O for H_2O did not increase the carbonate-dependent light emission, suggesting that $^1O_2$ is not an intermediate (368). Excited compounds also can be formed by peroxidase-catalyzed reactions (76,353). Fenton's reagent (ferrous sulfate + H_2O_2) emits light which is enhanced by tryptophan (14). This light emission is inhibited by ·OH and $^1O_2$ scavengers and is increased by D_2O, suggesting the requirement for both ·OH and $^1O_2$.

An additional consideration in the evaluation of the role of $^1O_2$ in light emission is the area of peak activity in the emission spectrum of $^1O_2$ in relation to the sensitivity of the photomultiplier tubes generally used for the detection of chemiluminescence. The predominant peaks are in the red and near-infrared region where standard photomultiplier tubes are relatively insensitive. Of particular value would be the detection of the major peak in the near-infrared region at 1270 nm resulting from the single molecule transition of $^1\Delta gO_2$. Recently, a sensitive near-infrared spectrophotometer has been developed which can detect the $^1\Delta gO_2 \rightarrow ^3\Delta gO_2$ 1270-nm emission band (240). Its application to the chemiluminescence of phagocytes would be of interest.

In summary, although chemiluminescence by stimulated phagocytes indicates the formation of electronically excited states, a contribution by $^1O_2$ to the light emission has not been demonstrated. The emission spectrum is not that of $^1O_2$ decay. However, the absence of a $^1O_2$ spectrum does not necessarily exclude a direct contribution by $^1O_2$ to the light emission, since its contribution would be hidden in the decay resulting from secondary excitations initiated by $^1O_2$ or other products of the respiratory burst.

Detection by Product Analysis

The detection of $^1O_2$ formation by product analysis requires the addition to granulocytes of a compound which reacts with $^1O_2$ to form a specific product and the demonstration of the formation of that product by the stimulated phagocytes. Chemical traps for $^1O_2$, however, are generally nonspecific. Furans have been extensively used for this purpose in cell-free systems; however, the $^1O_2$ product can be formed by a number of other oxidants. Phagocytosing PMNs oxidized methionine to methionine sulfoxide, a reaction that can occur by a $^1O_2$ mechanism (452). Formation of methionine sulfoxide by PMNs was inhibited by $^1O_2$-quenchers and stimulated by D_2O, results compatible with the involvement of $^1O_2$. However, as noted by the authors, the nonspecific nature of the conversion leaves open the possibility of another mechanism. The most specific chemical trap is cholesterol, which reacts with $^1O_2$ to yield 3β-hydroxy-5α-cholest-6-ene-5-hydroperoxide, a product different from those produced by radical oxidation (274). Cholesterol, however, is an inefficient $^1O_2$ scavenger as compared to other less specific traps. In one study, the specific $^1O_2$ product could not be detected on the uptake of mineral oil droplets containing ^{14}C-cholesterol by PMNs (137). The sensitivity of the assay was such that less than 1.6% of the oxygen consumed was released as $^1O_2$. Similarly, in preliminary experiments, cholesterol on the surface of polystyrene beads was not converted to its $^1O_2$ product on ingestion by rat lung macrophages.

TOXICITY OF $^1O_2$

Model Systems

That $^1O_2$ can be toxic to cells is suggested by the photodynamic action of dyes (135,155,204,265,427). Certain dyes in the presence of light and oxygen are toxic to cells. The dye absorbs light and is converted to a sensitized triplet state, which can initiate damage to a variety of targets by two mechanisms. In type I reactions the sensitized dye reacts directly with target molecules, whereas in type II reactions the sensitized dye reacts initially with oxygen. The most common consequence of the latter interaction is the excitation of oxygen to produce the electronically excited singlet state. Electron transfer from the sensitized dye to oxygen with the formation of O_2^- also can occur, although this reaction is considerably less efficient than is energy transfer to form $^1O_2$. The $^1O_2$ so formed is believed to be primarily responsible for oxygen-dependent dye-sensitized photooxygenation reactions (134,139,228,346) and thus for the toxicity of these systems on microorganisms and other cells (96,203,266,268,301,302,420). Singlet oxygen also has been implicated in the toxicity to intact cells produced by the xanthine oxidase system (233,385) and by the photoreduction of riboflavin at 365 nm in the presence of a hydrogen donor (322).

Phagocytes

The evidence for $^1O_2$ involvement in the microbicidal or cytotoxic activity of phagocytes is inconclusive. It is clear that $^1O_2$ can initiate a number of chemical reactions that produce damage to cells. Furthermore, evidence is accumulating that is compatible with the generation of $^1O_2$ by cytotoxic systems which appear to be operative in phagocytes, although this evidence is by no means conclusive. The generation of $^1O_2$ by intact phagocytes has not been demonstrated. Indirect evidence implicating $^1O_2$ in the toxic activity of phagocytes has appeared. Thus, for example, carotenoid-containing wild-type *Sarcina lutea* are less readily killed by human PMNs than are mutant pigmentless organisms (272). Since carotenoid pigments are very efficient singlet oxygen quenchers (136,138), one possible mechanism for this difference in sensitivity is the $^1O_2$-quenching effect of the carotenoid pigments *in situ.* However, other mechanisms are possible. Thus, the question of a role for $^1O_2$ in the microbicidal activity of phagocytes remains unresolved.

ACKNOWLEDGMENTS

The author gratefully acknowledges the collaboration of a number of colleagues in some of the studies reviewed in this paper, the very generous grant support from the National Institutes of Health, the Rockefeller Foundation and the Edna Mc-Connell Clark Foundation, and the secretarial assistance of Caroline Wilson in the preparation of the manuscript.

REFERENCES

1. Ackerman, G. A., and Clark, M. A. (1971): Ultrastructural localization of peroxidase activity in human basophil leukocytes. *Acta Haematol.*, 45:280–284.
2. Agner, K. (1941): Verdoperoxidase. A ferment isolated from leukocytes. *Acta Physiol. Scand.*, 2(Suppl. 8):1–62.
3. Agner, K. (1958): Peroxidative oxidation of chloride ions. *Proc. 4th Int. Congr. Biochem., Vienna*, 15:64.
4. Agner, K. (1972): Biological effects of hypochlorous acid formed by "MPO" peroxidation in the presence of chloride ions. In: *Structure and Function of Oxidation-Reduction Enzymes*, edited by A. Akeson and A. Ehrenberg, Vol. 18, pp. 329–335. Pergamon Press, New York.
5. Albrich, J. M., McCarthy, C. A., and Hurst, J. K. (1981): Biological reactivity of hypochlorous acid: implications for microbicidal mechanisms of leukocyte myeloperoxidase. *Proc. Natl. Acad. Sci. U.S.A.*, 78:210–214.
6. Allen, R. C. (1975): Halide dependence of the myeloperoxidase-mediated antimicrobial system of the polymorphonuclear leukocyte in the phenomenon of electronic excitation. *Biochem. Biophys. Res. Commun.*, 63:675–683.
7. Allen, R. C. (1975): The role of pH in the chemiluminescent response of the myeloperoxidase-halide-HOOH antimicrobial system. *Biochem. Biophys. Res. Commun.*, 63:684–691.
8. Allen, R. C. (1980): Free-radical production by reticuloendothelial cells. In: *The Reticuloendothelial System. A Comprehensive Treatise 2. Biochemistry and Metabolism*, edited by A. J. Sbarra and R. R. Strauss, pp. 309–338. Plenum Press, New York.
9. Allen, R. C., and Loose, L. D. (1976): Phagocytic activation of a luminol-dependent chemiluminescence in rabbit alveolar and peritoneal macrophages. *Biochem. Biophys. Res. Commun.*, 69:245–252.
10. Allen, R. C., Stjernholm, R. L., and Steele, R. H. (1972): Evidence for the generation of an electronic excitation state(s) in human polymorphonuclear leukocytes and its participation in bactericidal activity. *Biochem. Biophys. Res. Commun.*, 47:679–684.
11. Allen, R. C., Yevich, S. J., Orth, R. W., and Steele, R. H. (1974): The superoxide anion and singlet molecular oxygen: their role in the microbicidal activity of the polymorphonuclear leukocyte. *Biochem. Biophys. Res. Commun.*, 60:909–917.
12. Allison, F., Lancaster, M. G., and Crosthwaite, J. L. (1963): Studies on the pathogenesis of acute inflammation. V. An assessment of factors that influence *in vitro* the phagocytic and adhesive properties of leukocytes obtained from rabbit peritoneal exudate. *Am. J. Pathol.*, 43:775–795.
13. Ambruso, D. R., and Johnston, R. B., Jr. (1981): Lactoferrin enhances hydroxyl radical production by human neutrophils, neutrophil particulate fractions, and an enzymatic generating system. *J. Clin. Invest.*, 67:352–360.
14. Andersen, B. R., and Horvath, L. (1979): Light generation with Fenton's reagent. Its relationship to granulocyte chemiluminescence. *Biochim. Biophys. Acta*, 584:164–173.
15. Andersen, B. R., Brendzel, A. M., and Lint, T. F. (1977): Chemiluminescence spectra of human myeloperoxidase and polymorphonuclear leukocytes. *Infect. Immun.*, 17:62–66.
16. Andersen, B. R., Lint, T. F., and Brendzel, A. M. (1978). Chemically shifted singlet oxygen spectrum. *Biochim. Biophys. Acta*, 542:527–536.
17. Ando, M., Dannenberg, A. M., Jr., and Shima, K. (1972). Macrophage accumulation, division, maturation and digestion and microbicidal capacities in tuberculous lesions. II. Rate at which

mononuclear cells enter and divide in primary BCG lesions and those of reinfection. *J. Immunol.*, 109:8–19.

18. Archer, G. T., and Hirsch, J. G. (1963): Isolation of granules from eosinophil leucocytes and study of their enzyme content. *J. Exp. Med.*, 118:277–286.

19. Archer, G. T., Air, G., Jackas, M., and Morell, D. B. (1965): Studies on rat eosinophil peroxidase. *Biochim. Biophys. Acta*, 99:96–101.

20. Arneson, R. M. (1970): Substrate-induced chemiluminescence of xanthine oxidase and aldehyde oxidase. *Arch. Biochem. Biophys.*, 136:352–360.

21. Atwal, O. S. (1971): Cytoenzymological behavior in peritoneal exudate cells of rat *in vivo*. 1. Histochemical study of enzymatic function of peroxidase. *J. Reticuloendothel. Soc.*, 10:163–172.

22. Auclair, C., and Lecomte, M. -C. (1978): Singlet oxygen production associated with hydroperoxide induced lipid peroxidation in liver microsomes. *Biochem. Biophys. Res. Commun.*, 85:946–951.

23. Aune, T. M., and Thomas, E. L. (1977): Accumulation of hypothiocyanite ion during peroxidase-catalyzed oxidation of thiocyanate ion. *Eur. J. Biochem.*, 80:209–214.

24. Babior, B. M. (1978): Oxygen-dependent microbial killing by phagocytes. *N. Engl. J. Med.*, 298:659–668; 721–725.

25. Babior, B. M. (1979): Superoxide production by phagocytes. Another look at the effect of cytochrome C on oxygen uptake by stimulated neutrophils. *Biochem. Biophys. Res. Commun.*, 91:222–226.

26. Babior, B. M. (1980): The role of oxygen radicals in microbial killing by phagocytes. In: *The Reticuloendothelial System. A Comprehensive Treatise. 2. Biochemistry and Metabolism*, edited by A. J. Sbarra and R. R. Strauss, pp. 339–354. Plenum Press, New York.

27. Babior, B. M., and Kipnes, R. S. (1977): Superoxide-forming enzyme from human neutrophils: evidence for a flavin requirement. *Blood*, 50:517–524.

28. Babior, B. M., Curnutte, J. T., and Kipnes, R. S. (1975): Biological defense mechanisms. Evidence for the participation of superoxide in bacterial killing by xanthine oxidase. *J. Lab. Clin. Med.*, 85:235–244.

29. Babior, B. M., Kipnes, R. S., and Curnutte, J. T. (1973): Biological defense mechanisms. The production by leukocytes of superoxide, a potential bactericidal agent. *J. Clin. Invest.*, 52:741–744.

30. Badwey, J. A., and Karnovsky, M. L. (1980): Active oxygen species and the functions of phagocytic leukocytes. *Ann. Rev. Biochem.*, 49:695–726.

31. Baehner, R. L., and Johnston, R. B., Jr. (1971): Metabolic and bactericidal activities of human eosinophils. *Br. J. Haematol.*, 20:277–285.

32. Baehner, R. L., and Johnston, R. B., Jr. (1972): Monocyte function in children with neutropenia and chronic infections. *Blood*, 40:31–41.

33. Baehner, R. L., Boxer, L. A., Allen, J. M., and Davis, J. (1977): Autooxidation as a basis for altered function by polymorphonuclear leukocytes. *Blood*, 50:327–335.

34. Bainton, D. F. (1980): Changes in peroxidase distribution within organelles of blood monocytes and peritoneal macrophages after surface adherence *in vitro* and *in vivo*. In: *Mononuclear Phagocytes. Functional Aspects*, edited by R. van Furth, pp. 61–86. Martinus Nijhoff Publishers, The Hague.

35. Bainton, D. F., and Farquhar, M. G. (1970): Segregation and packaging of granule enzymes in eosinophilic leukocytes. *J. Cell Biol.*, 45:54–73.

36. Bainton, D. F., and Golde, D. W. (1978): Differentiation of macrophages from normal human bone marrow in liquid culture. Electron microscopy and cytochemistry. *J. Clin. Invest.*, 61:1555–1569.

37. Bakkenist, A. R. J., De Boer, J. E. G., Plat, H., and Wever, R. (1980): The halide complexes of myeloperoxidase and the mechanism of the halogenation reactions. *Biochim. Biophys. Acta*, 613:337–348.

38. Baldridge, C. W., and Gerard, R. W. (1933): The extra respiration of phagocytosis. *Am. J. Physiol.*, 103:235–236.

39. Bass, D. A., and Szejda, P. (1979): Eosinophils versus neutrophils in host defense. Killing of newborn larvae of *Trichinella spiralis* by human granulocytes *in vitro*. *J. Clin. Invest.*, 64:1415–1422.

40. Bass, D. A., and Szejda, P. (1979): Mechanisms of killi.   f newborn larvae of *Trichinella spiralis* by neutrophils and eosinophils. Killing by generators of hydrogen peroxide *in vitro*. *J. Clin. Invest.*, 64:1558–1564.

41. Bayliss, C. E., and Waites, W. M. (1976): Effect of hydrogen peroxide on spores of *Clostridium bifermentans*. *J. Gen. Microbiol.*, 96:401–407.
42. Bayliss, C. E., and Waites, W. M. (1979): The synergistic killing of *Bacillus subtilis* by hydrogen peroxide and ultra-violet light irradiation. *FEMS Microbiol. Lett.*, 5:331–333.
43. Beall, G. D., Repine, J. E., Hoidal, J. R., and Rasp, F. L. (1977): Chemiluminescence by human alveolar macrophages: stimulation with heat-killed bacteria or phorbol myristate acetate. *Infect. Immun.*, 17:117–120.
44. Beauchamp, C., and Fridovich, I. (1970). Mechanism for the production of ethylene from methional. Generation of the hydroxyl radical by xanthine oxidase. *J. Biol. Chem.*, 245: 4641–4646.
45. Becker, H., Munder, G., and Fischer, H. (1958): Über den Leukocytenstoffsechsel bei der Phagocytose. *Hoppe Seylers Z. Physiol. Chem.*, 313:266–275.
46. Beelen, R. H. J., Fluitsma, D. M., van der Meer, J. W. M., and Hoefsmit, E. C. M. (1980): Development of exudate-resident macrophages on the basis of the pattern of peroxidatic activity *in vivo* and *in vitro*. In: *Mononuclear Phagocytes. Functional Aspects*, edited by R. van Furth, pp. 87–112. Martinus Nijhoff Publishers, The Hague.
47. Behar, D., Czapski, G., Rabani, J., Dorfman, L. M., and Schwarz, H. A. (1970): The acid dissociation constant and decay kinetics of the perhydroxyl radical. *J. Phys. Chem.*, 74:3209–3213.
48. Belding, M. E., Klebanoff, S. J., and Ray, C. G. (1970). Peroxidase-mediated virucidal systems. *Science*, 167:195–196.
49. Bentfeld, M. E., Nichols, B. A., and Bainton, D. F. (1977): Ultrastructural localization of peroxidase in leukocytes of rat bone marrow and blood. *Anat. Rec.*, 187:219–240.
50. Bielski, B. H. J., and Allen, A. O. (1977): Mechanism of the disproportionation of superoxide radicals. *J. Phys. Chem.*, 81:1048–1050.
51. Bielski, B. H. J., and Shiue, G. G. (1979): Reaction rates of superoxide radicals with the essential amino acids. In: *Oxygen Free Radicals and Tissue Damage, Ciba Foundation Symposium 65*, pp. 43–48. Excerpta Medica, Amsterdam.
52. Biggar, W. D., and Sturgess, J. M. (1976): Peroxidase activity in alveolar macrophages. *Lab. Invest.*, 34:31–42.
53. Biggar, W. D., Buron, S., and Holmes, B. (1976): Bactericidal mechanisms in rabbit alveolar macrophages: evidence against peroxidase and hydrogen peroxide bactericidal mechanisms. *Infect. Immun.*, 14:6–10.
54. Biggar, W. D., Holmes, B., Page, A. R., Deinard, A. S., L'Esperance, P., and Good, R. A. (1974): Metabolic and functional studies of monocytes in congenital neutropenia. *Br. J. Haematol.*, 28:233–243.
55. Bodel, P. T., Nichols, B. A., and Bainton, D. F. (1977): Appearance of peroxidase activity within the rough endoplasmic reticulum of blood monocytes after surface adherence. *J. Exp. Med.*, 145:264–274.
56. Bodel, P. T., Nichols, B. A., and Bainton, D. F. (1978): Difference in peroxidase localization of rabbit peritoneal macrophages after surface adherence. *Am. J. Pathol.*, 91:107–117.
57. Borregaard, N., and Johansen, K. S. (1979): Cytochrome b and chronic granulomatous disease. *Lancet*, 1:1397–1398.
58. Borregaard, N., Johansen, K. S., Taudorff, E., and Wandall, J. H. (1979): Cytochrome b is present in neutrophils from patients with chronic granulomatous disease. *Lancet*, 1:949–951.
59. Bors, W., Lengfelder, E., Saran, M., Fuchs, C., and Michel, C. (1976): Reactions of oxygen radical species with methional: a pulse radiolysis study. *Biochem. Biophys. Res. Commun.*, 70:81–87.
60. Bors, W., Michel, C., and Saran, M. (1979): Superoxide anions do not react with hydroperoxides. *FEBS Lett.*, 107:403–406.
61. Bors, W., Michel, C., and Saran, M. (1979): On the nature of biochemically generated hydroxyl radicals. Studies of *p*-nitrosodimethylaniline as a direct assay method. *Eur. J. Biochem.*, 95:621–627.
62. Bors. W., Saran, M., Lengfelder, E., Michel, C., Fuchs, C., and Frenzel, C. (1978): Detection of oxygen radicals in biological reactions. *Photochem. Photobiol.*, 28:629–638.
63. Bos, A., Wever, R., and Roos, D. (1978): Characterization and quantification of the peroxidase in human monocytes. *Biochim. Biophys. Acta*, 525:37–44.
64. Breton-Gorius, J., Guichard, J., Vainchenker, W., and Vilde, J. L. (1980): Ultrastructural and cytochemical changes induced by short and prolonged culture of human monocytes. *J. Reticuloendothel. Soc.*, 27:289–301.

65. Briggs, R. T., Karnovsky, M. L., and Karnovsky, M. J. (1975): Cytochemical demonstration of hydrogen peroxide in the polymorphonuclear leukocyte phagosomes. *J. Cell Biol.*, 64:254–260.
66. Browne, R. J., and Ogryzlo, E. A. (1964): Chemiluminescence from the reaction of chlorine with aqueous hydrogen peroxide. *Proc. Chem. Soc. (Lond.)*, 117.
67. Browne, R. J. and Ogryzlo, E. A. (1965): The yield of singlet oxygen in the reaction of chlorine with hydrogen peroxide. *Can. J. Chem.*, 43:2915–2916.
68. Buettner, G. R., Oberley, L. W., and Leuthauser, S. W. H. C. (1978): The effect of iron on the distribution of superoxide and hydroxyl radicals as seen by spin trapping and on the superoxide dismutase assay. *Photochem. Photobiol.*, 28:693–695.
69. Cadet, J., and Teoule, R. (1978): Comparative study of oxidation of nucleic acid components by hydroxyl radicals, singlet oxygen and superoxide anion radicals. *Photochem. Photobiol.*, 28:661–667.
70. Cahill, A. E., and Taube, H. (1952): The use of heavy oxygen in the study of reactions of hydrogen peroxide. *J. Am. Chem. Soc.*, 74:2312–2318.
71. Capsoni, F., Meroni, P. L., Ciboddo, G. F., and Colombo, G. (1979): Cytotoxic mechanism in white blood cells. *N. Engl. J. Med.*, 300:44.
72. Carp, H., and Janoff, A. (1980): Potential mediator of inflammation. Phagocyte-derived oxidants suppress the elastase-inhibitory capacity of alpha$_1$-proteinase inhibitor *in vitro*. *J. Clin. Invest.*, 66:987–995.
73. Cederbaum, A. I., Dicker, E., and Cohen, G. (1980): Role of hydroxyl radicals in the iron-ethylenediaminetetraacetic acid mediated stimulation of microsomal oxidation of ethanol. *Biochemistry*, 19:3698–3704.
74. Chang, K. -P. (1981): Leishmanicidal mechanisms of human polymorphonuclear phagocytes. *Am. J. Trop. Med. Hyg.*, 30:322–333.
75. Cheson, B. D., Christensen, R. L., Sperling, R., Kohler, B. E., and Babior, B. M. (1976): The origin of the chemiluminescence of phagocytosing granulocytes. *J. Clin. Invest.*, 58:789–796.
76. Cilento, G., Duran, N., Zinner, K., Vidigal, C. C., Faria Oliveira, O. M. M., Haun, M., Falioni, A., Augusto, O., Casadei de Baptista, R., and Bechara, E. J. H. (1978): Chemienergized species in peroxidase systems. *Photochem. Photobiol.*, 28:445–451.
77. Clark, R. A. (1980): Chemotactic factor inactivation by stimulated neutrophils via secretion of myeloperoxidase and H$_2$O$_2$. *Fed. Proc.*, 39:699.
78. Clark, R. A., and Klebanoff, S. J. (1975): Neutrophil-mediated tumor cell cytotoxicity: role of the peroxidase system. *J. Exp. Med.*, 141:1442–1447.
79. Clark, R. A., and Klebanoff, S. J. (1977): Myeloperoxidase-H$_2$O$_2$-halide system: cytotoxic effect on human blood leukocytes. *Blood*, 50:65–70.
80. Clark, R. A., and Klebanoff, S. J. (1977): Studies on the mechanism of antibody-dependent polymorphonuclear leukocyte-mediated cytotoxicity. *J. Immunol.*, 119:1413–1418.
81. Clark, R. A., and Klebanoff, S. J. (1979): Myeloperoxidase-mediated platelet release reaction. *J. Clin. Invest.*, 63:177–183.
82. Clark, R. A., and Klebanoff, S. J. (1979): Chemotactic factor inactivation by the myeloperoxidase-hydrogen peroxide-halide system. An inflammatory control mechanism. *J. Clin. Invest.*, 64:913–920.
83. Clark, R. A., and Klebanoff, S. J. (1979): Role of the myeloperoxidase-H$_2$O$_2$-halide system in concanavalin A-induced tumor cell killing by human neutrophils. *J. Immunol.*, 122:2605–2610.
84. Clark, R. A., and Klebanoff, S. J. (1980): Neutrophil-platelet interaction mediated by myeloperoxidase and hydrogen peroxide. *J. Immunol.*, 124:399–405.
85. Clark, R. A., and Szot, S. (1981): The myeloperoxidase-hydrogen peroxide-halide system as effector of neurophil-mediated tumor cell cytotoxicity. *J. Immunol.*, 126:1295–1301.
86. Clark, R. A., Klebanoff, S. J., Einstein, A. B., and Fefer, A. (1975): Peroxidase-H$_2$O$_2$-halide system: cytotoxic effect on mammalian tumor cells. *Blood*, 45:161–170.
87. Clark, R. A., Stone, P. J., El Hag, A., Calore, J. D., and Franzblau, C. (1981): Myeloperoxidase-catalyzed inactivation of α$_1$-protease inhibitor by human neutrophils. *J. Biol. Chem.*, 256:3348–3353.
88. Clark, R. A., Szot, S., Venkatasubramanian, K., and Schiffmann, E. (1980): Chemotactic factor inactivation by myeloperoxidase-mediated oxidation of methionine. *J. Immunol.*, 124:2020–2026.
89. Cline, M. J. (1970): Bactericidal activity of human macrophages: Analysis of factors influencing the killing of *Listeria monocytogenes*. *Infect. Immun.*, 2:156–161.
90. Cline, M. J., and Lehrer, R. I. (1968). Phagocytosis by human monocytes. *Blood*, 32:423–435.
91. Cline, M. J., Hanifin, J., and Lehrer, R. I. (1968): Phagocytosis by human eosinophils. *Blood*, 32:922–934.

92. Cohen, G. (1978): The generation of hydroxyl radicals in biologic systems: toxicological aspects. *Photochem. Photobiol.*, 28:675–699.
93. Cohen, A. B., and Cline, M. J. (1971): The human alveolar macrophage: isolation, cultivation *in vitro*, and studies of morphologic and functional characteristics. *J. Clin. Invest.*, 50:1390–1398.
94. Cohen, H. J., Newburger, P. E., and Chovaniec, M. E. (1980): NAD(P)H-dependent superoxide production by phagocytic vesicles from guinea pig and human granulocytes. *J. Biol. Chem.*, 255:6584–6588.
95. Cohn, Z. A., and Morse, S. I. (1960): Functional and metabolic properties of polymorphonuclear leucocytes. 1. Observations on the requirements and consequences of particle ingestion. *J. Exp. Med.*, 111:667–687.
96. Cohn, G. E., and Tseng, H. Y. (1977): Photodynamic inactivation of yeast sensitized by eosin Y. *Photochem. Photobiol.*, 26:465–474.
97. Cone, R., Hasan, S. K., Lown, J. W., and Morgan, A. R. (1976): The mechanism of the degradation of DNA by streptonigrin. *Can. J. Biochem.*, 54:219–223.
98. Corey, E. J., and Taylor, W. C. (1964): Peroxidation of organic compounds by externally generated singlet oxygen molecules. *J. Am. Chem. Soc.*, 86:3881–3882.
99. Cotran, R. S., and Litt, M. (1969): The entry of granule-associated peroxidase into the phagocytic vacuole of eosinophils. *J. Exp. Med.*, 129:1291–1306.
100. Czapski, G., and Ilan, Y. A. (1978): On the generation of the hydroxylation agent from the superoxide radical. Can the Haber-Weiss reaction be the source of ·OH radicals? *Photochem. Photobiol.*, 28:651–653.
101. Daems, W. Th., and Brederoo, P. (1971): The fine structure and peroxidase activity of resident and exudate peritoneal macrophages in the guinea pig. In: *The Reticuloendothelial System and Immune Phenomena*, edited by N. R. DiLuzio and K. Flemming. pp. 19–31, Plenum Press, New York.
102. Daems, W. Th., and Brederoo, P. (1973): Electron microscopic studies on the structure, phagocytic properties and peroxidatic activity of resident and exudate peritoneal macrophages in the guinea pig. *Z. Zellforsch.*, 144:247–297.
103. Daems, W. Th., and van der Rhee, H. J. (1980): Peroxidase and catalase in monocytes, macrophages, epithelioid cells and giant cells of the rat. In: *Mononuclear Phagocytes. Functional Aspects*, edited by R. van Furth, pp. 43–60. Martinus Nijhoff Publishers, The Hague.
104. Daems, W. Th., Koerten, H. K., and Soranzo, M. R. (1976): Differences between monocyte-derived and tissue macrophages. In: *The Reticuloendothelial System in Health and Disease: Functions and Characteristics*, edited by S. M. Reichard, M. R. Escobar, and H. Friedman, pp. 27–40. Plenum Press, New York.
105. Daems, W. Th., Poelmann, R. E., and Brederoo, P. (1973): Peroxidatic activity in resident peritoneal macrophages and exudate monocytes of the guinea pig after ingestion of latex particles. *J. Histochem. Cytochem.*, 21:93–95.
106. Daems, W. Th., Wisse, E., Brederoo, P., and Emeis, J. J. (1975): Peroxidatic activity in monocytes and macrophages. In: *Mononuclear Phagocytes in Immunity, Infection, and Pathology*, edited by R. van Furth, pp. 57–77. Blackwell Scientific Publications Ltd., Oxford.
107. Danen, W. C., and Arudi, R. L. (1978): Generation of singlet oxygen in the reaction of superoxide anion radical with diacyl peroxides. *J. Am. Chem. Soc.*, 100:3944–3945.
108. Davis, W. C., Huber, H., Douglas, S. D., and Fudenberg, H. H. (1968): A defect in circulating mononuclear phagocytes in chronic granulomatous disease of childhood. *J. Immunol.*, 101:1093–1095.
109. DeChatelet, L. R. (1978): Initiation of the respiratory burst in human polymorphonuclear neutrophils: a critical review. *J. Reticuloendothel. Soc.*, 24:73–91.
110. DeChatelet, L. R., Cooper, M. R., and McCall, C. E. (1972): Stimulation of the hexose monophosphate shunt in human neutrophils by asorbic acid: mechanism of action. *Antimicrob. Agents Chemother.*, 1:12–16.
111. DeChatelet, L. R., Shirley, P. S., McPhail, L. C., Huntley, C. C., Muss, H. B., and Bass, D. A. (1977): Oxidative metabolism of the human eosinophil. *Blood*, 50:525–535.
112. Desser, R. K., Himmelhoch, S. R., Evans, W. H., Januska, M., Mage, M., and Shelton, E. (1972): Guinea pig heterophil and eosinophil peroxidase. *Arch. Biochem. Biophys.*, 148:452–465.
113. Diamond, R. D., and Krzesicki, R. (1978): Mechanisms of attachment of neutrophils to *Candida albicans* pseudohyphae in the absence of serum, and of subsequent damage to pseudohyphae by microbicidal processes of neutrophils *in vitro*. *J. Clin. Invest.*, 61:360–369.

114. Diamond, R. D., Clark, R. A., and Haudenschild, C. C. (1980): Damage to *Candida albicans* hyphae and pseudohyphae by the myeloperoxidase system and oxidative products of neutrophil metabolism *in vitro. J. Clin. Invest.*, 66:908–917.
115. Diamond, R. D., Root, R. K., and Bennett, J. E. (1972): Factors influencing killing of *Cryptococcus neoformans* by human leukocytes *in vitro. J. Infect. Dis.*, 125:367–376.
116. Dogon, I. L., Kerr, A. C., and Amdur, B. H. (1962): Characterization of an antibacterial factor in human parotid secretions, active against *Lactobacillus casei. Arch. Oral Biol.*, 7:81–90.
117. Dorfman, L. M., and Adams, G. E. (1973): *Reactivity of the hydroxyl radical in aqueous solutions.* National Standard Reference Data System, National Bureau of Standards, Number 46, pp. 1–59.
118. Drath, D. B., and Karnovsky, M. L. (1974): Bactericidal activity of metal-mediated peroxide-ascorbate systems. *Infect. Immun.*, 10:1077–1083.
119. Drath, D. B., and Karnovsky, M. L. (1975): Superoxide production by phagocytic leukocytes. *J. Exp. Med.*, 141:257–262.
120. Drath, D. B., Karnovsky, M. L., and Huber, G. L. (1979): Hydroxyl radical formation in phagocytic cells of the rat. *J. Appl. Physiol.*, 46:136–140.
121. Elstner, E. F., Saran, M., Bors, W., and Lengfelder, E. (1978): Oxygen activation in isolated chloroplasts. Mechanism of ferredoxin-dependent ethylene formation from methionine. *Eur. J. Biochem.*, 89:61–66.
122. Ericsson, Y., and Lundbeck, H. (1955): Antimicrobial effect *in vitro* on the ascorbic acid oxidation. 1. Effect on bacteria, fungi and viruses in pure culture. *Acta Pathol. Microbiol. Scand.*, 37:493–506.
123. Fabian, I., and Aronson, M.: (1975): Deamination of histamine by peroxidase of neutrophils and eosinophils. *J. Reticuloendothel. Soc.*, 17:141–145.
124. Fee, J. A., and Valentine, J. S. (1977): Chemical and physical properties of superoxide. In: *Superoxide and Superoxide Dismutases*, edited by A. M. Michelson, J. M. McCord, and I. Fridovich, pp. 19–60. Academic Press, New York.
125. Fenical, W., Kearns, D. R., and Radlick, P. (1969): Mechanism of the reaction of $^1\Delta g$ excited oxygen with olefins. II. Elimination of the concerted "ene" mechanism as the route to allylic hydroperoxides. *J. Am. Chem. Soc.*, 91:7771–7772.
126. Ferradini, C., Foos, J., Houee, C., and Pucheault, J. (1978): The reaction between superoxide anion and hydrogen peroxide. *Photochem. Photobiol.*, 28:697–700.
127. Finazzi Agrò, A., DeSole, P., Rotilio, G., and Mondovi, B. (1973): Influence of catalase and superoxide dismutase on side oxidations involving singlet oxygen. *Ital. J. Biochem.*, 22:217–231.
128. Finazzi Agrò, A., Giovagnoli, C., DeSole, P., Calabrese, L., Rotilio, G., and Mondovi, B. (1972): Erythrocuprein and singlet oxygen. *FEBS Lett.*, 21:183–185.
129. Finkelstein, E., Rosen, G. M., Rauckman, E. J., and Paxton, J. (1979): Spin trapping of superoxide. *Mol. Pharmacol.*, 16:676–685.
130. Finkelstein, E., Rosen, G. M., and Rauckman, E. J. (1980): Spin trapping. Kinetics of the reaction of superoxide and hydroxyl radicals with nitrones. *J. Am. Chem. Soc.*, 102:4994–4999.
131. Finkelstein, E., Rosen, G. M., and Rauckman, E. J. (1980): Spin trapping of superoxide and hydroxyl radical: practical aspects. *Arch. Biochem. Biophys.*, 200:1–16.
132. Fischer, L. J., and Hamburger, S. A. (1980): Inhibition of alloxan action in isolated pancreatic islets by superoxide dismutase, catalase, and a metal chelator. *Diabetes*, 29:213–216.
133. Fong, K.-L., McCay, P. B., Poyer, J. L., Keele, B. B., and Misra, H. (1973): Evidence that peroxidation of lysosomal membranes is initiated by hydroxyl free radicals produced during flavin enzyme activity. *J. Biol. Chem.*, 248:7792–7797.
134. Foote, C. S. (1968): Photosensitized oxygenations and the role of singlet oxygen. *Accounts Chem. Res.*, 1:104–110.
135. Foote, C. S. (1976): Photosensitized oxidation and singlet oxygen: consequences in biological systems. In: *Free Radicals in Biology, Vol. 2*, edited by W. A. Pryor, pp. 85–133, Academic Press, New York.
136. Foote, C. S. (1979): Quenching of singlet oxygen. In: *Singlet Oxygen*, edited by H. H. Wasserman, and R. W. Murray, pp. 139–171, Academic Press, New York.
137. Foote, C. S. (1979): Detection of singlet oxygen in complex systems: a critique: In: *Biochemical and Clinical Aspects of Oxygen*, edited by W. S. Caughey, pp. 603–625, Academic Press, New York.
138. Foote, C. S., and Denny, R. W. (1968): Chemistry of singlet oxygen. VII. Quenching by β-carotene. *J. Am. Chem. Soc.*, 90:6233–6235.

139. Foote, C. S., and Wecksler, S. (1964): Singlet oxygen. A probable intermediate in photosensitized autoxidations. *J. Am. Chem. Soc.*, 86:3880–3881.
140. Foote, C. S., Fujimoto, T. T., and Chang, Y. C. (1972): Chemistry of singlet oxygen. XV. Irrelevance of azide trapping to mechanism of the ene reaction. *Tetrahedron Lett.*, 1:45–48.
141. Foote, C. S., Shook, F. C., and Abakerli, R. A. (1980): Chemistry of superoxide anion. 4. Singlet oxygen is not a major product of dismutation. *J. Am. Chem. Soc.*, 102:2503–2504.
142. Fridovich, I. (1970): Quantitative aspects of the production of superoxide anion radical by milk xanthine oxidase. *J. Biol. Chem.*, 245:4053–4057.
143. Fridovich, I. (1975): Superoxide dismutases. *Ann. Rev. Biochem.*, 44:147–159.
144. Fridovich, I. (1976): Oxygen radicals, hydrogen peroxide, and oxygen toxicity. In: *Free Radicals in Biology, Vol. 1*, edited by W. A. Pryor, pp. 239–277, Academic Press, New York.
145. Fridovich, I. (1978): Superoxide radicals, superoxide dismutase and the aerobic lifestyle. *Photochem. Photobiol.*, 28:733–741.
146. Gabig, T. G.. and Babior, B. M. (1979): The O_2-forming oxidase responsible for the respiratory burst in human neutrophils. Properties of the solubilized enzyme. *J. Biol. Chem.*, 254:9070–9074.
147. Gabig, T. G., Kipnes, R. S., and Babior, B. M. (1978): Solubilization of the O_2^--forming activity responsible for the respiratory burst in human neutrophils. *J. Biol. Chem.*, 253:6663–6665.
148. Gee, J. B. L., Kaskin, J., Duncombe, M. P., and Vassallo, C. L. (1974): The effects of ethanol on some metabolic features of phagocytosis in the alveolar macrophage. *J. Reticuloendothel. Soc.*, 15:61–68.
149. Gee, J. B. L., Vassallo, C. L., Bell, P., Kaskin, J., Basford, R. E., and Field, J. B. (1970): Catalase-dependent peroxidative metabolism in the alveolar macrophage during phagocytosis. *J. Clin. Invest.*, 49:1280–1287.
150. Gibian, M. J., and Ungermann, T. (1979): The unlikelihood of an electron-transfer (Haber-Weiss) reaction between superoxide and peroxides. *J. Am. Chem. Soc.*, 101:1291–1293.
151. Gilbert, B. C., Norman, R. O. C., and Sealy, R. C. (1975): Electron spin resonance studies. Part XLIII. Reaction of dimethyl sulfoxide with hydroxyl radicals. *J. Chem. Soc.* (Perkin Trans. II),:303–308.
152. Goda, K., Chu, J. -W., Kimura, T., and Schaap, A. P. (1973): Cytochrome C enhancement of singlet molecular oxygen production by the NADPH-dependent adrenodoxin reductase-adrenodoxin system: the role of singlet oxygen in damaging adrenal mitochondrial membranes. *Biochem. Biophys. Res. Commun.*, 52:1300–1306.
153. Goda, K.. Kimura, T., Thayer, A. L., Kees, K., and Schaap, A. P. (1974): Singlet molecular oxygen in biological systems: non-quenching of singlet oxygen-mediated chemiluminescence by superoxide dismutase. *Biochem. Biophys. Res. Commun.*, 58:660–666.
154. Goldstein. I. M., Cerqueira, M., Lind, S., and Kaplan, H. B. (1977): Evidence that the superoxide-generating system of human leukocytes is associated with the cell surface. *J. Clin. Invest.*, 59:249–254.
155. Gollnick, K. (1975): Chemical aspects of photodynamic action in the presence of molecular oxygen. In: *Radiation Research: Biomedical, Chemical and Physical Perspectives*, edited by O. F. Nygaard, H. I. Adler, and W. K. Sinclair, pp. 590–611. Academic Press, New York.
156. Gorman, A. A., and Rodgers, M. A. J. (1978): Lifetime and reactivity of singlet oxygen in an aqueous micellar system: a pulsed nitrogen laser study. *Chem. Phys. Lett.*, 55:52–54.
157. Green, D. E., and Pauli, R. (1943): The anti-bacterial action of the xanthine oxidase system. *Proc. Soc. Exp. Biol. Med.*, 54:148–150.
158. Green, M. R., Hill, H. A. O., Okolow-Zubkowska, M. J., and Segal, A. W. (1979): The production of hydroxyl and superoxide radicals by stimulated human neutrophils. Measurements by EPR spectroscopy. *FEBS Lett.*, 100:23–26.
159. Green, T. R., Schaefer, R. E., and Makler, M. T. (1980): Significance of O_2 availability and cycling on the respiratory burst response of human PMNs exposed to cytochrome C and superoxide dismutase. *Biochem. Biophys. Res. Commun.*, 94:1213–1220.
160. Greenlee, L., Fridovich, I., and Handler, P. (1962): Chemiluminescence induced by operation of iron-flavoproteins. *Biochemistry*, 1:779–783.
161. Greenwald, R. A., and Moy, W. W. (1979): Inhibition of collagen gelation by action of the superoxide radical. *Arthritis Rheum.*, 22:251–259.
162. Greenwald, R. A., and Moy, W. W. (1980): Effect of oxygen-derived free radicals on hyaluronic acid. *Arthritis Rheum.*, 23:455–463.
163. Gregory, E. M., and Fridovich, I. (1973): Induction of superoxide dismutase by molecular oxygen. *J. Bacteriol.*, 114:543–548.

164. Gregory, E. M., and Fridovich, I. (1973): Oxygen toxicity and the superoxide dismutase. *J. Bacteriol.*, 114:1193–1197.
165. Gregory, E. M., and Fridovich, I. (1974): Oxygen metabolism in *Lactobacillus plantarum*. *J. Bacteriol.*, 117:166–169.
166. Gregory, E. M., Moore, W. E. C., and Holdeman, L. V. (1978): Superoxide dismutase in anaerobes: survey. *Appl. Environment. Microbiol.*, 35:988–991.
167. Gregory, E. M., Yost, F. J., Jr., and Fridovich, I. (1973): Superoxide dismutases of *Escherichia coli*. Intracellular localization and functions. *J. Bacteriol.*, 115:987–991.
168. Grignaschi, V. J., Sperperato, A. M., Etcheverry, M. J., and Macario, A. J. L. (1963): Un nuevo cuadro citoquimico: negatividad expontanea de las reacciones de peroxidasas, oxidasas y lipido en la progenie neutrofila y en los monocitos de dos hermanos. *Rev. Asoc. Méd. Argent.* 77:218–221.
169. Guiraud, H. J., and Foote, C. S. (1976): Chemistry of superoxide anion. III. Quenching of singlet oxygen. *J. Am. Chem. Soc.*, 98:1984–1986.
170. Gutteridge, J. M. C., Richmond, R., and Halliwell, B. (1979): Inhibition of the iron-catalyzed formation of hydroxyl radicals from superoxide and of lipid peroxidation by desferrioxamine. *Biochem. J.*, 184:469–472.
171. Haber, F., and Weiss, J. (1934): The catalytic decomposition of hydrogen peroxide by iron salts. *Proc. R. Soc. London [A]*, 147:332–351.
172. Hafeman, D. G., and Lucas, J. J. (1979): Polymorphonuclear leukocyte-mediated, antibody-dependent, cellular cytotoxicity against tumor cells: dependence on oxygen and the respiratory burst. *J. Immunol.*, 123:55–62.
173. Halliwell, B. (1976): An attempt to demonstrate a reaction between superoxide and hydrogen peroxide. *FEBS Lett.*, 72:8–10.
174. Halliwell, B. (1977): Hydroxylation of aromatic compounds by reduced nicotinamide-adenine dinucleotide and phenazine methosulphate requires hydrogen peroxide and hydroxyl radicals, but not superoxide. *Biochem. J.*, 167:317–320.
175. Halliwell, B. (1978): Superoxide-dependent formation of hydroxyl radicals in the presence of iron chelates: is it a mechanism for hydroxyl radical production in biochemical systems? *FEBS Lett.*, 92:321–326.
176. Halliwell, B. (1978): Superoxide-dependent formation of hydroxyl radicals in the presence of iron salts. Its role in degradation of hyaluronic acid by a superoxide-generating system. *FEBS Lett.*, 96:238–242.
177. Hamon, C. B., and Klebanoff, S. J. (1973): A peroxidase-mediated, *Streptococcus mitis*-dependent antimicrobial system in saliva. *J. Exp. Med.*, 137:438–450.
178. Harbour, J. R., Chow, V., and Bolton, J. R. (1974): An electron spin resonance study of the spin adducts of OH and HO_2 radicals with nitrones in the ultraviolet photolysis of aqueous hydrogen peroxide solutions. *Can. J. Chem.*, 52:3549–3553.
179. Harrison, J. E., and Schultz, J. (1976): Studies on the chlorinating activity of myeloperoxidase. *J. Biol. Chem.*, 251:1371–1374.
180. Harrison, J. E., Watson, B. D., and Schultz, J. (1978): Myeloperoxidase and singlet oxygen: a reappraisal. *FEBS Lett.*, 92:327–332.
181. Hassain, M. Z., and Bhatnagar, R. S. (1979): Involvement of superoxide in the paraquat-induced enhancement of lung collagen synthesis in organ culture. *Biochem. Biophys. Res. Commun.*, 89:71–76.
182. Hassan, H. M., and Fridovich, I. (1978): Superoxide radical and the oxygen enhancement of the toxicity of paraquat in *Escherichia coli*. *J. Biol. Chem.*, 253:8143–8148.
183. Hassan, H. M., and Fridovich, I. (1979): Paraquat and *Escherichia coli*. Mechanism of production of extracellular superoxide radical. *J. Biol. Chem.*, 254:10846–10852.
184. Hasty, N., Merkel, P. B., Radlick, P., and Kearns, D. R. (1972): Role of azide in singlet oxygen reactions: reaction of azide with singlet oxygen. *Tetrahedron Lett.*, 1:49–52.
185. Hatch, G. E., Gardner, D. E., and Menzel, D. B. (1978): Chemiluminescence of phagocytic cells caused by *N*-formylmethionyl peptides. *J. Exp. Med.*, 147:182–195.
186. Hattori, H. (1961): Studies on the labile, stable Nadi oxidase and peroxidase staining reactions in the isolated particles of horse granulocyte. *Nagoya J. Med. Sci.*, 23:362–378.
187. Heifets, L., Imai, K., and Goren, M. B. (1980): Expression of peroxidase-dependent iodination by macrophages ingesting neutrophil debris. *J. Reticuloendothel. Soc.*, 28:391–404.
188. Held, A. M., and Hurst, J. K. (1978): Ambiguity associated with use of singlet oxygen trapping agents in myeloperoxidase-catalyzed oxidations. *Biochim. Biophys. Res. Commun.*, 81:878–885.

189. Henderson, W. R., and Kaliner, M. (1978): Immunologic and nonimmunologic generation of superoxide from mast cells and basophils. *J. Clin. Invest.*, 61:187–196.
190. Henderson, W. R., and Kaliner, M. (1979): Mast cell granule peroxidase: location, secretion and SRS-A inactivation. *J. Immunol.*, 122:1322–1328.
191. Henderson, W. R., Chi, E. Y., and Klebanoff, S. J. (1980): Eosinophil peroxidase-induced mast cell secretion. *J. Exp. Med.*, 152:265–279.
192. Henderson, W. R., Chi, E. Y., Jong, E.C., and Klebanoff, S. J. (1981): Mast cell mediated tumor cell cytotoxicity: role of the peroxidase system. *J. Exp. Med.*, 153:520–533.
193. Henderson, W. R., Jong, E. C., and Klebanoff, S. J. (1980): Binding of eosinophil peroxidase to mast cell granules with retention of peroxidatic activity. *J. Immunol.*, 124:1383–1388.
194. Hewitt, J., and Morris, J. G. (1975): Superoxide dismutase in some obligately anaerobic bacteria. *FEBS Lett.*, 50:315–318.
195. Hodgson, E. K., and Fridovich, I. (1974): The production of superoxide radical during the decomposition of potassium peroxochromate (V). *Biochemistry*, 13:3811–3815.
196. Hodgson, E. K., and Fridovich, I. (1976): The mechanism of the activity-dependent luminescence of xanthine oxidase. *Arch. Biochem. Biophys.*, 172:202–205.
197. Holmes, B., Page, A. R., and Good, R. A. (1967): Studies of the metabolic activity of leukocytes from patients with a genetic abnormality of phagocytic function. *J. Clin. Invest.*, 46:1422–1432.
198. Holmes, B., Page, A. R., Windhorst, D. B., Quie, P. G., White, J. G., and Good, R. A. (1968): The metabolic pattern and phagocytic function of leukocytes from children with chronic granulomatous disease. *Ann. N.Y. Acad. Sci.*, 155:888–901.
199. Holmes, B., Quie, P. G., Windhorst, D. B., and Good, R. A. (1966): Fatal granulomatous disease of childhood. An inborn abnormality of phagocytic function. *Lancet*, 1:1225–1228.
200. Hoogendoorn, H., Piessens, J. P., Scholtes, W., and Stoddard, L. A. (1977): Hypothiocyanite ion: the inhibitor formed by the system lactoperoxidase-thiocyanate-hydrogen peroxide. 1. Identification of the inhibiting compound. *Caries Res.*, 11:77–84.
201. Howard. D. H. (1973): Fate of *Histoplasma capsulatum* in guinea pig polymorphonuclear leukocytes. *Infect. Immun.*, 8:412–419.
202. Ismail, G., Sawyer, W. D., and Wegener, W. S. (1977): Effect of hydrogen peroxide and superoxide radical on viability of *Neisseria gonorrhoeae* and related bacteria. *Proc. Soc. Exp. Biol. Med.*, 155:264–269.
203. Ito, T. (1977): Toluidine blue: the mode of photodynamic action in yeast cells. *Photochem. Photobiol.*, 25:47–53.
204. Ito, T. (1978): Cellular and subcellular mechanisms of photodynamic action: the $^1O_2$ hypothesis as a driving force in recent research. *Photochem. Photobiol.*, 28:493–508.
205. Iyer, G. Y. N., Islam, D. M. F., and Quastel, J. H. (1961): Biochemical aspects of phagocytosis. *Nature (London)*, 192:535–541.
206. Jacobs, A. A., Low, I. E., Paul, B. B., Strauss, R. R., and Sbarra, A. J. (1972): Mycoplasmacidal activity of peroxidase-H_2O_2-halide systems. *Infect. Immun.*, 5:127–131.
207. Jago, G. R., and Morrison, M. (1962): Antistreptococcal activity of lactoperoxidase III. *Proc. Soc. Exp. Biol. Med.*, 111:585–588.
208. Jandl, R. C., André-Schwartz, J., Borges-Dubois, L., Kipnes, R. S., McMurrich, B. J., and Babior, B. M. (1978): Termination of the respiratory burst in human neutrophils. *J. Clin. Invest.*, 61:1176–1177.
209. Janzen, E. G. (1980): A critical review of spin trapping in biological systems. In: *Free Radicals in Biology*, Vol. 4, edited by W. A. Pryor, pp. 115–154. Academic Press, New York.
210. Janzen, E. G., Nutter, D. E., Jr., Davis, E. R., Blackburn, B. J., Poyer, J. L., and McCay, P. B. (1978): On spin trapping hydroxyl and hydroperoxyl radicals. *Can. J. Chem.*, 56:2237–2242.
211. Jensen, M. S., and Bainton, D. F. (1973): Temporal changes in pH within the phagocytic vacuole of the polymorphonuclear neutrophilic leukocyte. *J. Cell Biol.*, 56:379–388.
212. Johnson, D., and Travis, J. (1978): Structural evidence for methionine at the active site of human α-1-proteinase inhibitor. *J. Biol. Chem.*, 253:7142–7144.
213. Johnson, D., and Travis, J. (1979): The oxidative inactivation of human α-1-proteinase inhibitor. Further evidence for methionine at the reactive center. *J. Biol. Chem.*, 254:4022–4026.
214. Johnston, R. B., Jr., and Baehner, R. L. (1970): Improvement of leukocyte bactericidal activity in chronic granulomatous disease. *Blood*, 35:350–355.
215. Johnston, R. B., Jr., Chadwick, D. A., and Pabst, M. J. (1980): Release of superoxide anion by macrophages: effect of *in vivo* and *in vitro* priming. In: *Mononuclear Phagocytes. Functional Aspects*, edited by R. van Furth, pp. 1143–1158. Martinus Nijhoff Publishers, The Hague.

216. Johnston, R. B., Jr., Godzik, C. A., and Cohn, Z. A. (1978): Increased superoxide production by immunologically activated and chemically elicited macrophages. *J. Exp. Med.*, 148:115–127.
217. Johnston, R. B., Jr., Keele, B. B., Jr., Misra, H. P., Lehmeyer, J. E., Webb, L. S., Baehner, R. L., and Rajagopalan, K. V. (1975): The role of superoxide anion generation in phagocytic bactericidal activity. Studies with normal and chronic granulomatous disease leukocytes. *J. Clin. Invest.*, 55:1357–1372.
218. Johnston, R. B., Jr., Lehmeyer, J. E., and Guthrie, L. A. (1976): Generation of superoxide anion and chemiluminescence by human monocytes during phagocytosis and on contact with surface-bound immunoglobulin G. *J. Exp. Med.*, 143:1551–1556.
219. Jong, E. C., and Klebanoff, S. J. (1980): Eosinophil-mediated mammalian tumor cell cytotoxicity: role of the peroxidase system. *J. Immunol.*, 124:1949–1953.
220. Jong, E. C., Henderson, W. R., and Klebanoff, S. J. (1980): Bactericidal activity of eosinophil peroxidase. *J. Immunol.*, 124:1378–1382.
221. Jong, E. C., Mahmoud, A. A. F., and Klebanoff, S. J. (1981): Peroxidase-mediated toxicity to schistosomula of *Schistosoma mansoni*. *J. Immunol.*, 126:468–471.
222. Kajiwara, T., and Kearns, D. R. (1973): Direct spectroscopic evidence for a deuterium solvent effect on the lifetime of singlet oxygen in water. *J. Am. Chem. Soc.*, 95:5886–5890.
223. Karnovsky, M. L. (1973): Chronic granulomatous disease—pieces of a cellular and molecular puzzle. *Fed. Proc.*, 32:1527–1533.
224. Karnovsky, M. L. (1975): Biochemical aspects of the functions of polymorphonuclear and mononuclear leukocytes. In: *The Phagocytic Cell in Host Resistance*, edited by J. A. Bellanti and D. H. Dayton, pp. 25–43. Raven Press, New York.
225. Kasha, M., and Brabham, D. E. (1979): Singlet oxygen electronic structure and photosensitization. In: *Singlet Oxygen*, edited by H. H. Wasserman and R. W. Murray, pp. 1–33. Academic Press, New York.
226. Kasha, M., and Khan, A. U. (1970): The physics, chemistry and biology of singlet molecular oxygen. *Ann. N.Y. Acad. Sci.*, 171:5–23.
227. Katz, P., Simone, C. B., Henkart, P. A., and Fauci, A. S. (1980): Mechanisms of antibody-dependent cellular cytotoxicity. The use of effector cells from chronic granulomatous disease patients as investigative probes. *J.Clin. Invest.*, 65:55–63.
228. Kautsky, H. (1937): Die Wechselwirkung zwischen Sensibilisatoren und Sauerstoff im Licht. *Biochem. Z.*, 291:271–284.
229. Kearns, D. R. (1971): Physical and chemical properties of singlet molecular oxygen. *Chem. Rev.*, 71:395–427.
230. Kearns, D. R. (1979): Solvent and solvent isotope effects on the lifetime of singlet oxygen. In: *Singlet Oxygen*, edited by H. H. Wasserman and R. W. Murray, pp. 115–137. Academic Press, New York.
231. Kearns, D. R., Fenical, W., and Radlick, P. (1970): Experimental and quantum chemical investigation of singlet oxygen reactions. *Ann. N.Y. Acad. Med.*, 171:34–48.
232. Kellogg, E. W., III, and Fridovich, I. (1975): Superoxide, hydrogen peroxide, and singlet oxygen in lipid peroxidation by a xanthine oxidase system. *J. Biol. Chem.*, 250:8812–8817.
233. Kellogg, E. W., III, and Fridovich, I. (1977): Liposome oxidation and erythrocyte lysis by enzymically generated superoxide and hydrogen peroxide. *J. Biol. Chem.*, 252:6721–6728.
234. Kellogg, E. W., III, Yost, M. G., Barthakur, N., and Kreuger, A. P. (1979): Superoxide involvement in the bactericidal effects of negative air ions on *Staphylococcus albus*. *Nature (London)*, 281:400–401.
235. Khan, A. U. (1970): Singlet molecular oxygen from superoxide anion and sensitized fluorescence of organic molecules. *Science*, 168:476–477.
236. Khan, A. U. (1976): Singlet molecular oxygen. A new kind of oxygen. *J. Phys. Chem.*, 80:2219–2228.
237. Khan, A. U. (1977): Theory of electron transfer generation and quenching of singlet oxygen [$^1\Sigma_g^+$ and $^1\Delta g$] by superoxide anion. The role of water in the dismutation of O_2. *J. Am. Chem. Soc.*, 99:370–371.
238. Khan, A. U. (1978): Activated oxygen: singlet molecular oxygen and superoxide anion. *Photochem. Photobiol.*, 28:615–627.
239. Khan, A. U., and Kasha, M. (1963): Red chemiluminescence of molecular oxygen in aqueous solution. *J. Chem. Phys.*, 39:2105–2106.
240. Khan, A. U., and Kasha, M. (1979): Direct spectroscopic observation of singlet oxygen emission at 1268 nm excited by sensitizing dyes of biological interest in liquid solution. *Proc. Natl. Acad. Sci. U.S.A.*, 76:6047–6049.

241. Klebanoff, S. J. (1967): Iodination of bacteria: a bactericidal mechanism. *J. Exp. Med.*, 126:1063–1078.
242. Klebanoff, S. J. (1968): Myeloperoxidase-halide-hydrogen peroxide antibacterial system. *J. Bacteriol.*, 95:2131–2138.
243. Klebanoff, S. J. (1969): Antimicrobial activity of catalase at acid pH. *Proc. Soc. Exp. Biol. Med.*, 132:571–574.
244. Klebanoff, S. J. (1970): Myeloperoxidase-mediated antimicrobial systems and their role in leukocyte function. In: *Biochemistry of the Phagocytic Process*, edited by J. Schultz, pp. 89–110. North-Holland Publ. Co., Amsterdam.
245. Klebanoff, S. J. (1970): Myeloperoxidase: contribution to the microbicidal activity of intact leukocytes. *Science*, 169:1095–1097.
246. Klebanoff, S. J. (1975): Antimicrobial mechanisms in neutrophilic polymorphonuclear leukocytes. *Semin. Hematol.*, 12:117–142.
247. Klebanoff, S. J. (1975): Antimicrobial systems of the polymorphonuclear leukocyte. In: *The Phagocytic Cell in Host Resistance*, edited by J. A. Bellanti and D. H. Dayton, pp. 45–56. Raven Press, New York.
248. Klebanoff, S. J. (1979): Effect of estrogens on the myeloperoxidase-mediated antimicrobial system. *Infect. Immun.*, 25:153–156.
249. Klebanoff, S. J. (1980): Oxygen intermediates and the microbicidal event. In: *Mononuclear Phagocytes. Functional Aspects*, edited by R. van Furth, pp. 1105–1137. Martinus Nijhoff Publishers, The Hague.
250. Klebanoff, S. J. (1980): Myeloperoxidase-mediated cytotoxic systems. In: *The Reticuloendothelial System, Volume 2, Biochemistry and Metabolism*, edited by A. J. Sbarra and R. R. Strauss, pp. 279–308. Plenum Press, New York.
251. Klebanoff, S. J., and Clark, R. A. (1975): Hemolysis and iodination of erythrocyte components by a myeloperoxidase-mediated system. *Blood*, 45:699–707.
252. Klebanoff, S. J., and Clark, R. A. (1977): Iodination by human polymorphonuclear leukocytes: a re-evaluation. *J. Lab. Clin. Med.*, 89:675–686.
253. Klebanoff, S. J., and Clark, R. A. (1978): *The Neutrophil: Function and Clinical Disorders.* North-Holland Publishing Co., Amsterdam.
254. Klebanoff, S. J., and Green, W. L. (1973): Degradation of thyroid hormones by phagocytosing human leukocytes. *J. Clin. Invest.*, 52:60–72.
255. Klebanoff, S. J., and Hamon, C. B. (1972): Role of myeloperoxidase-mediated antimicrobial systems in intact leukocytes. *J. Reticuloendothel. Soc.*, 12:170–196.
256. Klebanoff, S. J., and Hamon, C. B. (1975): Antimicrobial systems of mononuclear phagocytes. In: *Mononuclear Phagocytes in Immunity, Infection and Pathology*, pp. 507:531. Blackwell Scientific Publications, Oxford.
257. Klebanoff, S. J., and Luebke, R. G. (1965): The antilactobacillus system of saliva. Role of salivary peroxidase. *Proc. Soc. Exp. Biol. Med.*, 118:483–486.
258. Klebanoff, S. J., and Pincus, S. H. (1971): Hydrogen peroxide utilization in myeloperoxidase-deficient leukocytes: a possible microbicidal control mechanism. *J. Clin. Invest.*, 50:2226–2229.
259. Klebanoff, S. J., and Rosen, H. (1978): Ethylene formation by polymorphonuclear leukocytes. Role of myeloperoxidase. *J. Exp. Med.*, 148:490–506.
260. Klebanoff, S. J., and Smith, D. C. (1970): The source of H_2O_2 for the uterine fluid-mediated sperm-inhibitory system. *Biol. Reprod.*, 3:236–242.
261. Klebanoff, S. J., and White, L. R. (1969): Iodination defect in the leukocytes of a patient with chronic granulomatous disease of children. *N. Engl. J. Med.*, 280:460–466.
262. Klebanoff, S. J., Clem, W. H., and Luebke, R. G. (1966): The peroxidase-thiocyanate-hydrogen peroxide antimicrobial system. *Biochim. Biophys. Acta*, 117:63–72.
263. Klebanoff, S. J., Durack, D. T., Rosen, H., and Clark, R. A. (1977): Functional studies on human peritoneal eosinophils. *Infect. Immun.*, 17:167–173.
264. Klein, S. M., Cohen, G., and Cederbaum, A. I. (1980): The interaction of hydroxyl radicals with dimethylsulfoxide produces formaldehyde. *FEBS Lett.*, 116:220–222.
265. Knowles, A. (1975): The effects of photodynamic action involving oxygen upon biological systems. In: *Radiation Research: Biomedical, Chemical and Physical Perspectives*, edited by O. F. Nygaard, H. I. Adler, and W. K. Sinclair, pp. 612–622. Academic Press, New York.
266. Kobayashi, K. (1978): Effect of sodium azide on photodynamic induction of genetic changes in yeast. *Photochem. Photobiol.*, 28:535–538.

267. Kobayashi, S., and Ando, W. (1979): Co-oxidations of 1,3-diphenylisobenzofuran by the Haber-Weiss reaction. Is singlet oxygen concerned in this oxidation. *Biochem. Biophys, Res. Commun.*, 88:676–681.

268. Kobayashi, K., and Ito, T., (1976): Further *in vivo* studies on the participation of singlet oxygen in the photodynamic inactivation and induction of genetic changes in *Saccharomyces cerevisiae*. *Photochem. Photobiol.*, 23:21–28.

269. Koppenol, W. H. (1976): Reactions involving singlet oxygen and the superoxide anion. *Nature (London)*, 262:420–421.

270. Koppenol, W. H., and Butler, J. (1977): Mechanism of reactions involving singlet oxygen and the superoxide anion. *FEBS Lett.*, 83:1–6.

271. Koppenol, W. H., Butler, J., and van Leeuwen, J. W. (1978): The Haber-Weiss cycle. *Photochem. Photobiol.*, 28:655–660.

272. Krinsky, N. I. (1974): Singlet excited oxygen as a mediator of the antibacterial action of leukocytes. *Science*, 186:363–365.

273. Krinsky, N. I. (1979): Biological roles of singlet oxyten. In: *Singlet Oxygen*, edited by H. H. Wasserman and R. W. Murray, pp. 597–641. Academic Press, New York.

274. Kulig, M. J., and Smith, L. L. (1973): Sterol metabolism. XXV. Cholesterol oxidation by singlet molecular oxygen. *J. Org. Chem.*, 38:3639–3642.

275. Lee, D. C. -S., and Wilson, T. (1973): Oxygen in chemiluminescence. A competitive pathway of dioxetane decomposition catalyzed by electron donors. In: *Chemiluminescence and Bioluminescence*, edited by M. J. Cormier, D. M. Hercules, and J. Lee, pp. 265–283. Plenum Press, New York.

276. Lee-Ruff, E. (1977): The organic chemistry of superoxide. *Chem. Soc. Rev.*, 6:195–214.

277. Lehrer, R. I. (1969): Antifungal effects of peroxidase systems. *J. Bacteriol.* 99:361–365.

278. Lehrer, R. I. (1971): Measurement of candidacidal activity of specific leukocyte types in mixed cell populations. II. Normal and chronic granulomatous disease eosinophils. *Infect. Immun.*,3:800–802.

279. Lehrer, R. I. (1972): Functional aspects of a second mechanism of candidacidal activity by human neutrophils. *J. Clin. Invest.*, 51:2566–2572.

280. Lehrer, R. I. (1975): Fungicidal mechanism of human monocytes. 1. Evidence for myeloperoxidase-linked and myeloperoxidase-independent candidacidal mechanism. *J. Clin. Invest.*, 55:338–346.

281. Lehrer, R. I., and Cline, M. J. (1969): Leukocyte myeloperoxidase deficiency and disseminated candidiasis: the role of myeloperoxidase in resistance to *Candida* infection. *J. Clin. Invest.*, 48:1478–1488.

282. Lehrer, R. I., and Cline, M. J. (1969): Interaction of *Candida albicans* with human leukocytes and serum. *J. Bacteriol.*, 98:996–1004.

283. Lehrer, R. I., and Jan, R. G. (1970): Interaction of *Aspergillus fumigatus* spores with human leukocytes and serum. *Infect. Immun.*, 1:345–350.

284. Lehrer, R. I., Hanifin, J., and Cline, M. J. (1969): Defective bactericidal activity in myeloperoxidase-deficient human neutrophils. *Nature (London)*, 223:78–79.

285. Lemarbre, P., Hoidal, J., Vesella, R., and Rinehart, J. (1980): Human pulmonary macrophage tumor cell cytotoxicity. *Blood*, 55:612–617.

286. Lesko, S. A., Lorentzen, R. J., and Ts'o, P.O.P. (1980). Role of superoxide in deoxyribonucleic acid strand scission. *Biochemistry*, 19:3023–3028.

287. Lindig, B A., and Rodgers, M. A. J. (1979): Laser photolysis studies of singlet molecular oxygen in aqueous micellar dispersions. *J. Phys. Chem.*, 83:1683–1688.

288. Lindig, B A., Rodgers, M. A. J., and Schaap, A. P. (1980): Determination of the lifetime of singlet oxygen in D_2O using 9,10-anthracenedipropionic acid, a water soluble probe. *J. Am. Chem. Soc.*, 102: 5590–5593.

289. Lipmann, F., and Owen, C. R. (1943): The anti-bacterial effect of enzymatic xanthine oxidation. *Science*, 98:246–248.

290. Litchfield, W. J., and Wells, W. W. (1978): Effect of galactose on free radical reactions of polymorphonuclear leukocytes. *Arch. Biochem. Biophys.*, 188:26–30.

291. Long, C. A., and Kearns, D. R. (1975): Radiationless decay of singlet molecular oxygen in solution. II. Temperature dependence and solvent effects. *J. Am. Chem Soc.*, 97:2018–2020.

292. Lown, J. W., Begleitter, A., Johnson, D., and Morgan, J. R. (1976): Studies related to antitumor antibiotics. Part V. Reactions of mitomycin C with DNA examined by ethidium fluorescence assay. *Can. J. Biochem.*, 54:110–119.

293. Lynch, R. E., and Fridovich, I. (1978): Effects of superoxide on the erythrocyte membrane. *J. Biol. Chem.*, 253:1838–1845.

294. Lynch, R. E., and Fridovich, I. (1978): Permeation of the erythrocyte stroma by superoxide radical. *J. Biol. Chem.*, 253:4697–4699.

295. Mandell, G. L. (1974): Bactericidal activity of aerobic and anaerobic polymorphonuclear neutrophils. *Infect. Immun.*, 9:337–341.

296. Mandell, G. L. (1975): Catalase, superoxide dismutase, and virulence of *Staphylococcus aureus*. *In vitro* and *in vivo* studies with emphasis on staphylococcal-leukocyte interaction. *J. Clin. Invest.*, 55:561–566.

297. Mandell, G. L., and Hook, E. W. (1969): Leukocyte bactericidal activity in chronic granulomatous disease: correlation of bacterial hydrogen peroxide production and susceptibility to intracellular killing. *J. Bacteriol.*, 100:531–532.

298. Massey, V., Strickland, S., Mayhew, S. G., Howell, L. G., Engel, P. C., Matthews, R. G., Schuman, M., and Sullivan, P. A. (1969): The production of superoxide anion radicals in the reaction of reduced flavins and flavoproteins with molecular oxygen. *Biochem. Biophys. Res. Comun.*, 36:891–897.

299. Matheson, I. B. C., Lee, J., and King. A. D. (1978): The lifetime of singlet oxygen ($^1\Delta g$) in heavy water, a revised value. *Chem. Phys. Lett.*, 55:49–51.

300. Matheson, N. R., Wong, P. S., and Travis, J. (1979): Enzymatic inactivation of human alpha-1-proteinase inhibitor by neutrophil myeloperoxidase. *Biochem. Biophys. Res. Commun.*, 88:402–409.

301. Mathews-Roth, M. M., and Krinsky, N. I. (1970): Studies on the protective function of the carotenoid pigments of *Sarcina lutea*. *Photochem. Photobiol.*, 11:419–428.

302. Mathews-Roth, M. M., Wilson, T., Fujimori, E., and Krinsky, N. I. (1974): Carotenoid chromophore length and protection against photosensitization. *Photochem. Photobiol.*, 19:217–222.

303. Mayeda, E. A., and Bard, A. J. (1974): Singlet oxygen. The suppression of its production in dismutation of superoxide ion by superoxide dismutase. *J. Am. Chem. Soc.*, 96:4023–4024.

304. McCapra, F., and Hann, R. A. (1969): The chemiluminescent reaction of singlet oxygen with 10,10'-dimethyl-9,9'-biacridylidene. *Chem. Commun.*, 442–443.

305. McCay, P. B., Noguchi, T., Fong, K.-L., Lai, E. K., and Poyer, J. L. (1980): Production of radicals from enzyme systems and the use of spin traps. In: *Free Radicals in Biology, Vol. 4*, edited by W. A. Pryor, pp. 155–186. Academic Press, New York.

306. McClune, G. J., and Fee, J. A. (1976): Stopped flow spectrophotometric observation of superoxide dismutation in aqueous solution. *FEBS Lett.*, 67:294–298.

307. McCord, J. M. (1974): Free radicals and inflammation: protection of synovial fluid by superoxide dismutase. *Science*, 185:529–531.

308. McCord, J. M., and Day, E. D., Jr. (1978): Superoxide-dependent production of hydroxyl radical catalyzed by iron-EDTA complex. *FEBS Lett.*, 86:139–142.

309. McCord, J. M., and Fridovich, I. (1969): Superoxide dismutase. An enzymic function for erythrocuprein (hemocuprein). *J. Biol. Chem.*, 244:6049–6055.

310. McCord, J. M., Keele, B. B., Jr., and Fridovich, I. (1971): An enzyme-based theory of obligate anaerobiosis: the physiological function of superoxide dismutase. *Proc. Natl. Acad. Sci. U.S.A.*, 68:1024–1027.

311. McKeown, E., and Waters, W. A. (1966): The oxidation of organic compounds by "singlet" oxygen. *J. Chem. Soc. B.*, 1040–1046.

312. McLaren, D. J., Mackenzie, C. D., and Ramalho-Pinto, F. J. (1977). Ultrastructural observations on the *in vitro* interaction between rat eosinophils and some parasitic helminths (*Schistosoma mansoni, Trichinella spiralis* and *Nippostrongylus brasiliensis*). *Clin. Exp. Immunol.*, 30:105–118.

313. McLaren, D. J., Ramalho-Pinto, F. J., and Smithers, S. R. (1978): Ultrastructural evidence for complement and antibody-dependent damage to schistosomula of *Schistosoma mansoni* by rat eosinophils *in vitro*. *Parasitology*, 77:313–324.

314. McLennan, G., Oberley, L. W., and Autor, A. P. (1980): The role of oxygen-derived free radicals in radiation induced damage and death of nondividing eucaryotic cells. *Radiat. Res.*, 84:122–132.

315. McRipley, R. J., and Sbarra, A. J. (1967): Role of the phagocyte in host-parasite interactions. XI. Relationship between stimulated oxidative metabolism and hydrogen peroxide formation, and intracellular killing. *J. Bacteriol.*, 94:1417–1424.

316. McRipley, R. J., and Sbarra, A. J. (1967): Role of the phagocyte in host-parasite interactions. XII. Hydrogen peroxide-myeloperoxidase bactericidal system in the phagocyte. *J. Bacteriol.*, 94:1425–1430.

317. Melhuish, W. H., and Sutton, H. C. (1978): Studies of the Haber-Weiss reaction using a sensitive method for detection of OH radicals. *J. Chem. Soc. Chem. Commun.*, 22:970–971.
318. Merkel, P. B., and Kearns, D. R. (1972): Remarkable solvent effects on the lifetime of $^1\Delta g$ oxygen. *J. Am. Chem. Soc.*, 94:1029–1030.
319. Merkel, P. B., Nilsson, R., and Kearns, D. R. (1972): Deuterium effects on singlet oxygen lifetimes in solutions. A new test of singlet oxygen reactions. *J. Am. Chem. Soc.*, 94:1030–1031.
320. Metzger, Z., Hoffeld, J. T., and Oppenheim, J. J. (1980): Macrophage-mediated suppression. 1. Evidence for participation of both hydrogen peroxide and prostaglandins in suppression of murine lymphocyte proliferation. *J. Immunol.*, 124:983–988.
321. Michelson, A. M. (1974): Is singlet oxygen a substrate for superoxide dismutase? No. *FEBS Lett.*, 44:97–100.
322. Michelson, A. M., and Durosay, P. (1977): Hemolysis of human erythrocytes by activated oxygen species. *Photochem. Photobiol.*, 25:55–63.
323. Migler, R., and DeChatelet, L. R. (1978): Human eosinophilic peroxidase: biochemical characterization. *Biochem. Med.*, 19:16–26.
324. Migler, R., DeChatelet, L. R., and Bass, D. A. (1978): Human eosinophilic peroxidase: role in bactericidal activity. *Blood*, 51:445–456.
325. Miles, P. R., Lee, P., Trush, M. A., and Van Dyke, K. (1977): Chemiluminescence associated with phagocytosis of foreign particles in rabbit alveolar macrophages. *Life Sci.*, 20:165–170.
326. Miller, T. E. (1969): Killing and lysis of gram negative bacteria through the synergistic effect of hydrogen peroxide, ascorbic acid, and lysozyme. *J. Bacteriol.*, 98:949–955.
327. Miller, T. E. (1971): Metabolic event involved in the bactericidal activity of normal mouse macrophages. *Infect. Immun.*, 3:390–397.
328. Misra, H. P., and Fridovich, I. (1976): Superoxide dismutase and the oxygen enhancement of radiation lethality. *Arch. Biochem. Biophys.*, 176:577–581.
329. Morrison, M., Allen, P. Z., Bright, J., and Jayasinghe, W. (1965): Lactoperoxidase V. Identification and isolation of lactoperoxidase from salivary gland. *Arch. Biochem. Biophys.*, 111:126–133.
330. Murray, R. W. (1979): Chemical sources of singlet oxygen. In: *Singlet Oxygen*, edited by H. H. Wasserman and R. W. Murray, pp. 59–114. Academic Press, New York.
331. Murray, H. W., and Cohn, Z. A. (1979): Macrophage oxygen-dependent antimicrobial activity. I. Susceptibility of *Toxoplasma gondii* to oxygen intermediates. *J. Exp. Med.*, 150:938–949.
332. Murray, H. W., and Cohn, Z. A. (1980): Macrophage oxygen-dependent antimicrobial activity. III. Enhanced oxidative metabolism as an expression of macrophage activation. *J. Exp. Med.*, 152:1596–1609.
333. Murray, H. W., Juangbhanich, C. W., Nathan, C. F., and Cohn, Z. A. (1979): Macrophage oxygen-dependent antimicrobial activity. II. The role of oxygen intermediates. *J. Exp. Med.*, 150:950–964.
334. Murray, H. W., Nathan, C. F., and Cohn, Z. A. (1980): Macrophage oxygen-dependent antimicrobial activity. IV. Role of endogenous scavengers of oxygen intermediates. *J. Exp. Med.*, 152:1610–1624.
335. Nakae, T., Nakano, M., and Saito, K. (1967): Metabolic study of intracellular killing of bacteria by mouse macrophages. *Jap. J. Microbiol.*, 11:189–201.
336. Nakano, M., Noguchi, T., Sugioka, K., Fukuyama, H., and Sato, M. (1975): Spectroscopic evidence for the generation of singlet oxygen in the reduced nicotinamide adenine dinucleotide phosphate-dependent microsomal lipid peroxidation system. *J. Biol. Chem.*, 250:2404–2406.
337. Nathan, C. F. (1980): The release of hydrogen peroxide from mononuclear phagocytes and its role in extracellular cytolysis. In: *Mononuclear Phagocytes. Functional Aspects*, edited by R. van Furth, pp. 1165–1182. Martinus Nijhoff Publishers, The Hague.
338. Nathan, C., and Cohn, Z. (1980): Role of oxygen-dependent mechanisms in antibody-induced lysis of tumor cells by activated macrophages. *J. Exp. Med.*, 152:198–208.
339. Nathan, C. F., and Root, R. K. (1977): Hydrogen peroxide release from mouse peritoneal macrophages. Dependence on sequential activation and triggering. *J. Exp. Med.*, 146:1648–1662.
340. Nathan, C. F., Brukner, L. H., Silverstein, S. C., and Cohn, Z. A. (1979): Extracellular cytolysis by activated macrophages and granulocytes. I. Pharmacologic triggering of effector cells and the release of hydrogen peroxide. *J. Exp. Med.*, 149:84–99.
341. Nathan, C., Nogueira, N., Juangbhanich, C., Ellis, J., and Cohn, Z. (1979): Activation of macrophages *in vivo* and *in vitro*. Correlation between hydrogen peroxide release and killing of *Trypanosoma cruzi*. *J. Exp. Med.*, 149:1056–1068.

342. Nathan, C. F., Silverstein, S. C., Brukner, L. H., and Cohn, Z. A. (1979): Extracellular cytolysis by activated macrophages and granulocytes. II. Hydrogen peroxide as a mediator of cytotoxicity. *J. Exp. Med.*, 149:100–113.
343. Nelson, R. D., Mills, E. L., Simmons, R. L., and Quie, P. G. (1976): Chemiluminescence response of phagocytizing human monocytes. *Infect. Immun.*, 14:129–134.
344. Nichols, B. A., Bainton, D. F., and Farquhar, M. G. (1971): Differentiation of monocytes. Origin, nature and fate of their azurophil granules. *J. Cell Biol.*, 50:498–515.
345. Nilsson, R., and Kearns, D. R. (1974): Role of singlet oxygen in some chemiluminescence and enzyme oxidation reactions. *J. Phys. Chem.*, 78:1681–1683.
346. Nilsson, R., Merkel, P. B., and Kearns, D. R. (1972): Unambiguous evidence for the participation of singlet oxygen ($^1\Delta$) in photodynamic oxidation of amino acids. *Photochem. Photobiol.*, 16:117–124.
347. Nilsson, R., Pick, F. M., and Bray, R. C. (1969): EPR studies on reduction of oxygen to superoxide by some biochemical systems. *Biochim. Biophys. Acta*, 192:145–148.
348. North, R. J. (1970): The relative importance of blood monocytes and fixed macrophages to the expression of cell-mediated immunity to infection. *J. Exp. Med.*, 132:521–534.
349. Oberley, L. W., Lingren, A. L., Baker, S. A., and Stevens, R. H. (1976): Superoxide ion as the cause of the oxygen effect. *Radiat. Res.*, 68:320–328.
350. Ogryzlo, E. A. (1979): Gaseous singlet oxygen. In: *Singlet Oxygen*, edited by H. H. Wasserman and R. W. Murray, pp. 35–58. Academic Press, New York.
351. Ohmori, H., Komoriya, K., Azuma, A., Kurozumi, S., and Oto, Y. H. (1978): Xanthine oxidase-induced histamine release from isolated rat peritoneal mast cells: involvement of hydrogen peroxide. *Biochem. Pharmacol.*, 28:333–334.
352. Ohmori, H., Yamamoto, I., Akagi, M., and Tasaka, K. (1980): Properties of hydrogen peroxide-induced histamine release from rat mast cells. *Biochem. Pharmacol.*, 29:741–745.
353. Oliveira. O. M. M. F., Haun, M., Durán, N., O'Brien, P. J., O'Brien, C. R., Bechara, E. J. H., and Cilento, G. (1978): Enzyme-generated electronically excited carbonyl compounds. Acetone phosphorescence during the peroxidase-catalyzed aerobic oxidation of isobutanol. *J. Biol. Chem.*, 253:4707–4712.
354. Oren, R., Farnham, A. E., Saito, K., Milofsky, E., and Karnovsky, M. L. (1963): Metabolic patterns in three types of phagocytizing cells. *J. Cell Biol.*, 17:487–501.
355. Ouchi, E., Selvaraj, R. J., and Sbarra, A. J. (1965): The biochemical activities of rabbit alveolar macrophages during phagocytosis. Exp. Cell Res., 40:456–468.
356. Paschen, W., and Weser, U. (1973): Singlet oxygen decontaminating activity of erythrocuprein (superoxide dismutase). *Biochim. Biophys. Acta*, 327:217–222.
357. Paschen, W., and Weser, U. (1975): Problems concerning the biochemical action of superoxide dismutase (erythrocuprein). *Hoppe Seylers Z. Physiol. Chem.*, 356:727–737.
358. Paul, B. B., Strauss, R. R., Selvaraj, R. J., and Sbarra, A. J. (1973): Peroxidase mediated antimicrobial activities of alveolar macrophage granules. *Science*, 181:849–850.
359. Pederson, T. C., and Aust, S. D. (1973): The role of superoxide and singlet oxygen in lipid peroxidation promoted by xanthine oxidase. *Biochem. Biophys. Res. Commun.*, 52:1071–1078.
360. Peters, J. W., and Foote, C. S. (1976): Chemistry of superoxide anion. II. Reaction with hydroperoxides. *J. Am. Chem. Soc.*, 98:873–875.
361. Petrone, W. F., English, D. K., Wong, K., and McCord, J. M. (1980): Free radicals and inflammation: superoxide-dependent activation of a neutrophil chemotactic factor in plasma. *Proc. Natl. Acad. Sci. U.S.A.*, 77:1159–1163.
362. Piatt, J. F., and O'Brien, P. J. (1979): Singlet oxygen formation by a peroxidase H_2O_2 and halide system. *Eur. J. Biochem.*, 93:323–332.
363. Piatt, J. F., Cheema, A. S., and O'Brien, P. J. (1977): Peroxidase catalyzed singlet oxygen formation from hydrogen peroxide. *FEBS Lett.*, 74:251–254.
364. Poupko, R., and Rosenthal, I. (1973): Electron transfer interactions between superoxide ion and organic compounds. *J. Phys. Chem.*, 77:1722–1724.
365. Pruitt, K. M., Adamson, M., and Arnold, R. (1979): Lactoperoxidase binding to streptococci. *Infect. Immun.*, 25:304–309.
366. Pryor, W. A. (1978): The formation of free radicals and the consequences of their reactions *in vivo*. *Photochem. Photobiol.*, 28:787–801.
367. Pryor, W. A., and Tang, R. H. (1978): Ethylene formation from methional. *Biochim. Biophys. Res. Commun.*, 81:498–503.

368. Puget, K., and Michelson, A. M. (1976): Oxidation of luminol by the xanthine oxidase system in presence of carbonate anions. *Photochem. Photobiol.*, 24:499–501.
369. Quie, P. G., White, J. G., Holmes, B., and Good, R. A. (1967): *In vitro* bactericidal capacity of human polymorphonuclear leukocytes: diminished activity in chronic granulomatous disease in childhood. *J. Clin. Invest.*, 46:668–679.
370. Rabani, J., Klug, D., and Fridovich, I. (1972): Decay of the HO_2 and O_2 radicals catalyzed by superoxide dismutase. A pulse radiolytic investigation. *Israel J. Chem.*, 10:1095–1106.
371. Ramsey, P. G., Martin, T., Chi, E., and Klebanoff, S. J. (1982): Arming of mononuclear phagocytes by eosinophil peroxidase bound to *Staphylococcus aureus*. *J. Immunol., (in press)*.
372. Reiss, M., and Roos, D. (1978): Differences in oxygen metabolism of phagocytosing monocytes and neutrophils. *J. Clin. Invest.*, 61:480–488.
373. Reiter, B., Pickering, A., and Oram, J. D. (1964): An inhibitory system—lactoperoxidase/thiocyanate/peroxide—in raw milk. In: *Proceedings of the Fourth International Symposium on Food Microbiology*, pp. 297–305, Göteborg, Sweden.
374. Repine, J. E., Eaton, J. W., Anders, M. W., Hoidal, J. R., and Fox, R. B. (1979): Generation of hydroxyl radical by enzymes, chemicals and human phagocytes *in vitro*. Detection with the anti-inflammatory agent, dimethyl sulfoxide. *J. Clin. Invest.*, 64:1642–1651.
375. Rest, R. F., and Spitznagel, J. K. (1977): Subcellular distribution of superoxide dismutases in human neutrophils. Influence of myeloperoxidase on the measurement of superoxide dismutase activity. *Biochem. J.*, 166:145–153.
376. Reuvers, A. P., Greenstock, C. L., Borsa, J., and Chapman, J. D. (1973): Studies on the mechanism of chemical radioprotection by dimethyl sulfoxide. *Int. J. Radiat. Biol.*, 24:533–536.
377. Richter, C., Wendel, A., Weser, U., and Azzi, A. (1975): Inhibition by superoxide dismutase of linoleic acid peroxidation induced by lipoxidase. *FEBS Lett.*, 51:300–303.
378. Rigo, A., Stevanato, R., Finazzi-Agrò, A., and Rotilio, G. (1977): An attempt to evaluate the rate of the Haber-Weiss reaction by using ·OH radical scavengers. *FEBS Lett.*, 80:130–132.
379. Rodey, G. E., Park, B. H., Windhorst, D. B., and Good, R. A. (1969): Defective bactericidal activity of monocytes in fatal granulomatous disease. *Blood*, 33:813–820.
380. Roos, D., and Balm, A. J. M. (1980): The oxidative metabolism of monocytes. In: *The Reticuloendothelial System. A Comprehensive Treatise 2. Biochemistry and Metabolism*, edited by A. J. Sbarra and R. R. Strauss, pp. 189–229. Plenum Press, New York.
381. Root, R. K. (1974): Correction of the function of chronic granulomatous disease (CGD) granulocytes (PMN) with extracellular H_2O_2. *Clin. Res.*, 22:452A.
382. Rosen, H., and Klebanoff, S. J. (1976): Chemiluminescence and superoxide production by myeloperoxidase-deficient leukocytes. *J. Clin. Invest.*, 58:50–60.
383. Rosen, H., and Klebanoff, S. J. (1977): Formation of singlet oxygen by the myeloperoxidase-mediated antimicrobial system. *J. Biol. Chem.*, 252:4803–4810.
384. Rosen, H., and Klebanoff, S. J. (1979): Hydroxyl radical generation by polymorphonuclear leukocytes measured by electron spin resonance spectroscopy. *J. Clin. Invest.*, 64:1725–1729.
385. Rosen, H., and Klebanoff, S. J. (1979): Bactericidal activity of a superoxide anion generating system. A model for the polymorphonuclear leukocyte. *J. Exp. Med.*, 149:27–39.
386. Rosen, H., and Klebanoff, S. J. (1981): Role of iron and ethylenediaminetetraacetic acid in the bactericidal activity of a superoxide anion generating system. *Arch Biochem. Biophys.*, 208:512–519.
387. Rosenthal, I. (1975): Singlet molecular oxygen and superoxide radical anion. *Israel J. Chem.*, 13:86–90.
388. Ross. R., and Klebanoff, S. J. (1966): The eosinophil leukocyte. Fine structure studies of changes in the uterus during the estrous cycle. *J. Exp. Med.*, 124:653–659.
389. Rossi, F., Patriarca, P., and Romeo, D. (1980): Metabolic changes accompanying phagocytosis. In: *The Reticuloendothelial System. A Comprehensive Treatise 2. Biochemistry and Metabolism*, edited by A. J. Sbarra and R. R. Strauss, pp. 153–188. Plenum Press, New York.
390. Rossi, F., Zabucchi, G., and Romeo, D. (1975): Metabolism of phagocytosing mononuclear phagocytes. In: *Mononuclear Phagocytes in Immunity, Infection and Pathology*, edited by R. van Furth, pp. 441–460. Blackwell Scientific Publications, Oxford.
391. Ruco, L. P., and Meltzer, M. S. (1978): Macrophage activation for tumor cytotoxicity: increased lymphokine responsiveness of peritoneal macrophages during acute inflammation. *J. Immunol.*, 120:1054–1062.
392. Rumyantseva, G. V., Weiner, L. M., Molin, Y. N., and Budker, V. G. 1979: Permeation of liposome membrane by superoxide radical. *FEBS Lett.*, 108:477–480.

393. Sachs, T., Moldow, C. F., Craddock, P. R., Bowers, T. K., and Jacob, H. S. (1978): Oxygen radicals mediate endothelial cell damage by complement-stimulated granulocytes. *J. Clin. Invest.*, 61:1161–1167.
394. Sagone, A. L., Jr., Decker, M. A., Wells, R. M., and DeMocko, C. 1980: A new method for the detection of hydroxyl radical production by phagocytic cells. *Biochim. Biophys. Acta*, 628:90–97.
395. Sagone, A. L., Jr., Kamps, S., and Campbell, R. (1978): The effect of oxidant injury on the lymphoblastic transformation of human lymphocytes. *Photochem. Photobiol.*, 28:909–915.
396. Sagone, A. L., Jr., King, G. W., and Metz, E. N. (1976): A comparison of the metabolic response to phagocytosis in human granulocytes and monocytes. *J. Clin. Invest.*, 57:1352–1358.
397. Sagone, A. L., Jr., Mendelson, D. S., and Metz, E. N. (1977): The effect of sodium azide on the chemiluminescence of granulocytes—evidence for the generation of multiple oxygen radicals. *J. Lab. Clin. Med.*, 89:1333–1340.
398. Salin, M. L., and McCord, J. M. (1974): Superoxide dismutase in polymorphonuclear leukocytes. J. Clin. Invest., 54:1005–1009.
399. Salin, M. L., and McCord, J. M. (1975): Free radicals and inflammation. Protection of phagocytosing leukocytes by superoxide dismutase. *J. Clin. Invest.*, 56:1319–1323.
400. Salin, M. L., and McCord, J. M. (1977): Free radicals in leukocyte metabolism and inflammation. In: *Superoxide and Superoxide Dismutases*, edited by A. M. Michelson, J. M. McCord, and I. Fridovich, pp. 257–270. Academic Press, New York.
401. Salmon, S. E., Cline, M. J., Schultz, J., and Lehrer, R. I. (1970): Myeloperoxidase deficiency. Immunologic study of a genetic leucocyte defect. *N. Engl. J. Med.*, 282:250–253.
402. Samuni, A., and Czapski, G. (1978): Radiation-induced damage in *Escherichia coli B*: the effect of superoxide radicals and molecular oxygen. *Radiat. Res.*, 76:624–632.
403. Saran, M., Bors, W., Michel, C., and Elstner, E. F. (1980): Formation of ethylene from methionine. Reactivity of radiolytically produced oxygen radicals and effect of substrate activation. *Int. J. Radiat. Biol.*, 37:521–527.
404. Sawyer, D. T., and Gibian, M. J. (1979): The chemistry of superoxide ion. *Tetrahedron*, 35:1471–1481.
405. Sbarra, A. J., and Karnovsky, M. L. (1959): The biochemical basis of phagocytosis. I. Metabolic changes during the ingestion of particles by polymorphonuclear leukocytes. *J. Biol. Chem.*, 234:1355–1362.
406. Sbarra, A. J., and Shirley, W. (1963): Phagocytosis inhibition and reversal. I. Effect of glycolytic intermediates and nucleotides on particle uptake. *J. Bacteriol.*, 86:259–265.
407. Schaap, A. P., Thayer, A. L., Faler, G. R., Goda, K., and Kimura, T. (1974): Singlet molecular oxygen and superoxide dismutase. *J. Am. Chem. Soc.*, 96:4025–4026.
408. Schultz, J. (1980): Myeloperoxidase. In: *The Reticuloendothelial System. A Comprehensive Treatise 2. Biochemistry and Metabolism*, edited by A. J. Sbarra and R. R. Strauss, pp. 231–254. Plenum Press, New York.
409. Segal, A. W., and Jones, O. T. G. (1978): Novel cytochrome b system in phagocytic vacuoles of human granulocytes. *Nature (London)*, 276:515–517.
410. Segal, A. W., and Jones, O. T. G. (1979): The subcellular distribution and some properties of the cytochrome b component of the microbicidal oxidase system of human neutrophils. *Biochem. J.*, 182:181–188.
411. Segal, A. W., and Jones. O. T. G. (1979): Reduction and subsequent oxidation of a cytochrome b of human neutrophils after stimulation with phorbol myristate acetate. *Biochem. Biophys. Res. Commun.*, 88:130–134.
412. Segal, A. W., and Jones, O. T. G. (1980); Absence of cytochrome b reduction in stimulated neutrophils from both female and male patients with chronic granulomatous disease. *FEBS. Lett.*, 110:111–114.
413. Segal, A. W., and Meshulam, T. (1979): Production of superoxide by neutrophils: a reappraisal. *FEBS Lett.*, 100:27–32.
414. Segal, A. W., Jones, O. T. G., Webster, D., and Allison, A. C. (1978): Absence of a newly described cytochrome b from neutrophils of patients with chronic granulomatous disease. *Lancet*, 2:446–449.
415. Seliger, H. H. (1960): A photoelectric method for the measurement of spectra of light sources of rapidly varying intensities. *Anal. Biochem.*, 1:60–65.
416. Selvaraj, R. J., and Sbarra, A. J. (1966): Relationship of glycolytic and oxidative metabolism to particle entry and destruction in phagocytosing cells. *Nature (London)*, 211:1272–1276.

417. Selvaraj, R. J., Zgliczynski, J. M., Paul, B. B., and Sbarra, A. J. (1978): Enhanced killing of myeloperoxidase-coated bacteria in the myeloperoxidase-H₂O₂-Cl⁻ system. *J. Infect. Dis.*, 137:481–485.

418. Selvaraj, R. J., Zgliczynski, J. M., Paul, B. B., and Sbarra, A. J. (1980): Chlorination of reduced nicotinamide adenine dinucleotides by myeloperoxidase: a novel bactericidal mechanism. *J. Reticuloendothel. Soc.*, 27:31–38.

419. Shakhashiri, B. Z., and Williams, L. G. (1976): Singlet oxygen in aqueous solution: a lecture demonstration. *J. Chem. Educ.*, 53:358–361.

420. Shimizu, M., Egashira, T., and Takahama, U. (1979): Inactivation of *Neurospora crassa* conidia by singlet molecular oxygen generated by a photosensitized reaction. *J. Bacteriol.*, 138:293–296.

421. Shinagawa, Y., Tanaka, C., Teraoka, A., and Shinagawa, Y. (1966): A new cytochrome in neutrophilic granules of rabbit leucocyte. *J. Biochem.*, 59:622–624.

422. Simmons, S. R., and Karnovsky, M. L. (1973): Iodinating ability of various leukocytes and their bactericidal activity. *J. Exp. Med.*, 138:44–63.

423. Slivka, A., LoBuglio, A. F., and Weiss, S. J. (1980): A potential role for hypochlorous acid in granulocyte-mediated tumor cell cytotoxicity. *Blood*, 55:347–350.

424. Smith, D. C., and Klebanoff, S. J. (1970): A uterine fluid-mediated sperm-inhibitory system. *Biol. Reprod.*, 3:229–235.

425. Smith, L. L., and Kulig, M. J. (1976): Singlet molecular oxygen from hydrogen peroxide disproportionation. *J. Am. Chem. Soc.*, 98:1027–1029.

426. Spector, W. G. (1969): The granulomatous inflammatory exudate. *Int. Rev. Exp. Pathol.*, 8:1–36.

427. Spikes, J. (1975): Porphyrins and related compounds as photodynamic sensitizers. *Ann. N.Y. Acad. Sci.*, 244:496–508.

428. Stankovich, M. T., Schopfer, L. M., and Massey, V. (1978): Determination of glucose oxidase oxidation-reduction potentials and the oxygen reactivity of fully reduced and semiquinoid forms. *J. Biol. Chem.*, 253:4971–4979.

429. Stanley, J. P. (1980): Reactions of superoxide with peroxides. *J. Org. Chem.*, 45:1413–1418.

430. Stauff, J., Sander, U., and Jaeschke, W. (1973): Chemiluminescence of perhydroxyl- and carbonate-radicals. In: *Chemiluminescence and Bioluminescence*, edited by M. J. Cormier, D. M. Hercules, and J. Lee, pp. 131–140. Plenum Press, New York.

431. Stauff, J., Schmidkunz, H., and Hartmann, G. (1963): Weak chemiluminescence of oxidation reactions. *Nature (London)*, 198:281–282.

432. Steele, W. F., and Morrison, M. (1969): Antistreptococcal activity of lactoperoxidase. *J. Bacteriol.*, 97:635–639.

433. Steinman, R. M., and Cohn, Z. A. (1972): The interaction of soluble horseradish peroxidase with mouse peritoneal macrophages *in vitro. J. Cell Biol.*, 55:186–204.

434. Stelmaszynska, T., and Zgliczynski, J. M. (1978): N-(2-oxoacyl) amino acids and nitriles as final products of dipeptide chlorination mediated by the myeloperoxidase/H₂O₂/Cl⁻ system. *Eur. J. Biochem.*, 92:301–308.

435. Stjernholm, R. L., Allen, R. C., Steele, R. H., Waring, W. W., and Harris, J. A. (1973): Impaired chemiluminescence during phagocytosis of opsonized bacteria. *Infect. Immun.*, 7:313–314.

436. Stokes, S. H., Davis, W. B., and Sorber, W. A. (1978): Effect of phagocytosis on superoxide anion production and superoxide dismutase levels in BCG activated and normal rabbit alveolar macrophages. *J. Reticuloendothel. Soc.*, 24:101–106.

437. Stossel, T. P., Mason, R. J., Pollard, T. D., and Vaughan, M. (1972): Isolation and properties of phagocytic vesicles. II. Alveolar macrophages. *J. Clin. Invest.*, 51:604–614.

438. Sugioka, K., and Nakano, M. (1976): A possible mechanism of the generation of singlet molecular oxygen in NADPH-dependent microsomal lipid peroxidation. *Biochim. Biophys. Acta*, 423:203–216.

439. Svingen, B. A., O'Neal, F. O., and Aust, S. D. (1978): The role of superoxide and singlet oxygen in lipid peroxidation. *Photochem. Photobiol.*, 28:803–809.

440. Tally, F. P., Goldin, B. R., Jacobus, N. V., and Gorbach, S. L. (1977): Superoxide dismutase in anaerobic bacteria of clinical significance. *Infect. Immun.*, 16:20–25.

441. Tauber, A. I., and Babior, B. M. (1977): Evidence for hydroxyl radical production by human neutrophils. *J. Clin. Invest.*, 60:374–379.

442. Tauber, A. I., and Goetzl, E. J. (1979): Structural and catalytic properties of the solubilized superoxide-generating activity of human polymorphonuclear leukocytes. Solubilization, stabilization in solution and partial characterization. *Biochemistry*, 18:5576–5584.

443. Tauber, A. I., Gabig, T. G., and Babior, B. M. (1979): Evidence for production of oxidizing radicals by the particulate O_2^--forming system from human neutrophils. *Blood*, 53:666–67444.
444. Tauber, A. I., Goetzl, E. J., and Babior, B. M. (1976): The production of superoxide (O_2^-) by human eosinophils. *Blood*, 48:968.
445. Thalinger, K. K., and Mandell, G. L. (1971): Bactericidal activity of macrophages in an anaerobic environment. *J. Reticuloendothel. Soc.*, 9:393–396.
446. Thomas, E. L. (1979): Myeloperoxidase, hydrogen peroxide, chloride antimicrobial system: nitrogen-chloride derivatives of bacterial components in bacterial action against *Escherichia coli*. *Infect. Immun.*, 23:522–531.
447. Thomas, E. L. (1979): Myeloperoxidase-hydrogen peroxide-chloride antimicrobial system: effect of exogenous amines on antibacterial action against *Escherichia coli*. *Infect. Immun.*, 25:110–116.
448. Thomas, E. L., and Aune, T. M. (1978): Cofactor role of iodide in peroxidase antimicrobial action against *Escherichia coli*. *Antimicrob. Agents Chemother.*, 13:1000–1005.
449. Thomas, E. L., and Aune, T. M. (1978): Oxidation of *Escherichia coli* sulfhydryl components by the peroxidase-hydrogen peroxide-iodide antimicrobial system. *Antimicrob. Agents Chemother.*, 13:1006–1010.
450. Thomas, M. J., Mehl, K. S., and Pryor, W. A. (1978): The role of the superoxide anion in the xanthine oxidase-induced autoxidation of linoleic acid. *Biochem. Biophys. Res. Commun.*, 83:927–932.
451. Thorne, K. J. I., Svvennsen, R. J., and Franks, D. (1978): Role of hydrogen peroxide and peroxidase in the cytotoxicity of *Trypanosoma dionisii* by human granulocytes. *Infect. Immun.*, 21:798–805.
452. Tsan, M. F., and Chen, J. W. (1980): Oxidation of methionine by human polymorphonuclear leukocytes. *J. Clin. Invest.*, 65:1041–1050.
453. Tsan, M. -F., and Denison, R. C. (1980): Phorbol myristate acetate-induced neutrophil autotoxicity. A comparison with H_2O_2 toxicity. *Inflammation*, 4:371–380.
454. Ushijima, Y., and Nakano, M. (1980): No or little production of singlet molecular oxygen in HOCl or HOCl/H_2O_2. A model system for myeloperoxidase/H_2O_2/Cl$^-$. *Biochem. Biophys. Res. Commun.*, 93:1232–1237.
455. van der Meer, J. W. M., Beelen, R. H. J., Fluitsma, D. M., and van Furth, R. (1979): Ultrastructure of mononuclear phagocytes developing in liquid bone marrow cultures. A study on peroxidatic activity. *J. Exp. Med.*, 149:17–26.
456. van Furth, R., Hirsch, J. G., and Fedorko, M. E. (1970): Morphology and peroxidase cytochemistry of mouse promonocytes, monocytes and macrophages. *J. Exp. Med.*, 132:794–812.
457. van Hemmen, J. J., and Meuling, W. J. A. (1975): Inactivation of biologically active DNA by X-ray-induced superoxide radicals and their dismutation products, singlet molecular oxygen and hydrogen peroxide. *Biochim. Biophys. Acta*, 402:133–141.
458. van Hemmen, J. J., and Meuling, W. J. A. (1977): Inactivation of *Escherichia coli* by superoxide radicals and their dismutation products. *Arch. Biochem. Biophys.*, 182:743–748.
459. Vidigal-Martinelli, C., Zinner, K., Kachar, B., Dufan, N., and Cilento, G. (1979): Emission from singlet oxygen during the peroxidase-catalyzed oxidation of malonaldehyde. *FEBS Lett.*, 108:266–268.
460. Walling, C. (1975): Fenton's reagent revisited. *Accounts Chem. Res.*, 8:125–131.
461. Wasserman, H. H., and Murray, R. W., editors (1979): *Singlet Oxygen*. Academic Press, New York.
462. Webb, L. S., Keele, B. B., Jr., and Johnston, R. B., Jr. (1974): Inhibition of phagocytosis-associated chemiluminescence by superoxide dismutase. *Infect. Immun.*, 9:1051–1056.
463. Weinstein, J., and Bielski, B. H. J. (1979): Kinetics of the interaction of HO_2 and O_2^- radicals with hydrogen peroxide. The Haber-Weiss reaction. *J. Am. Chem. Soc.*, 101:58–62.
464. Weiss, S. J., King, G. W., and LoBuglio, A. F. (1977): Evidence for hydroxyl radical generation by human monocytes. *J. Clin. Invest.*, 60:370–373.
465. Weiss, S. J., King, G. W., and LoBuglio, A. F. (1978): Superoxide generation by human monocytes and macrophages. *Am. J. Hematol.*, 4:1–8.
466. Weiss, S. J., LoBuglio, A. F., and Kessler, H. B. (1980): Oxidative mechanisms of monocyte-mediated cytotoxicity. *Proc. Natl. Acad. Sci. U.S.A.*, 77:584–587.

467. Weiss, S. J., Rustagi, P. K., and LoBuglio, A. F. (1978): Human granulocyte generation of hydroxyl radical. *J. Exp. Med.*, 147:316–323.
468. Welch, W. D., Graham, C. W., Zaccari, J., and Thrupp, L. D. (1980): Analysis and comparison of the luminol-dependent chemiluminescence responses of alveolar macrophages and neutrophils. *J. Reticuloendothel. Soc.*, 28:275–283.
469. Weser, U., Paschen, W., and Younes, M. (1975): Singlet oxygen and superoxide dismutase (cuprein). *Biochem. Biophys. Res. Commun.*, 66:769–777.
470. Wilson, T., and Hastings, J. W. (1970): Chemical and biological aspects of singlet excited molecular oxygen. *Photophysiology*, 5:49–95.
471. Wilson, T., and Schaap, A. P. (1971): The chemiluminescence from *cis*-diethyl-1,2-dioxetane. An unexpected effect of oxygen. *J. Am. Chem. Soc.*, 93:4126–4136.
472. Woeber, K. A., and Ingbar, S. H. (1973): Metabolism of L-thyroxine by phagocytosing human leukocytes. *J. Clin. Invest.*, 52:1796–1803.
473. Wright, J. R., Rumbaugh, R. C., Colby, H. D., and Miles, P. R. (1979): The relationship between chemiluminescence and lipid peroxidation in rat hepatic microsomes. *Arch. Biochem. Biophys.*, 192:344–351.
474. Yang, S. F. (1967): Biosynthesis of ethylene. Ethylene formation from methional by horseradish peroxidase. *Arch. Biochem. Biophys.*, 122:481–487.
475. Yang, S. F. (1969): Further studies on ethylene formation from α-keto-γ-methylthiobutyric acid or β-methylthiopropionaldehyde by peroxidase in the presence of sulfite and oxygen. *J. Biol. Chem.*, 244:4360–4365.
476. Yong, E. C., Kuo, C. C., and Klebanoff, S. J. (1980): Toxic effect of the myeloperoxidase antimicrobial system on *Chlamydia trachomatis*. *Am. Soc. Microbiol. Abst. Annual Meeting*, p. 38.
477. Zeldow, B. J. (1963): Studies on the antibacterial action of human saliva. III. Cofactor requirements of a lactobacillus bactericidin. *J. Immunol.*, 90:12–16.
478. Zgliczynski, J. M. (1980): Characteristics of myeloperoxidase from neutrophils and other peroxidases from different cell types. In: *The Reticuloendothelial System. A Comprehensive Treatise 2. Biochemistry and Metabolism*, edited by A. J. Sbarra and R. R. Strauss, pp. 255–278. Plenum Press, New York.
479. Zgliczynski, J. M., and Stelmaszynska, T. (1979): Hydrogen cyanide and cyanogen chloride formation by the myeloperoxidase-H_2O_2-Cl$^-$ system. *Biochim. Biophys. Acta*, 567:309–314.
480. Zgliczynski, J. M., Selvaraj, R. J., Paul, B. B., Stelmaszynska, T., Poskitt, P. K. F., and Sbarra, A. J. (1977): Chlorination by the myeloperoxidase-H_2O_2-Cl$^-$ anti-microbial system at acid and neutral pH. *Proc. Soc. Exp. Biol. Med.*, 154:418–422.

Advances in Host Defense Mechanisms, Vol. 1,
edited by John I. Gallin and Anthony S. Fauci,
Raven Press, New York © 1982.

Neutrophil Dysfunction and Recurrent Infection

Paul G. Quie

University of Minnesota Medical School, Minneapolis, Minnesota 55455

A normally functioning phagocytic system is essential for host defense against infectious disease, since most species of bacteria and fungi are resistant to non-phagocytic cell microbicidal mechanisms. Patients with abnormal phagocytic cell microbicidal function and recurrent severe infection were first described in 1967 when intracellular survival of staphylococci in neutrophils was discovered (82). This abnormality of neutrophil function was discovered in patients with a clinical syndrome characterized by normal or increased immunoglobulins, normal numbers of circulating phagocytic cells and recurrent abscesses involving subcutaneous tissue, reticuloendothelial system, and lungs (55,17). This syndrome has come to be known as chronic granulomatous disease (CGD). Patients with CGD frequently suffer recurrent severe disease from microbial species which are usually considered to have little virulence. In addition, these patients often do not respond to what is adequate antimicrobial therapy in persons with normal host-defense mechanisms. Therefore, laboratory investigation of phagocytic cell function has become essential for evaluation of patients with suspected abnormal host defense.

During the past decade it has become increasingly appreciated that disorders of several functions of neutrophils including adherence, locomotion, response to chemotactic stimuli, and phagocytosis as well as microbicidal function may be associated with increased susceptibility to infection. Emphasis in this chapter will be on disorders of neutrophil locomotion and microbicidal capacity.

Neutrophil-directed locomotion (chemotaxis) is regulated by a complex interaction of cellular and humoral constituents. Chemoattractants include products of invading microbes as well as serum components which may be activated during inflammatory responses. The most thoroughly studied chemoattractants are C5a and small-molecular-weight synthetic peptides derived from gram-negative bacterial species or produced synthetically. Complement component C5 is a chemotaxinogen, which is activated via either the alternative or classical pathways to C5a, an active chemoattractant (chemotaxin).

Miles and co-workers (70) reported in 1957 that delay of migration of neutrophils into experimental infections for as little as 2 hr enhanced capacity of bacteria to produce severe lesions by as much as 10,000-fold. These early experimental observations have been supported by clinical experience in patients with disorders of granulocyte chemotaxis. Patients with defective leukocyte chemotaxis have purulent lesions, and indeed there may be polymorphonuclear leukocytes and copious fluid in abscesses involving subcutaneous tissue or lungs. Delay in accumulation of phagocytic cells is probably involved in the pathogenesis of abscesses, but systemic spread may be prevented by eventual migration of granulocytes and monocytes into the lesions. Infectious lesions in these patients most frequently involve the skin, subcutaneous tissue, and regional lymph nodes. Pneumonia is also a frequent complication; however, septicemia and osteomyelitis are uncommon.

DEFICIENCY OF CHEMOTACTIC FACTORS

A patient with Klinefelter's syndrome with a history of repeated pyogenic infections and a low serum C3 level was found to lack serum chemotactic factor activity; activity could be restored by addition of normal serum, but not by purified C3 (5). The abnormal function in this patient was due to the congenital absence of a C3 regulatory protein normally present in plasma.

Patients with congenital absence of the third component of complement have serious infections with staphylococci and gram-negative bacteria, since these sera lack opsonic and bactericidal activity as well as chemotactic activity.

A 19-year-old female patient with C5 deficiency and lupus erythematosus since age 11 years has recently been described (88). The patient's infections included oral and vaginal moniliasis, infected cutaneous and subcutaneous ulcers, chronically draining sinus tracts, sepsis, and meningitis. A markedly impaired ability to generate chemotactic activity was demonstrated in her serum. Family members heterozygous for C5 deficiency were able to generate chemotactic activity normally. Elucidation of the role of the complement system in host defense against microbicidal disease has been one of the most dramatic advances of the past decade, and a recent review by Frank (43) is recommended to the interested reader.

DEFECTIVE NEUTROPHIL CHEMOTAXIS

Ward and Schlegel (99) first described a patient with defective neutrophil locomotion and suggested possible association with recurrent infections. The neutrophils from this patient were deficient in bactericidal capacity for gram-negative bacteria as well as defective in chemotaxis, and the clinical syndrome described was similar to chronic granulomatous disease so the contribution of abnormal neutrophil locomotion was uncertain. Two children with neutropenia, depressed neutrophil locomotion, and recurrent infections were described by Miller and co-workers (72), and "lazy leukocyte syndrome" was used to identify these associated clinical and laboratory findings. The children were severely neutropenic but had normal myeloid precursors and mature neutrophils in their bone marrow. Their illnesses were characterized by gingivitis and stomatitis and recurrent upper respiratory infections. The only immunologic or inflammatory abnormality identified in these children was defective locomotion of their neutrophils. This neutrophil abnormality could not be corrected by fresh normal plasma, and there was no lack of chemotactic factors, suggesting a primary cellular defect. Table 1 lists several clinical entities with disordered neutrophil locomotion and increased susceptibility to infection. Assay of neutrophil locomotion has become a part of the laboratory evaluation of patients with recurrent infections.

A 58-year-old male was reported by Singh and colleagues (92) with recurrent severe protracted subcutaneous infections, wound healing, and defective neutrophil chemotaxis. He also had defective neutrophil bactericidal capacity and absent nitroblue tetrazolium (NBT) reduction during phagocytosis. Chromosome analysis revealed deletion of a segment of chromosome 16.

Still another combination of intrinsic neutrophil functional defects was identified in a 4-year-old boy with recurrent severe pulmonary infections (94). Laboratory studies revealed abnormal phagocytosis of staphylococci and defective granulocyte chemotaxis. There was a paucity of neutrophils in lesions, and markedly delayed wound healing complicated his clinical course. The patient also had X-linked hypogammaglobulinemia, and severe susceptibility to infections was probably a consequence of defective humoral as well as phagocytic function.

TABLE 1. *Clinical conditions with abnormal neutrophil locomotion*

Lazy leukocyte syndrome
Actin dysfunction syndrome
Kartagener's syndrome
Schwachman syndrome
Chediak-Higashi syndrome
Felty's syndrome
Anchor disease
Hyperimmunoglobulin E (Job's syndrome)
Acrodermatitis enteropathica
Mucocutaneous candidiasis
Behçet's disease
Icthyosis
Mannosidosis
Down's syndrome
Diabetes mellitus
Newborn infants
Malignancy
Overwhelming infections
Viral infections
Severe trauma
Severe burns
Periodontitis
Bone marrow transplant
Immobile ciliary syndrome
Microtubule abnormality

CHEDIAK-HIGASHI SYNDROME

Patients with Chediak-Higashi syndrome (CHS) have several functional abnormalities of their neutrophils including defective chemotaxis (27). The diagnosis of CHS is made by identification of leukocytes with giant cytoplasmic lysosomal granules, and the chemotactic defect has been postulated to result from the giant granules preventing the neutrophils from squeezing through small spaces. Recent evidence, however, suggests that there may be a metabolic defect in Chediak-Higashi leukocytes as well which inhibits neutrophil migration. Extremely elevated levels of intracellular cyclic adenosine monophosphate (AMP) have been reported in leukocytes of a patient with CHS (16). Ascorbic acid at a 200-mg daily dose brought about a sharp reduction in the levels of leukocyte cyclic AMP in this patient, and there was convincing improvement in the patient's neutrophil chemotactic responsiveness.

MANNOSIDOSIS

Abnormal chemotactic responsiveness was found in a child with mannosidosis (39,44). This storage disease results from deficiency of acidic α-mannosidase activity, and mannose-rich material accumulates in cells, including the circulating leukocytes. Chronic otitis media, with marked hearing loss and severe upper respiratory infections and nearly continuous hospitalization characterized this child's first three years of life. Her terminal illness was severe infiltrative lung disease with progressive respiratory failure. Viral cultures revealed adenovirus Type 7 from urine, stool, and throat cultures and from lung tissue obtained at autopsy.

There was a generally depressed immunologic response, with low immunoglobulin levels and decreased response of lymphocytes to phytohemagglutinin. A striking defect in neutrophil chemotactic responsiveness was identified and there was also delayed phagocytosis of *Staphylococcus aureus* and *Escherichia coli*. Normal neutrophil NBT reduction was found, suggesting a normal oxidative metabolic response during phagocytosis. It is interesting to speculate that abnormal mannose material in this patient may have interfered with leukocyte membrane function or with the process of cell locomotion.

ICHTHYOSIS

Patients with defective neutrophil chemotaxis frequently have severe dermatologic abnormalities (71,77). For example, patients with ichthyosis have severe subcutaneous abscesses from *S. aureus*, *Candida albicans*, *Trichophyton rubrum*, or gram-negative enteric bacteria. The frequent infections are undoubtedly related to the abnormal epidermal barrier, but the severity of the infectious process may have been related to defective neutrophil chemotaxis that has been described in these patients.

HYPERIMMUNOGLOBULIN E (JOB'S SYNDROME)

A clinical syndrome characterized by unusual susceptibility to serious staphylococcal disease, chronic skin lesions similar to eczema, and "cold" abscesses was reported in 1966 as Job's syndrome (36). Several years after this initial description Buckley and co-workers (21) reported two boys with chronic dermatitis and recurrent severe lung, skin, and joint abscesses primarily due to staphylococci. A striking elevation of serum immunoglobulin E (IgE) in these patients suggested an association between extremely elevated levels of IgE and susceptibility to infection.

Depressed neutrophil chemotaxis and extremely elevated levels of serum IgE was first described in a patient with recurrent staphylococcal pneumonia, lymph node abscesses and chronic candida by Clark and colleagues (28). Hill and Quie (51) described several children with depressed neutrophil chemotaxis, increased levels of serum IgE, and recurrent staphylococcal infections, suggesting an association between hyperimmunoglobulin E and neutrophil locomotion. The possibility that abnormally elevated IgE and neutrophil chemotactic dysfunction might be a genetic disorder was suggested when a mother and daughter with a severe staphylococcal disease were described (97). Both mother and daughter had depressed neutrophil chemotaxis. A father and son with hyperimmunoglobulin E and staphylococcal lesions have also been described but abnormal neutrophil chemotaxis was not a consistent finding (13). Hill and colleagues (50) studied patients with Job's syndrome originally described in 1966 and demonstrated extremely elevated IgE levels and abnormal neutrophil chemotaxis. The clinical association of extremely elevated levels of serum IgE and recurrent severe staphylococcal infections is now termed hyperimmunoglobulin E syndrome, which is probably identical with Job's syndrome.

NEUTROPHIL CHEMOTAXIS IN HYPERIMMUNOGLOBULIN E SYNDROME

Disordered neutrophil chemotaxis and recurrent staphylococcal disease is associated in most patients with hyperimmunoglobulin E syndrome; however, it is a highly variable finding.

When Gallin and co-workers (45) serially evaluated neutrophil chemotactic responsiveness in 10 patients with hyperimmunoglobulin E syndrome, a variable chemotactic response was observed; however, chemotactic responsiveness was either in the lower part of the normal range or depressed below the normal range. In 20 patients with hyperimmunoglobulin E syndrome reported by Buckley and colleagues (19) neutrophil chemotactic abnormality was not a prominent feature.

The molecular basis for depressed chemotaxis in the hyperimmunoglobulin E syndrome has not been defined, and, indeed, abnormal locomotion of phagocytic cells may be a secondary rather than primary dysfunction in these patients.

Lesions in patients with the hyperimmunoglobulin E syndrome do have granulocytes, but, in spite of these cells, there are viable staphylococci in the lesions and infections persist for weeks without specific treatment. It is postulated that delay in granulocyte accumulation may be related to pathogenesis of the lesions. The eventual accumulation of phagocytic cells may prevent systemic spread of the staphylococci but be insufficient to clear organisms and staphylococci or other microbes persist in lesions.

Patients with hyperimmunoglobulin E syndrome generally have onset of severe infection problems during the first weeks or months of life and infections are severe. Lung lesions are especially serious since pneumatoceles develop as a consequence of staphylococcal pneumonia and may persist for months and years. Surgical removal of the affected lung has frequently been necessary.

ANTISTAPHYLOCOCCAL IgE ANTIBODIES

The role of IgE in the pathogenesis of staphylococcal disease in patients with the hyperimmunoglobulin E syndrome was recently investigated. Schopfer and co-workers (89) demonstrated antibodies to *S. aureus* of the IgE class in sera from 7 patients with the hyperimmunoglobulin E syndrome. A radioimmunoassay was used for these studies with *S. aureus* Wood 46 as the solid phase. This particular strain of *S. aureus* was chosen, since it does not possess surface protein A, and, therefore, nonspecific binding of immunoglobulin via the Fc region is less of a technical problem. The patients with hyperimmunoglobulin E included in this study had chronic eczematoid skin lesions, severe recurrent staphylococcal infections, and intermittently depressed chemotaxis as well as serum IgE levels ranging from 4,500 to 17,000 international units. Control patients were healthy blood donors, patients with chronic parasitic infections and elevated IgE levels, and patients with chronic staphylococcal infections with normal levels of serum IgE. There was markedly increased binding of IgE to *S. aureus* Wood 46 in patients with hyperimmunoglobulin E syndrome. The binding percentage of IgE to *S. aureus* ranged from 12% to 32% in patients and less than 5% in healthy controls. Control patients with elevated IgE on the basis of seasonal allergy or parasitic disease had higher levels of IgE binding to *S. aureus* than healthy controls, but there was no overlap in binding percentage in these sera and sera from patients with hyperimmunoglobulin E syndrome. Furthermore, no IgE antistaphylococcal antibody could be detected in patients with chronic staphylococcal infections with normal serum IgE.

It is known that IgE mediates degranulation of mast cells in the presence of specific antibody (54). Histamine, released from mast cells by this mechanism, may inhibit granulocyte chemotaxis and other leukocyte functions and interfere with local defense mechanisms. It is interesting that abscesses in patients with the hyperimmunoglobulin E syndrome are localized primarily in subcutaneous tissue and the lungs, areas particularly rich in mast cells (93).

STAPHYLOCOCCAL ANTIGEN—IgE ANTIBODIES

The finding of increased levels of circulating IgE antistaphylococcal antibodies in patients with hyperimmunoglobulin E syndrome stimulated search for the antigenic specificity of these antibodies using purified cell-wall material from several strains of staphylococci (91). Sera from patients with the hyperimmunoglobulin E syndrome were studied and IgE antibody binding sites on staphylococci were associated with cell-wall peptidoglycan. There was no IgE binding when normal sera were incubated with staphylococcal cell walls, and the patients' IgE did not bind to cell wall preparations from streptococci or *Staphylococcus epidermidis*. Antistaphylococcal IgE antibodies in patients with hyperimmunoglobulin E syndrome therefore appear to have antigenic specificity for *S. aureus* cell-wall structures. Evidence was presented which suggests that these binding sites may be interpeptide bridges of peptidoglycan. This is the first report of specific antibacterial antibodies of the IgE class. Since patients with IgE antistaphylococcal antibodies are unusually susceptible to recurrent severe staphylococcal disease, the possible role of immune dysregulation and excessive amounts of IgE in susceptibility to staphylococcal disease is suggested.

Patients with the hyperimmunoglobulin E syndrome are susceptible to microbial species other than *S. aureus*, and frequently manifest superficial mucous membrane lesions with *C. albicans*. Indeed, this fungal species appears to stimulate immunoglobulin E antibodies in patients with the hyperimmunoglobulin E syndrome (12). Elevated levels of IgE antibodies to *C. albicans* were found in patients with hyperimmunoglobulin E syndrome and partial cross-reactivity between IgE antibodies to *S. aureus* and *C. albicans* was demonstrated. A variety of microbial species may be recovered from lesions in patients with hyperimmunoglobulin E syndrome (19).

LYMPHOCYTE RESPONSE IN HYPERIMMUNOGLOBULIN E SYNDROME

Delayed hypersensitivity skin-test response to several recall antigens was found to be absent in several patients with hyperimmunoglobulin E syndrome (45). Decreased lymphocyte response to antigen stimulation *in vitro* could also be demonstrated, and, in fact, an inverse relationship was found between serum levels of IgE and thymidine incorporation by stimulated lymphocytes. Buckley and Becker (20) also reported that patients with hyperimmunoglobulin E syndrome had depressed response to skin-test antigens and decreased lymphocyte proliferative response to antigens *in vitro*. The synthesis of IgE by leukocytes from patients with hyperimmunoglobulin E syndrome were suppressed by normal mononuclear cells, suggesting that IgE-suppressor activity is abnormal in patients with the hyperimmunoglobulin E syndrome.

PATIENTS WITH INCREASED SERUM IgE WITHOUT SERIOUS INFECTIONS

Antistaphylococcal IgE antibodies have been determined in patients with chronic atopic eczema without serious infections whose skin is heavily colonized with staphylococci (1). These patients may have superficial lesions and elevated serum IgE levels but do not have systemic staphylococcal infections, which characterize patients with the hyperimmunoglobulin E syndrome. The mean antistaphylococcal IgE binding in atopic eczema was 27% (compared with 34% in patients with the hyperimmunoglobulin E syndrome). Therefore, elevated levels of IgE antibodies to staphylococci may be related to increased staphylococcal colinization of skin in patients with eczema, which in turn suggests that IgE antibodies may develop against bacterial antigens as well as allergens in patients with atopic disease. Release of mast-cell histamine as a consequence of staphylococcal-IgE antibody interactions could result in increased neutrophil cyclic 5' AMP and depressed neutrophil locomotion (15). Normal neutrophil chemotaxis (32) and abnormal neutrophil chemotaxis (85) have been described in patients with atopic dermatitis and elevated serum IgE without severe staphylococcal infections, suggesting that patients with atopic disease have transiently abnormal neutrophil locomotion. Depressed neutrophil chemotaxis was found in patients with allergic rhinitis and recurrent staphylococcal furunculosis but only associated with allergic symptoms and not during active staphylococcal infection (52).

ABNORMAL CHEMOTAXIS ASSOCIATED WITH OTHER DISORDERS

Patients with Kartagener's syndrome have a primary defect in neutrophil locomotion (66). This syndrome includes situs inversus and abnormal ciliary function of the respiratory tract, and patients are highly susceptible to recurrent sinusitis and lower respiratory infections. Abnormal respiratory tract ciliary function and abnormal granulocyte chemotaxis may also be found in patients without situs inversus. Eliasson and co-workers (41) termed this constellation of findings immobile cilia syndrome. It seems probable that abnormality of neutrophil locomotion as well as defective ciliary activity may have a common physiological basis. Decreased numbers of microtubules in the pericentriolar region of granulocytes as well as respiratory ciliary cells and sperm cells have been described in patients with immobile cilia syndrome (2). These patients provide evidence that an intact microtubular system is necessary for normal phagocytic cell chemotactic responsiveness.

Hayward and colleagues (48) described abnormal neutrophil chemotaxis in infants with delayed separation of the umbilical cord and recurrent serious bacterial infections. The molecular basis for abnormal granulocyte locomotion was not established; however, ascorbic acid therapy was associated with improved chemotaxis and improvement in clinical response to infections in these infants. We have recently studied a similar patient with delayed cord separation and recurrent severe bacterial infections. The patient's neutrophils had delayed uptake of opsonized bacteria and delayed chemiluminescence and defective killing of bacteria as well as depressed chemotaxis (81).

Abnormal response to chemoattractants has also been described in a patient with defective neutrophil adherence (31). This has been termed Anchor disease, and is believed to be a consequence of absence of a glycoprotein normally present on the surface of neutrophils which is necessary for adherence to surfaces.

Abnormal neutrophil chemotaxis was found in 13 of 14 patients with Schwachman syndrome (3). Patients with this syndrome are susceptible to recurrent staphylococcal infections, pancreatic insufficiency and metaphyseal chondroplasia. The parents of children with Schwachman syndrome also have depressed granulocyte chemotaxis, suggesting this defect may be inherited as a recessive characteristic similar to other features of Schwachman syndrome. Patients with Schwachman syndrome provide additional evidence that abnormal granulocyte chemotaxis may be a primary defect in patients with increased susceptibility to recurrent infections with *S. aureus* and other microbes.

A patient with these clinical and laboratory findings was recently examined in our laboratory and was found to have a delayed granulocyte chemiluminescence response and delayed engulfment of opsonized bacteria in addition to depressed granulocyte chemotaxis. The bacterial infections in this patient included cellulitis and peritonitis with klebsiella and enterococcus and perirectal abscess with pseudomonas as well as enterococcus. Laboratory evaluation of the patient's granulocytes revealed markedly depressed chemotaxis, delayed uptake of opsonized *S. aureus* and *E. coli*, and delayed chemiluminescence after engulfment of opsonized zymosan. The delayed chemiluminescence was similar to that reported with granulocytes from patients with myeloperoxidase deficiency; however, myeloperoxidase activity was normal in this patient's granulocytes. There was normal chemiluminescence response of the patient's granulocytes when exposed to soluble stimulators phorbol myristate acetate (PMA) and calcium ionophore; therefore, the abnormality of granulocyte function appeared to be one of locomotion and engulfment rather than metabolic activity. The delayed chemiluminescence may be a consequence of delayed engulfment of zymosan which participates in the generation of chemiluminescence during phagocytosis.

Transient Disorders of Neutrophil Locomotion

Transient disorders of neutrophil chemotactic responsiveness have been reported in several of the clinical conditions listed in Table 1. For example, a marked depression of neutrophil random and directed locomotion was found in children with measles (8). Chemotactic function of patients' neutrophils returned to normal approximately 10 days after onset of measles, with resolution of the rash and clinical improvement.

Depressed neutrophil chemotaxis has been noted in bone marrow transplant recipients, especially during graft-versus-host reactions or when the patients are receiving antithymocyte globulin (26). Antithymocyte globulin depressed chemotaxis *in vitro*. Bone marrow transplant patients with defective chemotaxis were observed to suffer more severe bacterial infections than patients with normal chemotaxis.

Depressed neutrophil chemotactic responsiveness has been reported in patients with severe bacterial infections, especially when peripheral neutrophils have abnormal morphology such as toxic granules, Döhle bodies or cytoplasmic vacuoles (68). Neutrophil chemotaxis may be increased rather than depressed in usual types of bacterial infections (49). Increased neutrophil chemotactic responsiveness appears to be an early response to infection, which may become depressed in severe overwhelming infection.

Children with severe protein-calorie malnutrition have been reported to have depressed neutrophil locomotion (90). They have increased susceptibility to fungal and viral infections as well as staphylococci. Few polymorphonuclear neutrophil leukocytes (PMN) are present in lesions despite the presence of pyogenic micro-organisms. Since these children also have decreased antibody production, decreased cell-mediated immunity, low levels of complement components, and defective intra-leukocyte killing of bacteria and fungi, the role of phagocytic cell chemotactic defects in their susceptibility to staphylococcal infections is difficult to assess.

INHIBITORS OF NEUTROPHIL LOCOMOTION

Disorders of chemotaxis may be a consequence of circulating inhibitors of leu-kocyte locomotion or inhibitors of serum chemotactic factors. Inhibitors of neutro-phil chemotactic responsiveness have been identified in patients with Hodgkin's disease (98) and with hepatic cirrhosis (38). Patients with these conditions have greatly increased susceptibility to severe staphylococcal disease. Patients with Hodg-kin's disease and cirrhosis are frequently incapable of developing delayed skin hypersensitivity reactions to recall antigens, which may be related to inhibitors that prevent migration of leukocytes to antigenic sites.

An association between the presence of acute illnesses with leukocytosis, negative skin-test response to recall antigens, and a serum chemotaxis inhibitor has been noted (96). Sixteen patients demonstrated this combination of clinical and laboratory findings during illness, with return of normal neutrophil chemotactic activity and skin-test responsiveness when clinical improvement occurred. The serum fractions with inhibitor activity had characteristics associated with immunoglobulin A (IgA).

A patient with chronic mucocutaneous candidiasis had markedly depressed chem-otactic responsiveness of granulocytes suspended in her own plasma but not in control plasma (80). Normal neutrophils were also inhibited by the patient's plasma, and partial characterization of this inhibitor revealed that it had several properties in common with IgG. A 10-year-old black female with onset of eczema in the early months of life, recurrent staphylococcal abscesses, gonococcal conjunctivitis, and repeated episodes of bronchopneumonia was reported with depressed neutrophil chemotaxis (34). The patient's serum IgA was markedly elevated at 1.2 g/ml, and an IgA and IgM containing cryoglobulin was found in the patient's serum. There was no inhibition of chemotactic factors by the patient's serum, and the patient's neutrophil chemotaxis was restored by incubation in control plasma, suggesting a cell-directed inhibitor of chemotaxis.

Children with Wiskott-Aldrich syndrome have plasma which inhibits chemotaxis of normal monocytes (6). Lymphocytes from patients with Wiskott-Aldrich syn-drome produce much more lymphocyte-derived chemotactic factor than normal lymphocytes, and it is postulated that leukocytes in patients with Wiskott-Aldrich syndrome are constantly exposed to high levels of the lymphocyte-derived chem-otactic factor and are "deactivated."

There are several clinical situations that suggest that inhibitors of neutrophil chemotactic responsiveness may perturbate the neutrophil membrane. For example, burn patients frequently demonstrate abnormal granulocyte chemotaxis and serum which inhibits chemotactic responsiveness of neutrophils from control patients.

Circulating factors in the serum of burn patients may inhibit neutrophil chemotaxis by partial degranulation from abnormal chemotaxis, since decreased levels of neutrophil lysozyme and depressed chemotactic responsiveness have been associated in burn patients (35).

A patient with recurrent severe staphylococcal disease with a serum inhibitor of neutrophil response to chemotactic stimulation has been reported recently (63). The patient's neutrophils did not respond to chemotactic stimulation, and serum inhibited chemotactic response of normal neutrophils. A serum factor identified as IgG was cytotrophic for neutrophils and inhibited locomotion but not adherence or metabolic response. The patient had increased numbers of circulating neutrophils instead of the neutropenia that characterizes patients with leukocytic antibodies. The serum factor inhibited locomotion either by oxidizing membrane receptors or causing partial degranulation and deactivation.

Recent studies in our laboratory have provided evidence that neutrophil chemotactic responsiveness may be severely modified by products of inflammation (46). Chemotactic responsiveness of neutrophils was inhibited by extracts of material aspirated from experimental staphylococcal abscesses and from joint fluid of patients with septic arthritis. In addition, bacterial products including lipopolysaccharide, lipoteichoic acid, and extracts from dental plaque were highly inhibitory. Cationic polyelectrolytes and myeloperoxidase (MPO) were inhibitory; however, inhibition was reversible. These findings demonstrate that inflammatory products may influence chemotactic responsiveness and several cellular mechanisms may be involved. These include: a) change in surface charge; b) masking of receptors for chemoattractants; c) protease activity; d) lipid-phospholipid interaction; e) release of granulocyte-immobilizing factors; f) stimulation of granulocyte membranes with inactivation; and g) granulocyte agglutination. When abscess lesions are established, bacterial products and inflammatory factors may have a profound influence on neutrophil function and on local host defense.

DISORDERS OF NEUTROPHIL MICROBICIDAL FUNCTION

Patients with CGD have severe infections accompanied by generalized granulomatous processes and hypergammaglobulinemia. The chemotactic responsiveness of their neutrophils is normal, and capacity to engulf microbes is normal; however, there is defective triggering of oxidative metabolism during infection, and phagocytic cells do not kill intracellular organisms. Viable intracellular bacteria contribute to severe prolonged infectious lesions in these patients (78). Granulomas in patients with CGD consist of mononuclear cells, often containing lipochrome pigment, in juxtaposition with suppurative material in the lymph nodes, skin, lungs, liver, gastrointestinal tract, or bone (64).

METABOLIC ABNORMALITIES IN CGD GRANULOCYTES

The engulfment process in phagocytic cells is associated with increased anaerobic glycolysis and ATP consumption. In addition, there is a burst of respiratory oxidative activity, increased oxygen consumption, and a shift to glucose metabolism via the hexose-monophosphate shunt. In the resting state, only about 1% of glucose is metabolized by the hexose-monophosphate shunt, but during phagocytosis as much as 10% of glucose is oxidized by this route. As glucose is used by the leukocytes, reduced pyridine nucleotides (NADH and NADPH) accumulate, and leukocyte oxidase are activated. Leukocytes from patients with CGD do not respond to phagocytosis with increased oxygen uptake; there is little shift to the hexose-monophosphate shunt, and there is little accumulation of H_2O_2 (53).

Klebanoff (61) demonstrated that H_2O_2 in association with MPO and halide has a potent bactericidal action and suggested that the failure of CGD leukocytes to produce H_2O_2 may be a critical element of their bactericidal defect. Iodination of bacteria within phagocytic vacuoles occurs in normal neutrophils but not in neutrophils from CGD patients.

Diagnosis of CGD is not always confined to the pediatric age group. Several reports of abnormal neutrophil function discovered for the first time in adult patients have been published (11,24,40,47). These adult patients have usually had recurrent severe infections as children, and diagnosis was delayed; however, there appears to be a subgroup of patients with CGD with few infections that are easily controlled with antimicrobial agents. The patients with few infections have abnormal neutrophil function similar to patients with severe infections, which suggests they may have hypertrophy of other host-defense mechanisms such as cell-mediated immunity. Studies of monocyte microbicidal function in patients with CGD have been reported (37,84), and defects of oxidative metabolism and microbial killing are present in these cells as well as neutrophils. Since the monocyte-macrophage system provides back-up host defense in patients with CGD, it will be interesting to compare macrophage function in CGD patients with severe problems with infections with patients with less severe disease.

There is a remarkable lack of infections due to pneumococci and streptococci in patients with CGD, and in the laboratory CGD neutrophils kill these bacteria normally. These bacterial species are catalase-negative and produce H_2O_2; therefore the MPO-halide system is provided with bacterial H_2O_2, and intracellular bacteria are killed (60).

CLINICAL MANIFESTATIONS IN CGD

The areas of the body primarily involved in CGD are those that receive constant challenge from bacteria, such as the skin, lungs, and perianal tissue. The earliest lesions are staphylococcal infections of skin around the ears and nose. These progress to purulent dermatitis and enlarged local lymph nodes. With recurrences, tissue necrosis, granuloma formation, and suppurative adenopathy occur. Hepatosplenomegaly is a constant finding, suggesting spread of bacteria to the reticuloendothelial system (58).

Pulmonary disorders occur in nearly all children with CGD, and include hilar lymphadenopathy, bronchopneumonia, empyema, and lung abscess. Antibiotic treatment does not result in rapid clearing so that lung infiltrates persist for weeks or months. The chest x-ray may show reticulonodular densities, which represent areas of granuloma. In certain patients, areas of bronchopneumonia resolve into discrete areas of consolidation, termed "encapsulating pneumonia"; these are considered distinctive and diagnostic of CGD (102,22).

Gastrointestinal disorders are frequent in patients with CGD. These include obstruction, perianal fistula, vitamin B_{12} malabsorption, and steatorrhea. Rectal and jejeunal biopsies may reveal characteristic histiocytes (7).

Osteomyelitis occurs frequently in CGD, particularly of the small bones of the hands or feet. Although bony enlargement and destruction occur, there is minimal sclerosis, presumably because of the granulomatous cellular response. The bacteria recovered from the bone are similar to those recovered from suppurative lymph nodes or abscesses. Osteomyelitis may develop at multiple sites even during antibiotic therapy, but eventually, after prolonged therapy, complete healing of all affected bones occurs (101).

Patients with CGD are especially susceptible to fungal infections (29). Cohen and co-workers (29) have recently reviewed fungal complications in 245 patients with CGD. They reported 50 CGD patients (20% of those reviewed) with serious and frequently recurrent fungal disease. *Aspergillus* was the fungal species most frequently encountered in these patients and was associated with pneumonia, osteomyelitis, and soft-tissue lesions. *Candida* species and torulopsis were also causes of disseminated infections. The CGD patients responded to antifungal agents, i.e., amphotericin B, 5-flurocytosine, and other agents, and there was evidence in certain patients that granulocyte transfusions were associated with clinical response.

GENETIC ASPECTS OF CGD

The familial nature of CGD was clearly documented in a report of 13 patients with CGD in Los Angeles (23) and in 5 patients in Tennessee (57). When a defect in the bactericidal activity was noted in CGD leukocytes, it became possible to search for heterozygous carriers, since the mothers and some sisters of boys with CGD also have diminished bactericidal function. The NBT reduction test was used to show that mothers, grandmothers, and sisters of affected boys with CGD have abnormal leukocyte metabolism (100). Approximately 50% of the granulocytes of female carriers reduce NBT during phagocytosis, in contrast to 80% to 100% in normal individuals and 5% to 10% in male patients with CGD.

The leukocyte bactericidal defect present *in vitro* is not as profound in female carriers as in boys with the syndrome, but it is clearly distinguishable from the bactericidal activity of fathers and normal controls. In spite of this defect, the mothers of boys with CGD do not show symptoms of the syndrome or unusual susceptibility to infection. However, several of these mothers have demonstrated lesions of the skin diagnosed as discoid lupus erythematosus. The finding of discoid lupus in mothers of 5 patients with CGD suggests an association between autoimmune phenomenon and abnormal leukocyte function (65).

Kell X (K_x) is an antigen on the erythrocytes and leukocytes of all normal persons. Other related antigens are Kell k, K_p^a, and K_p^b. Nine male patients with CGD have been shown to lack any Kell antigen, i.e., $Kell_0$ on their leukocytes (67). The association between absent K_x antigen and a bactericidal defect in CGD is of particular interest, because the genetic loci controlling both reside on the X chromosome. The absence of Kell antigen on the erythrocytes of CGD patients may also influence ability to provide blood transfusion (18).

Female patients with CGD have clinical manifestations similar to those of male patients. Although genetic transmission in females has been postulated to be autosomal recessive, recent evidence using luminol amplified chemiluminescence suggests that female CGD patients may be carriers with extreme Lyonization (74).

LABORATORY FINDINGS

Laboratory findings in CGD include leukocytosis, anemia, elevated sedimentation rate, abnormal chest X-ray, and hypergammaglobulinemia. The leukocytosis is secondary to an increase of juvenile and segmented neutrophils. The anemia is usually microcytic or hypochromic, but occasionally it is normochromic. All three major immunoglobulins are elevated; IgE levels are variably increased. Antibody studies such as isohemagglutinin titers are normal. Skin tests for delayed hypersensitivity are positive (79). The CGD neutrophils demonstrate normal phagocytosis of bacteria but reduced intracellular bactericidal activity. This bactericidal assay remains the definitive diagnostic test for CGD. Eosinophils and mononuclear phagocytic cells in CGD also have abnormal bactericidal activity.

Baehner and Nathan (10) used NBT for a histochemical test to study oxidase activity of leukocytes during phagocytosis. Oxidized NBT is colorless, but when reduced, NBT precipitates in the cytoplasm as blue formazan. Although approximately 80% to 90% of normal leukocytes reduce NBT during phagocytosis of latex particles, only 10% of leukocytes from patients with CGD reduce NBT during phagocytosis. This is a simple and useful screening test for CGD.

A modified NBT procedure has been used to make a prenatal diagnosis of CGD, using fetal blood obtained at amniocentesis (76). Demonstration of an intracellular bactericidal defect is the most definitive laboratory test for diagnosis of CGD.

Allen and co-workers (4) showed that human neutrophils during phagocytosis produce chemiluminescence (chemically produced light). A direct correlation between chemiluminescence and intracellular bacterial killing was suggested when it was demonstrated that CGD granulocytes produced no chemiluminescence during phagocytosis of opsonized bacteria (95). During phagocytosis normal neutrophils and monocytes produce free-oxygen radicals, including singlet oxygen, hydroxyl radicals, superoxide, and hydrogen peroxide. These react with oxidizable substrates on microbes such as unsaturated lipids, nucleic acids, and peptides to form unstable intermediates. When these intermediates return to their ground state, light energy measurable as chemiluminescence is released. Since chemiluminescence is readily measured with a beta scintillation spectrometer, it has become a valuable assay of oxidative metabolism during phagocytosis and an aid in the diagnosis of CGD and in family studies to determine the carrier state (73).

MPO DEFICIENCY

In contrast to CGD neutrophils, oxygen consumption from patients with MPO deficiency and hexose-monophosphate shunt activity during phagocytosis have normal oxygen consumption. Like CGD leukocytes, there was little bacterial iodination and diminished bactericidal activity (53).

An adult male with myelomonocytic leukemia, candidiasis, pneumonia, and MPO deficiency was described by Davis and co-workers (33). His peripheral and bone marrow leukocytes showed no MPO activity. In addition, a partial bactericidal deficiency was present. After a 60-min incubation, few bacteria had been killed by the patient's leukocytes, whereas more than 90% had been killed by normal leukocytes. However, after a 4-hr incubation, the patient's leukocytes killed nearly 90% of the bacteria. Therefore, a decreased rate of intracellular bacteria killing was present, unlike the persistent defect of CGD leukocytes. Alternative intracellular bactericidal mechanisms appear to provide effective although delayed bactericidal capacity in the MPO-deficient leukocytes. Increased levels of H_2O_2 have been demonstrated in the leukocytes from patients with MPO deficiency, suggesting compensatory mechanisms.

Many patients have been identified with congenital MPO deficiency, and most of these patients are well and free from infection. Thus, the delayed-killing defect in MPO deficiency is clearly much less serious than the profound killing defect in granulocytes of CGD patients.

GLUCOSE-6-PHOSPHATE DEHYDROGENASE DEFICIENCY

Cooper and co-workers (30) described a white female with severe infections and complete absence of leukocyte glucose-6-phosphate dehydrogenase (G-6-PD) activity. Phagocytosis of particles by the patient's leukocytes was normal, but was accompanied by minimal stimulation of hexose-monophosphate shunt activity, and less than 25% of normal H_2O_2 production. The patient's leukocytes were unable to kill intracellular bacteria. However, patients with G-6-PD levels that are 25% of normal have normal leukocyte bactericidal activity. Patients with absent G-6-PD have deficient cellular NADH and NADPH, and there was little hexose-mono-phosphate shunt activity or H_2O_2 produced. The G-6-PD-deficient leukocytes do not kill *S. aureus*, *E. coli*, or *Serratia*, but do kill *Streptococcus faecalis* normally, suggesting a leukocyte bactericidal deficiency similar to that in CGD. Thus normal quantities of reduced pyridine nucleotides (NADH + NADPH), as well as oxygen and oxidase activity, may be necessary for normal hexose-monophosphate shunt and bactericidal activity (9).

DEFECTIVE GLUTATHIONE SYSTEM

The glutathione system of phagocytic cells has an essential role for detoxifying the reactive oxygen metabolites that are formed in abundance during phagocytosis.

Therefore, the indentification of a family with neutrophil glutathione reductase deficiency was of great interest (86). Neutrophils from affected members of this family had a normal initial burst of oxidative metabolism during phagocytosis, but after approximately 5 min there was an abrupt halt in metabolism. Neutrophil microbicidal activity was normal, an observation suggesting that the glutathione system may be more important in detoxification of metabolic products than in microbicidal activity. The patients' leukocytes accumulated large amounts of H_2O_2 during phagocytosis, which damaged the cells, and few circulating peripheral neutrophils were present during infections (86).

CHEDIAK-HIGASHI SYNDROME

Studies by Root and co-workers (87) demonstrated defective bactericidal activity in Chediak-Higashi neutrophils. They found that the neutrophils from 2 patients with CHS phagocytized *S. aureus* at normal rates, but there was defective intracellular bacterial killing of *S. aureus*. Streptococci and pneumococci were also killed at a slower rate than normal. The difference in intracellular killing of bacteria by CHS and control leukocytes occurred during the first 20 min of incubation; thereafter, the rate of killing was parallel in patients and controls. These authors also observed that the characteristic cytoplasmic inclusions of CHS leukocytes remain intact after phagocytosis, and, although seemingly incorporated into the phagocytic vacuole, do not discharge their contents into the vacuole. Resting CHS leukocytes had twice normal hexose-monophosphate shunt activity, as measured by oxidation of ^{14}C-glucose. There was a normal burst in oxygen consumption and increased H_2O_2 formation during phagocytosis.

The finding of a defect in intracellular killing despite normal hexose-monophosphate shunt activity suggests that there may be two phases of intracellular killing. The initial phase may be dependent on lysosomal factors (which are compromised in CHS); the late phase may be dependent on the respiratory oxidative response and activation of the MPO-H_2O_2-halide system (which is normal in CHS). The CGD leukocytes have a dual defect with little activation of respiratory metabolism or increase in intracellular H_2O_2, leading to a persistent intracellular killing defect.

Patients with CHS, like patients with CGD, suffer from frequent pyogenic infections. Unlike CGD, the diagnosis of CHS is relatively simple, since the patient's phagocytic cells contain characteristic large cytoplasmic inclusions.

The peripheral neutropenia in patients with CHS may be secondary to increased intramedullary destruction of granulocytes; the hypersplenism may result from the autophagocytic activity. On the basis of striking elevations of serum lysozyme activity and increased numbers of granulocytic precursors in the bone marrow, it has been suggested that an accelerated rate of neutrophil turnover is present in CHS (14).

TUFTSIN DEFICIENCY

Tuftsin deficiency is a congenital familial disorder (or an acquired disorder as a result of splenectomy) characterized by increased susceptibility to infection and defective granulocyte phagocytosis (75).

Tuftsin is a tetrapeptide (threonyl-lysyl-prolyl-arginine) synthesized by the spleen in the form of a cytophilic gammaglobulin termed leukokinin. Leukokinin binds to granulocytes and is cleaved by the granulocyte enzyme leukokininase to form tuftsin. Tuftsin, in turn, enhances the phagocytic ability of granulocytes.

Nine patients from four families have been described with hereditary tuftsin deficiency (75). Clinical findings include respiratory infections (bronchitis, pneumonia, bronchiectasis), enlarged and fluctuant lymph nodes, and seborrheic skin rashes. The usual organisms are *Pneumococcus*, *S. aureus*, and *Candida*. Immunoglobulins, complement, and NBT reduction are normal.

THERAPY IN PATIENTS WITH ABNORMAL GRANULOCYTE FUNCTION

Abnormalities of phagocytic cell chemotactic responsiveness are associated with susceptibility to infections, and although correlation between the phagocyte chemotactic disorder demonstrated *in vitro* and the pathogenesis of infection susceptibility is difficult, the primary clinical problem is prevention of infection and cure of infectious lesions. Vigorous diagnostic measures are needed for identification of infecting agents so that susceptibility to antimicrobial agents can be identified. Serious lesions caused by organisms of low virulence may occur in patients with granulocyte dysfunction.

The skin is frequently the portal of microbial entry since atopy or other underlying disorders of surface integrity are present. Efforts to improve skin health appear to be effective for preventing frequency of lesions, especially in patients with the hyperimmunoglobulin E syndrome. *S. aureus* is a primary pathogen in patients with this syndrome, and improved skin integrity as well as freedom from abscess lesions has coincided with prolonged antistaphylococcal therapy. However, susceptibility to a variety of gram-negative organisms as well as fungal agents prompts caution in this prophylactic approach.

There have been several reports of successful improvement of granulocyte locomotion when levamisole is incubated with abnormal granulocytes *in vitro*. A clinical study involving patients with hyperimmunoglobulin E syndrome has also suggested a role for this immunostimulating drug. The uncertainties about toxic effect from prolonged therapy, however, necessitates carefully controlled trials to determine if benefit outweighs risk. Therapy of patients with disorders of granulocyte function consists essentially of vigorous application of optimal medical and surgical modalities.

Specific therapy for patients with CGD and other phagocytic defects is not yet available. Leukocyte transfusions are only of temporary benefit and thus are used only during emergencies. Nevertheless, they can be life-saving under certain circumstances and can bring about successful control of severe infection (25,29,83,). McCullough and co-workers (69) showed that blood stored under standard blood-bank conditions contains polymorphonuclear leukocytes with excellent bactericidal activity for as long as 48 hr.

The identification of the bactericidal defect in CGD has resulted in a more rational use of antimicrobial therapy in this disease. High-doses of bactericidal antibiotics should be used to treat even mild infection. Prompt and complete surgical drainage of abscesses is essential. Prior to antibiotic therapy, attempts to culture the patient's infecting organisms should be made, so that antibiotic sensitivity can be assured.

Continuous antimicrobial therapy may be of value in the management of certain patients with CGD, especially the younger child with frequent staphylococcal infections (62,69). Johnston and co-workers (59) noted *in vitro* enhancement of bactericidal activity of CGD neutrophils following treatment with sulfisoxazole.

We prefer to stop antibiotics as soon as an infectious lesion is cleared completely, inasmuch as life-threatening infections often are secondary to bacteria resistant to most antimicrobial agents, i.e., *Pseudomonas* or *Aspergillus*. Most life-threatening infections in CGD patients result from delay in diagnosis or treatment.

It is not yet possible to achieve clinical benefit from measures that alter leukocyte metabolism. Although methylene blue increases hexose-monophosphate shunt activity, it has had no clinical benefit. Glucose oxidase is bound to latex particles, which are phagocytized by the CGD leukocytes and increase hexose-monophosphate shunt activity, but this cannot be used clinically (56).

A successful bone marrow transplantation has been accomplished in CGD. The patient, a 2½-year-old boy, was given 5.5×10^6 nucleated marrow cells from an HLA-identical unrelated female donor 4 days after receiving 60 mg/kg of cyclophosphamide (42). Evidence of successful engraftment of donor granulocyte precursors included clinical improvement for over 3 yr, and circulating NBT- positive cells. Aggressive antimicrobial therapy is our present mainstay of therapy, but bone marrow transplantation offers the hope of cure.

REFERENCES

1. Abramson, J. S., Dahl, M. V., Walsh, G., Blumenthal, M. N., Douglas, S. D., and Quie, P. G. (1981): Antistaphylococcal IgE in patients with eczema, hyperimmunoglobulin E and recurrent infections. *J. Am. Acad. Derm.*, (in press).
2. Afzelius, B. A., Ewetz, L., Palmblad, J., Uden, A. M., and Venizelos, N. (1980): Structure and function of neutrophil leukocytes from patients with immobile cilia syndrome. *Acta Med. Scand.*, 208:145–154.
3. Aggett, P. J., Harries, J. T., Harvey, B. A. M., and Foothill, J. F. (1979): An inherited defect of neutrophil mobility in Schwachman syndrome. *J. Pediatr.*, 94:391–394.
4. Allen, R. C., Stjernholm, R. L., and Steele, R. H. (1972): Evidence for the generation of an electronic excitation state in human polymorphonuclear leukocytes and its participation in bactericidal activity. *Biochem. Biophys. Res. Commun.*, 47:679–684.
5. Alper, C. A., Abramson, N., Johnston, R. B., Jr., Jandl, J. H., and Rosen, F. S. (1970): Increased susceptibility to infection associated with abnormalities of complement-mediated functions and of the third component of complement (C3). *N. Engl. J. Med.*, 282:349–358.
6. Altman, L. C., Snyderman, R., and Blaese, R. M. (1974): Abnormalities in chemotactic lymphokine synthesis and mononuclear leukocyte chemotaxis in Wiskott-Aldrich syndrome. *J. Clin. Invest.*, 54:486–493.

7. Ament, M. E., and Ochs, H. D. (1973): Gastrointestinal manifestations of chronic granulomatous disease. *N. Engl. J. Med.*, 288:382–387.
8. Anderson, R., Sher, R., Rabson, A. R., and Koornhof, H. J. (1974): Defective chemotaxis in measles patients. *S. Afr. Med. J.*, 48:1819–1820.
9. Baehner, R. L., Johnston, R. B., Jr., and Nathan, D. G. (1971): Reduction pyridine nucleotide (RPN) content in G-6-PD deficient granulocytes (PMN): An explanation for their defective bactericidal function. *Prog. Am. Soc. Clin. Invest.*, 13:4a.
10. Baehner, R. L., and Nathan, D. G. (1968): Quantitative nitroblue tetrazolium test in chronic granulomatous disease. *N. Engl. J. Med.*, 278:971–976.
11. Balfour, H. H., Shehan, J. J., Speicher, C. E., and Kauder, E. (1971): Chronic granulomatous disease of childhood in a 23-year-old man. *J. A. M. A.*, 217:960–961.
12. Berger, M., Kirkpatrick, C. H., and Gallin, J. I. (1980): IgE antibodies to *Staphylococcus aureus* and *Candida albicans* in patients with hyperimmunoglobulin E and recurrent infections. *J. Immunol.*, 125:2437–2443.
13. Blum, R., Geller, G., and Fish, L. A. (1977): Recurrent severe staphylococcal infections, eczematoid rash, extreme elevations of IgE, Eosinophilia and divergent chemotactic responses in two generations. *J. Pediatr.*, 90:607–609.
14. Blume, R. S., Bennett, J. M., Yankee, R. A., and Wolf, S. M. (1968): Defective granulocyte regulation in the Chediak-Higashi syndrome. *N. Engl. J. Med.*, 279:1009–1015.
15. Bourne, H. R., Melmon, K. L., and Lichtenstein, L. M. (1971): Histamine augments leukocyte adenosine $3'5'$ monophosphate and blocks antigenic histamine release. *Science*, 173:743–745.
16. Boxer, L. A., Watanabe, A. M., Rister, M., Besch, H. R., Jr., Allen, J., and Baehner, R. L. (1976): Correction of leukocyte function in Chediak-Higashi syndrome by ascorbate. *N. Engl. J. Med.*, 295:1041–1045.
17. Bridges, R. A., Berendes, H., and Good, R. A. (1959): A fatal granulomatous disease of childhood: The clinical, pathological and laboratory features of a new syndrome. *Am. J. Dis. Child.*, 97:387–408.
18. Brzica, S. M., Rhodes, K. H., Pineda, A. A., and Taswell, N. F. (1977): Chronic granulomatous disease and the McLeod phenotype: Successful treatment of infection with granulocyte transfusions resulting in subsequent hemolytic transfusion reaction. *Mayo Clin. Proc.*, 52:153–158.
19. Buckley, R. H. (1979): Hyperimmunoglobulin E, undue susceptibility to infection, and depressed immunologic function. In: *Pediatric Immunology*, edited by H. Hodes and B. M. Kagan, pp. 219–232. Science and Medicine, New York.
20. Buckley, R. H., and Becker, W. G. (1978): Abnormalities in regulation of human IgE synthesis. *Immunol. Rev.*, 41:288–314.
21. Buckley, R. H., Wray, B. B., and Belmaker, E. Z. (1972): Extreme hyperimmunoglobulin E and undue susceptibility to infection. *Pediatrics*, 49:59–70.
22. Caldicott, J. H., and Baehner, R. L. (1968): Chronic granulomatous disease of childhood. *Am. J. Roentgenol.*, 103:133–139.
23. Carson, M. J., Chadwick, D. L., Brubaker, C. A., Cleland, R. S., and Landing, B. H. (1965): Thirteen boys with progressive septic granulomatous disease. *Pediatrics*, 34:405–412.
24. Chusid, M. J., Parillo, J. E., and Fauci, A. S. (1975): Chronic granulomatous disease: Diagnosis in a 27-year-old man with mycobacterium fortuitum. *J. A. M. A.*, 233:1295–1296.
25. Chusid, M. J., and Tomasulo, P. A. (1978): Survival of transfused normal granulocytes in a patient with chronic granulomatous disease. *Pediatrics*, 61:556–559.
26. Clark, R. A., Johnson, F. L., Klebanoff, S. J., and Thomas, E. D. (1976): Defective neutrophil chemotaxis in bone marrow transplant patients. *J. Clin. Invest.*, 58:22–31.
27. Clark, R. A., and Kimball, H. R. (1971): Defective granulocyte chemotaxis in the Chediak-Higashi syndrome. *J. Clin. Invest.*, 50:2645–2652.
28. Clark, R. A., Root, R. K., Kimball, H. R., and Kirkpatrick, C. H. (1973): Defective neutrophil chemotaxis and cellular immunity in a child with recurrent infection. *Ann. Intern. Med.*, 78:515–519.
29. Cohen, M. S., Isturiz, R. E., Malech, H. L., Root, R. K., Wilfert, C. M., Gutman, L., and Buckley, R. H. (1981): Fungal infection in chronic granulomatous disease: The importance of the phagocyte in defense against fungi. *Am. J. Med.*, 71:59–66.
30. Cooper, M. R., McCall, C. E., and DeChatelet, L. R. (1971): Stimulation of leukocyte hexose monophosphate shunt activity by ascorbic acid. *Infect. Immun.*, 3:851–853.

31. Crowley, C. A., Curmitte, J. T., Rosin, R. E., Andre-Schwartz, J., Gallin, J. I., Klenysner, M., Snyderman, R., Southwick, R. S., Stossel, T. P., and Babior, B. (1980): An inherited abnormality of neutrophil adhesion. *New Engl. J. Med.*, 302:1163–1168.

32. Dahl, M. V., Cates, K. L., and Quie, P. G. (1978): Neutrophil chemotaxis in patients with atopic dermatitis without infection. *Arch. Dermatol.*, 114:546–554.

33. Davis, A. T., Brunning, R. D., and Quie, P. G. (1971): Polymorphonuclear leukocytes and mye-loperoxidase deficiency in a patient with myelomonocytic leukemia. *N. Engl. J. Med.*, 285:789–790.

34. Davis, A. T., Grady, P. G., Shapiro, E., and Pachman, L. M. (1977): PMN chemotactic inhibition associated with a cryoglobulin. *J. Pediatr.*, 90:225–229.

35. Davis, J. M., Dineen, P., and Gallin, J. I. (1980): Neutrophil degranulation and abnormal chem-otaxis after thermal injury. *J. Immunol.*, 124:1467–1471.

36. Davis, S. D., Schaller, J., and Wedgwood, R. J. (1966): Job's syndrome: Recurrent "cold" staph-ylococcal abscesses. *Lancet*, 1:1013–1015.

37. Davis, W. C., Huber, H., Douglas, S. D., and Fudenberg, H. H. (1968): A defect in circulating mononuclear phagocytes in chronic granulomatous disease of childhood. *J. Immunol.*, 101:1093–1095.

38. DeMeo, A. N., and Anderson, B. R. (1972): Defective chemotaxis associated with a serum in-hibitor in cirrhotic patients. *N. Engl. J. Med.*, 286:735–740.

39. Desnick, R. J., Sharp, H. L., Grabowski, G. A., Brunning, R. D., Quie, P. G., Sung, J. H., Gorlin, R. J., and Ikonne, J. U. (1976): Mannosidosis: Clinical, morphologic, immunologic, and biochemical studies. *Pediatr. Res.*, 10:985–996.

40. Dilworth, J. A., and Mandell, G. L. (1977): Adults with chronic granulomatous disease of child-hood. *Am. J. Med.*, 63:233–243.

41. Eliasson, R., Mossberg, B., Camner, P., and Afzelius, B. A. (1977): The immobile cilia syn-drome: A congenital ciliary abnormality as an etiologic factor in chronic airway infections and male sterility. *N. Engl. J. Med.*, 297:1–6.

42. Foroozonfar, N., Hobbs, J. R., and Hugh-Jones, K. (1977): Bone marrow transplant from an unrelated donor for chronic granulomatous disease. *Lancet*, 1:210–213.

43. Frank, M. M. (1980): Complement mediated defense mechanisms in the immune compromised host. In: *Infections in the Immunocompromised Host—Pathogenesis, Prevention and Therapy*, edited by J. Verhoef, P. K. Peterson, and P. G. Quie, pp. 23–36. Elsevier North-Holland Biomed-ical Press, New York and Amsterdam.

44. Gallin, J. I., Wright, D. G., Fauci, A. S., Rosenwasser, L. J., Chusid, M. J., Taylor, H. A., Thomas, G., Libaers, I., Shapiro, L. J., and Neufeld, E. F. (1976): Defective leukocyte chem-otaxis in mannosidosis. *Clin. Res.*, 24:344A.

45. Gallin, J. I., Wright, D. G., Malech, H. L., Davis, J. M., Klempner, M. S., and Kirkpatrick, C. H. (1980): Disorders of chemotaxis. *Ann. Intern. Med.*, 92:520–538.

46. Ginsburg, I., and Quie, P. G. (1980): Modulation of human polymorphonuclear leukocyte chem-otaxis by leukocyte extracts, bacterial products and polyelectrolyte. *Inflammation*, 4:301–311.

47. Godtfredsen, J., and Koch, C. (1972): Chronic granulomatous disease in a 19-year-old male. *Scand. J. Infect. Dis.*, 4:259–261.

48. Hayward, A. R., Leonard, J., Wood, C. B. S., Harvey, B. A. M., Greenwood, M. C., and Foothill, J. F. (1979): Delayed separation of the umbilical cord, widespread infections and defective neu-trophil mobility. *Lancet*, 1:1099–1101.

49. Hill, H. R., Gerrard, J. M., Hogan, N. A., and Quie, P. G. (1974): Hyperactivity of neutrophil leukotactic responses during active bacterial infection. *J. Clin. Invest.*, 53:996–1002.

50. Hill, H. R., Ochs, H. D., Quie, P. G., Clark, R. A., Pabst, H. F., Klebanoff, S. S., and Wedg-wood, R. J. (1974): Defect in neutrophil chemotaxis in Job's syndrome of recurrent "cold" staph-ylococcal abscesses. *Lancet*, 1:183–187.

51. Hill, H. R., and Quie, P. G. (1974): Raised serum IgE levels and defective neutrophil chemotaxis in three children with eczema and recurrent bacterial infections. *Lancet*, 1:193–197.

52. Hill, H. R., Williams, R. B., Krueger, G. G., and Janis, B. (1976): Recurrent staphylococcal abscesses associated with defective neutrophil chemotaxis and allergic rhinitis. *Ann. Intern. Med.*, 85:39–43.

53. Holmes, B., Page, A. R., and Good, R. A. (1967): Studies of the metabolic activity of leukocytes from patients with a genetic abnormality of phagocytic function. *J. Clin. Invest.*, 46:1422–1432.

54. Ishizaka, T., Ishizaka, K., and Tomioka, H. (1972): Release of histamine and slow reacting substances of anaphylaxis (SRS-A) by IgE anti IgE reactions on monkey mast cell. *J. Immunol.*, 108:513–519.
55. Janeway, C. A., Craig, J., Davidson, M., Downey, V. Y., Gitlin, D., and Sullivan, J. C. (1954): Hypergammaglobulinemia associated with severe recurrent and chronic non-specific infection. *Am. J. Dis. Child.*, 88:388–392.
56. Johnston, R. B.,Jr., and Baehner, R. L. (1970): Improvement of leukocyte bactericidal activity in chronic granulomatous disease. *Blood*, 35:350–355.
57. Johnston, R. B., Jr., and McMurray, J. S. (1967): Chronic familial granulomatosis: Report of five cases and review of the literature. *Am. J. Dis. Child.*, 114:370–378.
58. Johnston, R. B., Jr., and Newman, S. L. (1977): Chronic granulomatous disease. *Pediatr. Clin. North Am.*, 24:365–389.
59. Johnston, R. B.,Jr., Wilfert, C. M., Buckley, R. H., Webb, L. S., DeChatelet, L. R., and McCall, C. E. (1975): Enhanced bactericidal activity of phagocytes from patients with chronic granulomatous disease in the presence of sulphasoxazole. *Lancet*, 1:824–827.
60. Kaplan, E. L., Laxdal, T., and Quie, P. G. (1968): Studies of polymorphonuclear leukocytes from patients with chronic granulomatous disease of childhood: Bactericidal capacity for streptococci. *Pediatrics*, 41:591–599.
61. Klebanoff, S. J. (1971): Intraleukocytic microbicidal defects. *Annu. Rev. Med.*, 22:39–62.
62. Kobayashi, Y., Ameno, D., Ueda, K., Kayosaki, Y., and Usni, T. (1978): Treatment of seven cases of chronic granulomatous disease with sulfamethoxozole-trimethaprim (SMX-TMP). *Eur. J. Pediatr.*, 127:247–254.
63. Kramer, N., Perez, H. D., and Goldstein, I. M. (1980): An immunoglobulin (IgG) inhibitor of polymorphonuclear leukocyte motility in a patient with recurrent infection. *N. Engl. J. Med.*, 303:1253–1258.
64. Landing, B. H., and Shirkey, H. S. (1957): A syndrome of recurrent infection and infiltration of viscera by pigmented lipid histiocytes. *Pediatrics*, 20:431–438.
65. Macfarlane, P. S., Speirs, A. L., and Sommerville, R. G. (1967): Fatal granulomatous disease of childhood and benign lymphocytic infiltration of the skin (congenital dysphagocytosis). *Lancet*, 1:408–410.
66. Malech, H., Englander, L., and Zakhirek, B. (1979): Abnormal polymorphonuclear leukocyte function in Kartagener's syndrome. *Clin. Res.*, 27:290A.
67. Marsh, W. L., Uretsky, S. C., and Douglas, S. C. (1975): Antigens of the Kell blood group system on neutrophils and monocytes: Their relation to chronic granulomatous disease. *J. Pediatr.*, 87:1117–1120.
68. McCall, C. E., Caves, J., Cooper, R., and DeChatelet, L. (1971): Functional characteristics of human toxic neutrophils. *J. Infect. Dis.*, 124:68–75.
69. McCullough, J., Benson, S., Yunis, E. J., and Quie, P. G. (1969): Effect of blood bank storage on leukocyte function. *Lancet*, 2:1333–1337.
70. Miles, A. A., Miles, E. M., and Burke, J. (1957): The value and duration of defense reactions of the skin to the primary lodgment of bacteria. *Br. J. Exp. Pathol.*, 38:79–96.
71. Miller, M. E., Norman, M. E., Koblenzer, P. J., and Schonauer, T. (1973): A new familial defect of neutrophil movement. *J. Lab. Clin. Med.*, 82:1–8.
72. Miller, M. E., Oski, F. A., and Harris, M. B. (1971): Lazy-leukocyte syndrome: A new disorder of neutrophil function. *Lancet*, 1:665–669.
73. Mills, E. L., and Quie, P. G. (1980): Congenital disorders of the functions of polymorphonuclear neutrophils. *Rev. Infect. Dis.*, 2:505–517.
74. Mills, E. L., Rholl, K. S., and Quie, P. G. (1980): X-linked inheritance in females with chronic granulomatous disease. *J. Clin. Invest.*, 66:332–340.
75. Najjar, V. A. (1975): Defective phagocytosis due to deficiencies involving the tetrapeptide tuftsin. *J. Pediatr.*, 87:1121–1124.
76. Newburger, P. E., Cohen, H. J., Rothschild, S. B., Hobbin, J. C., Malawista, S. E., and Mahoney, M. J. (1979): Prenatal diagnosis of chronic granulomatous disease. *N. Engl. J. Med.*, 300:178–181.
77. Pincus, S. H., Thomas, I. T., Clark, R. A., and Ochs, H. D. (1975): Defective neutrophil chemotaxis with variant ichthyosis, hyperimmunoglobulinemia E, and recurrent infections. *J. Pediatr.*, 87:908–911.
78. Quie, P. G. (1969): Chronic granulomatous disease of childhood. *Adv. Pediatr.*, 16:287–300.

79. Quie, P. G. (1975): Pathology of bactericidal power of neutrophils. *Semin. Hematol.*, 12:143–160.
80. Quie, P. G., and Cates, K. L. (1978): Clinical manifestations of disorders of neutrophil chemotaxis. In: *Leukocyte Chemotaxis: Methods, Physiology, and Clinical Implications*, edited by J. I. Gallin and P. G. Quie, pp. 307–328. Raven Press, New York.
81. Quie, P. G., Mills, E. L., Yanai, M., and Abramson, J. (1980): Patients with congenital abnormalities of granulocyte microbicidal function: Clinical and laboratory observations. In: *Primary Immunodeficiencies in Serum, Symposium #16*, edited by M. Seligmann and W. H. Hitzig, pp. 339–351. Elsevier North-Holland Biomedical Press, New York and Amsterdam.
82. Quie, P. G., White, J. G., Holmes, B., and Good, R. A. (1967): In vitro bactericidal capacity of human polymorphonuclear leukocytes: Diminished activity in chronic granulomatous disease of childhood. *J. Clin. Invest.*, 46:668–679.
83. Raubitschek, A. A., Levin, A. S., Stites, D. P., Shaw, E. B., and Fudenberg, H. H. (1973): Normal granulocyte infusion therapy for aspergillosis in chronic granulomatous disease. *Pediatrics*, 51:230–233.
84. Rodey, C. E., Park, B. H., Windhorst, D. B., and Good, R. A. (1969): Defective bactericidal activity of monocytes in fatal granulomatous disease. *Blood*, 33:813–820.
85. Rogge, J. L., and Hanifin, J. M. (1976): Immunodeficiency in severe atopic dermatitis, depressed chemotaxis and lymphocyte transformation. *Arch. Dermatol.*, 112:1391–1396.
86. Roos, D., Weening, R. S., and Loos, I. A. (1979): The protective role of glutathione: The effect of congenital defects of glutathione metabolism on the function of erythrocytes eye lens cells and phagocytic leukocytes. A review and some personal observations. In: *Inborn Errors of Immunity and Phagocytosis*, edited by F. Guttler, J. W. T. Seakins, and R. A. Harkness, pp. 261–268. University Park Press, Baltimore.
87. Root, R. K., Rosenthal, A. S., and Balestra, D. J. (1972): Abnormal bactericidal, metabolic and lysosomal functions in Chediak-Higashi syndrome. *J. Clin. Invest.*, 51:649–665.
88. Rosenfeld, S. I., Kelly, M. E., and Leddy, J. P. (1976): Hereditary deficiency of the fifth component of complement in man. I. Clinical, immunochemical and family studies. *J. Clin. Invest.*, 57:1626–1634.
89. Schopfer, K., Baerlocher, K., Price, P., Krech, U., Quie, P. G., and Douglas, S. D. (1979): Staphylococcal IgG antibodies, hyperimmunoglobulinemia E and *Staphylococcus aureus* infections. *N. Engl. J. Med.*, 300:835–838.
90. Schopfer, K., and Douglas, S. D. (1976): Neutrophil function in children with kwashiorkor. *J. Lab. Clin. Med.*, 88:450–461.
91. Schopfer, K., Douglas, S. D., and Wilkinson, B. J. (1980): Immunoglobulin E antibodies against *Staphylococcus aureus* cell walls in the sera of patients with hyperimmunoglobulin E and recurrent staphylococcal infection. *Infect. Immun.*, 27:563–568.
92. Singh, H., Boyd, E., Hutton, M. M., Wilkinson, P. C., Peebles Brown, D. A., and Ferguson-Smith, M. A. (1972): Chromosomal mutation in bone marrow as cause of acquired granulomatous disease and refractory macrocytic anemia., *Lancet* 1:873–879.
93. Soter, N. A., and Austen, K. F. (1976): The diversity of mast cell derived mediators: Implications for acute, subacute, and chronic inflammatory disorders. *J. Invest. Dermatol.*, 64:313–319.
94. Steerman, R. L., Snyderman, R., Leikin, S. L., and Colten, H. R. (1971): Intrinsic defect of the polymorphonuclear leukocyte resulting in impaired chemotaxis and phagocytosis. *Clin. Exp. Immunol.*, 9:939–946.
95. Stjernholm, R. L., Allen, R. C., and Steele, R. H. (1973): Impaired chemiluminescence during phagocytosis of opsonized bacteria. *Infect. Immun.*, 7:313–314.
96. Van Epps, D. E., Palmer, D. L., and Williams, R. C., Jr. (1974): Characterization of serum inhibitors of neutrophil chemotaxis associated with anergy. *J. Immunol.*, 113:189–200.
97. Van Scoy, R. E., Hill, H. R., Ritts, R. E., and Quie, P. G. (1975): Familial neutrophil chemotaxis defect, recurrent bacterial infections, mucocutaneous candidiasis, and hyperimmunoglobulin E. *Ann. Intern. Med.*, 82:766–771.
98. Ward, P. A., and Bergenberg, J. L. (1974): Defective regulation of inflammatory mediators in Hodgkin's disease: Supernormal levels of chemotactic factor inactivator. *N. Engl. J. Med.*, 290:76–80.
99. Ward, P. A., and Schlegel, R. J. (1969): Impaired leukotactic responsiveness in a child with recurrent infections. *Lancet*, 2:344–347.

100. Windhorst, D. B., Page, A. R., Holmes, B., Quie, P. G., and Good, R. A. (1968): The pattern of genetic transmission of the leukocytes defect in fatal granulomatous disease of childhood. *J. Clin. Invest.*, 47:1026–1034.
101. Wolfson, J. J., Kane, W. J., Laxdal, S. D., Good, R. A., and Quie, P. G. (1969): Bone findings in chronic granulomatous disease of childhood. A genetic abnormality of leukocyte function. *J. Bone Joint Surg. (Am.)*, 51:1573–1583.
102. Wolfson, J. J., Quie, P. G., Laxdal, S., and Good, R. A. (1968): Roentgenologic manifestations in children with a genetic defect of polymorphonuclear leukocyte function: Chronic granulomatous disease of childhood. *Radiology*, 91:37–48.

Advances in Host Defense Mechanisms, Vol. 1,
edited by John I. Gallin and Anthony S. Fauci,
Raven Press, New York © 1982.

Antibiotic-Neutrophil Interactions in Microbial Killing

Edward L. Yourtee and Richard K. Root

*Department of Internal Medicine, Section of Infectious Diseases, Yale University
School of Medicine, New Haven, Connecticut 06510*

Phagocytic cells play a pivotal role in determining the outcome of most bacterial and some fungal infections. Since antibiotics and other antimicrobials are the mainstay of treatment of such infections, their potential interactions with phagocytic cells, especially neutrophils, have come under increasing scrutiny. This review summarizes the available information on the interaction of various antimicrobials with human phagocytic cells *in vitro* and *in vivo* and, where possible, relates it to the treatment of infection. Attention will be focused on the polymorphonuclear neutrophilic leukocyte (PMN), although abundant reference will be made to other phagocytic cell types.

Antibiotics can affect the interaction of leukocytes with microbes in several ways. Perhaps the most recognizable way clinically is through antibiotic-induced neutropenia, a topic beyond the scope of this review. Second, phagocytes may provide a protected environment for some microbes, in which the phagocyte itself is unable to kill the bacteria, yet antibiotics are either unable to reach the bacteria or are inactivated in the intracellular milieu. Third, antibiotics may affect phagocytes directly, either potentiating or inhibiting their migratory, phagocytic, and microbicidal functions. Finally, antibiotics may modify the microbe itself so that its phagocytosis and killing by neutrophils is altered.

This review will focus on these last three topics. In instances where information on neutrophils is unavailable, we will cite data obtained from the study of other phagocytic cells, or occasionally "nonprofessional" phagocyte systems. This is done with the proviso that there is no warranty of similarity between cell types in their interactions with antibiotics and microbes, and that an unknown degree of error is inherent in attributing to human neutrophils the phenomena observed in other cell types.

METHODOLOGIC CONSIDERATIONS

The encounter of a neutrophil with a microbe is functionally divided into the phases of attraction, binding, ingestion, and killing (112). Much of the confusion and contradiction in the early literature on antibiotic-phagocyte interactions in bacterial killing is the result of a failure to make a clear distinction between these phases with the use of appropriate experimental methodology.

For instance, visual evaluation of phagocytosis has been commonly used, yet such assays are notoriously difficult, and accuracy is limited both by the inability to distinguish between cell-bound and ingested microorganisms, and by the inability to accurately quantitate intracellular microbes. Likewise, estimation of phagocytic rates from the reduction in viable extracellular bacteria in incubation mixtures with cells does not distinguish between alterations due to phagocytosis and intracellular killing per se, and may be further confounded by factors such as intracellular multiplication of bacteria with consequent cell rupture and microbial release. In recent years the use of radiolabeled bacteria to measure cellular uptake has overcome some of these difficulties (112).

These methodologic problems in estimation of phagocytosis are paralleled by problems in the quantitation of bacterial killing. Accurate measurements of intracellular killing based on the recovery of live bacteria from phagocytic cells may be difficult because of the incomplete removal of noningested bacteria. When the investigation concerns the effects of antibiotics, killing or inhibition of growth of extracellular bacteria by the antibiotic may result in fewer bacteria available for ongoing phagocytosis, thus spuriously lowering the intracellular bacterial population. These difficulties, particularly vexing in long-term cell cultures, have been repeatedly recognized and forgotten (14,63,98). The most successful approaches to circumvent these problems have included the use of obligate intracellular parasites (20,55), the use of tissue culture medium which does not favor bacterial growth (81), or the use of enzymes such as lysostaphin (28,116) to destroy extracellular bacteria. Alternatively, bacterial killing may be assessed only during the lag period before bacterial division resumes (1–3).

A critical reading of experimental papers dealing with antibiotic-microbe-neutrophil interactions must include an evaluation of the above-mentioned problems. The ideal experiments are those which discriminate effects due to alterations in phagocytosis from those due to modification of killing of intracellular microbes.

The study of phagocyte chemotaxis also carries unique methodologic pitfalls. The plethora of techniques for evaluating neutrophil locomotion has been extensively described and reviewed (41,132). Most reports evaluating antibiotic effects have used the measurement of the net movement of a population of neutrophils. The advance of neutrophils through a semisolid medium may be quantitated (the under-agarose technique), or the migration through a micropore filter evaluated (Boyden-chamber technique). Variations of the latter include determining the distance moved in a specified time (leading front); measuring the accumulation of neutrophils at the opposite side of the filter; or measuring the accumulation of PMNs on a second filter beneath the first (either visually or by accumulation of ^{51}Cr-labeled PMNs). Each of these techniques carries its own technical hazards and problems in reproducibility; clearly, also, each method relies on a somewhat different interplay of neutrophil adherence, deformability, and speed of movement. Comparisons of results obtained by different methods are therefore hazardous, and the difficulty is compounded by the lack of a standardized method for reporting results and by the variety of chemotactic attractants (synthetic chemotactic peptides, endotoxin-treated serum, bacterial culture filtrates) used.

ANTIBIOTIC ENTRY INTO PHAGOCYTES

The initial observation of the protection from extracellular factors afforded by the intraphagocytic environment was made by Rous and Jones (102) in 1916 with the demonstration that *Bacillus typhosus* within guinea pig neutrophils were protected from the bactericidal action of serum. An important extension of such observations to antibiotics was made by Holmes and co-workers (54) who noted that staphylococci ingested by neutrophils from patients with chronic granulomatous disease (CGD) (congenitally defective in staphylocidal ability) were protected from the bactericidal action of extracellular penicillin and streptomycin. From their studies it was unclear whether this protection derived from a failure of the antibiotic to penetrate the cell, or from an arrest of the bacterial growth and division required for penicillin action (52). As it has turned out, both elements may be important. A summary of our current understanding of antibiotic penetration into phagocytes is presented in Table 1.

Penicillin

It was shown in 1956 that gonococci phagocytized by HeLa cells were not susceptible to killing by low concentrations of extracellular penicillin (117). Alexander and Good (5) later demonstrated that despite an initial additive effect on killing, PMNs protected staphylococci from the action of penicillin. Since these observations, it has been repeatedly demonstrated that, once ingested by PMNs,

TABLE 1. *Entry of some antibiotics into phagocytic cells[a]*

Poor[b]	Good[c]
Penicillins (13,61,72,79,93)	Tetracycline (13,30,61)
Cephalosporins (61,93)	Chloramphenicol (61,93)
Streptomycin (14,30)	Erythromycin (61,93)
Gentamicin (120)	Clindamycin (61,93)
Spectinomycin (18)	Rifampin (61,79,93)
Paraaminosalicylic acid (107)	Polymyxin B (13)
	Isoniazid (61,107)
	Cycloserine (107)
	Pyrazinamide (107)
	Ethambutol (61,93)

[a]Only those antibiotics which have been specifically studied are listed. References are noted in parentheses.

[b]Intracellular concentrations < 50% of simultaneous extracellular concentrations.

[c]Intracellular concentrations ≥ 100% of extracellular concentrations.

staphylococci are protected not only from penicillin (13,28) but also from cefazolin (28), and from combinations of penicillin and gentamicin (111) or penicillin and streptomycin (110). Similarly, *Escherichia coli* within macrophages are protected from ampicillin (68).

Initial efforts to quantitate penicillin entry into HeLa cells using ^{35}S-penicillin demonstrated a failure of these cells to concentrate the antibiotic (27). Later, using elegant techniques to discriminate between ^{14}C-penicillin in extracellular water and that in a PMN pellet, Mandell (79) found that all of the cell-associated penicillin was, in fact, in the extracellular water, i.e., no clear proof of PMN intracellular uptake of the drug could be found.

In the same studies, Mandell also noted that staphylococci within neutrophils bound only 13% as much penicillin as extracellular bacteria did (79). Subsequent investigators found that in the absence of phagocytosis, intracellular ^{14}C-penicillin concentration in mouse peritoneal macrophages was 13% of extracellular concentration (72). In these latter studies, the lack of an effect of metabolic inhibitors on penicillin uptake was interpreted as evidence that penicillin diffuses passively into cells. A rapid initial absorption, with a subsequent slow rise to a plateau, was found, followed by a rapid loss of penicillin when the drug was removed from the surrounding medium (72).

More recently, limited evidence suggests that the small amounts of penicillin that penetrate cells during phagocytosis can be bactericidal for bacteria that ordinarily might multiply within phagocytes. For example, in one study as little as 0.4 μg/ml of penicillin led to measurable inhibition of growth of gonococci within human PMNs (122). Similarly, others have shown that *Listeria monocytogenes* within activated macrophages is susceptible to penicillin when the extracellular concentration of penicillin is 3 to 4 times the minimum inhibitory concentration (MIC) (21). Division of *Salmonella typhosa* within a mouse fibroblast culture was halted promptly when penicillin was added to the medium (108).

Thus, it appears that penicillin enters cells poorly, and that penicillin activity against intracellular bacteria can be easily demonstrated only against bacteria that can multiply within cells.

Aminoglycosides

Considerable interest was initially focused on the penetration of streptomycin into cells because of its usefulness in suppressing bacterial overgrowth in tissue cultures. It was originally believed that streptomycin in low concentrations did not penetrate macrophages in culture and therefore did not inhibit intracellular tubercle bacilli (116), *Brucella* (74), or *Salmonella typhimurium* (29). However, it became apparent that high concentrations of streptomycin would inhibit these organisms (40,73,90,106), as well as other bacteria within fibroblasts (108), macrophages (13,59), and neutrophils (28). Streptomycin was also demonstrated to inhibit intracellular growth of *Pasturella tularensis* in alveolar macrophages (87) and *Mycobacterium lepraemurium* in tissue culture (20), two systems in which the bacteria are unable to grow extracellularly.

Quantitation of the relative protection from streptomycin afforded by an intracellular location within phagocytes was obtained by measuring the MIC for intracellular *Mycobacterium tuberculosis*; this was 200-fold higher than the MIC for extracellular organisms (107,115).

Direct measurement of streptomycin levels intracellularly has been performed only for macrophages. Bioassays of cellular lysates after a brief exposure to streptomycin (3 to 6 hr) demonstrated negligible (14) or low (30) intracellular levels, although after 24 hr the intracellular concentration was found to be twice that of the medium, and after 7 days it was five times that of the surroundings (12). Autoradiography localized its intracellular distribution to the cytoplasm (12), and cell fractionation studies of rat fibroblasts suggested that streptomycin is concentrated within lysosomes (119).

Phagocytes provide relative protection against a variety of other aminoglycoside antibiotics as well. Phagocytes protect bacteria against gentamicin in some studies (68,120), although not in others (13,28); the intracellular concentration of ^{14}C-gentamicin is about 20% of that in serum (120). Spectinomycin fails to kill intracellular gonococci (18).

Other Antimicrobials

Certain other antibiotics appear to penetrate phagocytes well and to exert an antimicrobial action within cells. The penetration of tetracycline into cells has been documented by the demonstration of fluorescence of PMN nuclei following antibiotic exposure (89). After incubation of human PMNs in tetracycline for 3 hr, intracellular concentrations range from 74% (13) up to 250% of extracellular levels (30). Other studies demonstrate that tetracycline may not penetrate into phagosomes of guinea pig peritoneal macrophages, since *E. coli* located in phagosomes will not fluoresce, unless the phagocytic cell dies (25). However, tetracycline inhibited division of *S. typhimurium* within macrophages (29).

Chloramphenicol enters fibroblasts readily to cure experimental rickettsial infections (55) or arrest division of salmonella (29,108). Brucella within human phagocytes appear to be protected at least partially from killing by chloramphenicol, although the experimental design did not permit evaluation of bacteriostatic activity (74). Radiolabeled chloramphenicol appears to be concentrated within human neutrophils by about twofold above extracellular levels (93).

Among the antituberculous drugs, INH, cycloserine, and pyrazinamide all showed an increase in the MIC for *M. tuberculosis* when it was in the intracellular as opposed to an extracellular location in a HeLa cell model (107,114). Conversely, paraaminosalicylic acid (PAS) has a markedly increased MIC for intracellular tubercle bacilli compared to its MIC for extracellular organisms (107). Radiolabeled ethambutol is concentrated approximately sevenfold in human neutrophils (93).

Particular interest has centered on rifampin, a highly lipid-soluble drug. Rifampin readily kills intracellular staphylococci (28,80,111) and *E. coli* (68) at 37° C, although it appears to be inactive against intracellular staphylococci at 5°C, despite being concentrated to twice the extracellular concentration (79,93).

A method has recently been developed for the measurement of radiolabeled intracellular antibiotics, using rapid separation of neutrophils from incubation medium by centrifugation through a layer of silicone oil (61). Observations with this technique indicate that erythromycin and clindamycin are both markedly concentrated within human neutrophils (65,93). It has been suggested that this may be a means of delivering these antibiotics to sites of infection (65).

ANTIBIOTIC INACTIVATION BY PHAGOCYTES

There is a paucity of data regarding the question of antibiotic inactivation by phagocytes. For example, although gentamicin is known to be inactive at the acid pH (104) that prevails in neutrophil phagosomes (60,78), there is no good data available to indicate an actual loss of its biologic activity within phagocytes, nor its chemical degradation. Cephalosporins and penicillins have been shown to be inactivated by human pus, but this appears to result from the accumulation of bacterial beta-lactamase in the exudate (16). Gentamicin is also inactivated in human pus, by reversibly binding to chromatin DNA liberated during neutrophil death and lysis (15,121). Neither of these mechanisms appears to apply to the possible inactivation of these antibiotics within neutrophils, however, and the significance of these observations to the activity of these drugs in clinical situations remains to be determined.

ANTIBIOTIC MODIFICATION OF LEUKOCYTES

Chemotactic Response

Some antibiotics have been shown to stimulate chemotaxis of neutrophils (Table 2). Bacitracin is a chemoattractant for rabbit peritoneal PMNs, and competes with radiolabeled chemoattractant peptides such as F-Met-Leu-Phe for the same membrane receptor (8). Chloramphenicol was noted to stimulate chemotaxis at a variety of concentrations (76), although in another laboratory chloramphenicol depressed chemotaxis (36). Nafcillin at low concentrations stimulated chemotaxis, although at suprapharmacologic concentrations it had an inhibitory effect (76).

A number of authors have reported that tetracyclines at therapeutic concentrations inhibit both chemotaxis and random migration *in vitro* (10,31,36,45,75,76,81) and for up to 48 hr after *in vivo* administration (especially with doxycycline) (10,81). Effects on chemotaxis persist far longer than detectable amounts of tetracycline in the serum (10). *In vivo* patch tests with an irritant demonstrate that oral tetracycline administration decreases the local inflammatory response, a crude functional assay of multiple aspects of the inflammatory response (92). In one study, however, in which mycoplasma antigen was used as the chemoattractant, tetracycline was found to stimulate chemotaxis in concentrations from 30 to 300 μg/ml, independent of the presence of serum (81).

Neutrophils washed free of tetracycline display normal chemotactic behavior (75). The addition of tetracycline to a chemoattractant mixture (after incubation of serum

TABLE 2. *Direct effects of some antibiotics on neutrophil function*[a]

Function	Increase	Decrease	No effect
Chemotaxis	Nafcillin (76)	Tetracyclines (10,31,36,45,75, 76,81)	Penicillin G (31,36,42)
	Bacitracin (8) Lincomycin (42)	Rifampin (36,49)	Oxacillin (76) Cephalosporins (36,76,77)
	Clindamycin (42,76) Chloramphenicol (76)	Clindamycin (31) Chloramphenicol (36)	Clindamycin (36) Chloramphenicol (42)
		Erythromycin (31)	Erythromycin (36,42)
		Gentamicin (47, 64,105)	Gentamicin (36,76)
		Amphotericin B (11)	Colistin (36) Sulfonamides (31,36) 5FC (11) Miconazole (11)
Phagocytic activity		Tetracyclines (37,46,84)	Tetracycline (53)
		Polymyxin B (24)	Cephalosporins (83)
		Amphotericin B (19)	Gentamicin (83,105) Trimethoprim (83) Rifampin (53) Polymyxin B (53)
Oxidative metabolism		Tetracyclines (103)	Tetracycline (82)
		Sulfonamides (66)	Sulfonamides (82)
		Polymyxin B[b] (9)	Polymyxin B (24)
		Amphotericin B (11)	Chloramphenicol (62,67,82) Gentamicin (105) 5FC (11) Miconazole (11)
Microbicidal activity		Sulfonamides (66) Aminoglycosides (32)	

[a]Only those antibiotics which have been both specifically studied and the effects noted at usual therapeutic concentrations are listed. See text for details. References are noted in parentheses. Where conflicting data exist, multiple entries for the antibiotic are listed, with references.
[b]Blocks activation of neutrophils by endotoxin-activated serum.

with endotoxin to generate chemoattractants) was found to decrease the chemotaxis of normal neutrophils (75). This study was interpreted as demonstrating binding of chemoattractants by tetracycline; it is not evident, however, whether adequate controls were performed to exclude cation chelation or an effect of residual tetracycline in the chemoattractant mixture on the PMNs during migration.

The effect of tetracycline has been hypothesized to be secondary to chelation of divalent cations (48,76). Experimental support for this concept comes from the demonstration that inhibition of leukocyte migration by tetracycline was reversed by cation ionophores, which permit free entry of Ca^{2+} into the cell (48). These by cation ionophores, which permit free entry of Ca^{2+} into the cell (48). These data support the hypothesis that the effect of tetracycline is due to chelation of intracellular Ca^{2+}.

Other drugs have been noted to depress chemotaxis, including erythromycin (31) and clindamycin (31), although this effect has not been seen in other laboratories (36). Likewise, amphotericin B caused reversible inhibition of PMN chemotaxis in one study (11). A variety of other antibiotics tested, including cephalosporins, penicillins, and sulfonamide derivatives all appear to have no effect on chemotaxis at levels therapeutically achievable (31,36,42,76,77).

The effect of aminoglycosides on chemotaxis is less clear. In general, chemotaxis is unchanged (76) or only slightly decreased (47,105) by solutions of gentamicin or amikacin powders, but a significant decrease in chemotaxis attributable to the preservative in parenteral gentamicin has been seen (47,64). Cells obtained after the administration of parenteral gentamicin in one study showed decreased chemotaxis, increased random movement, and increased PMN adherence (64).

Rifampin has been found to decrease chemotaxis (36,49). Curiously, however, rifampin also is capable of reversing the "deactivation" of chemotaxis seen with very high concentrations of synthetic chemoattractants, suggesting a possible competition for chemoattractant receptors (49).

Phagocytic Activity

The phagocytosis of microorganisms usually depends on the interplay of serum factors which coat the organism (opsonins) and the activity of the phagocytic cells themselves. Antibiotics could affect either of these phases by altering the organism or the phagocyte. The discussion below will be centered on the latter possibility (Table 2).

Considerable attention has focused on the effects of tetracycline on phagocytosis, although engulfment and attachment have not been clearly separated in the interpretations. In an early study, rats with upper respiratory infections were noted to have increased clearance of bloodstream particulates by the reticuloendothelial system; this heightened activity was abolished by the administration of tetracycline (7). An *in vitro* study measuring the removal of viable *S. aureus* by human PMNs failed to show an effect of tetracycline on phagocytosis (53). However, visual assays of cell-associated bacteria (phagocytosis) have shown that tetracycline and doxycycline inhibit the phagocytosis of yeast and *E. coli in vitro* (37,46,84); a similar result was seen when uptake of radiolabeled bacteria was used (83). This inhibition was noted even when the neutrophils were preincubated with tetracycline and then washed, implying that the effect is not reversible (37). Decreased phagocytosis has also been noted in leukocytes from donors who had taken oral tetracycline (37). Scanning electron micrographs of doxycycline-treated neutrophils showed that the PMN surface was smoother than normal, with fewer pseudopods than normal cells, and that bacteria tended to adhere to the cell surface rather than actually being ingested (46). No reports have directly addressed the possible significance for phagocytosis of cation chelation by tetracycline. The clinical consequences of these *in vitro* observations remain to be established.

Scattered reports indicate a depressive effect of certain other antibiotics on phagocytosis. Bacitracin and polymyxin in massive doses (24) led to decreased phagocytosis of *S. aureus* and latex by guinea pig PMNs in a visual assay; in these cells, bacteria were found to be attached to the periphery of cells rather than spread throughout the cytoplasm. At therapeutic levels, however, polymyxin and rifampin were found not to alter engulfment of pneumococci and *E. coli*, respectively (53). Amphotericin B at 1 μg/ml has also been shown to inhibit phagocytosis of *Candida* by neutrophils (19). The mechanism of these effects has yet to be elucidated.

Postphagocytic Events

Degranulation

Some antibiotics may be capable of inhibiting postphagocytic lysosomal fusion (degranulation). The only report in this regard pertains to chloramphenicol in massive amounts (1,000 μg/ml or more) and its effects on cultured human monocytes (88). Although exposure of the cells to these concentrations of chloramphenicol caused decreased digestion of phagocytized *Candida*, the clinical importance of this observation is not likely to be significant because of the dosages used.

Polymyxin B can modify a related phenomenon, the extracellular release of lysosomal enzymes from neutrophils which results when PMNs are exposed to endotoxin-activated serum (9). Pretreatment of neutrophils with polymyxin B protects the PMNs from activation by endotoxin in serum. As a consequence, polymyxin B inhibits both the release of lysosomal enzymes and the associated activation of the hexose-monophosphate shunt under these conditions (9). Whether this phenomenon influences neutrophil bactericidal capacity for gram-negative bacilli remains to be investigated.

Neutrophil Metabolism and Microbicidal Activity

Antibiotics may affect other postphagocytic events, including metabolism and microbicidal mechanisms. The effects of antibiotics on the postphagocytic metabolic events in PMNs have been examined in a variety of ways (Table 2). In some cases, effects have been demonstrable only at antimicrobial levels far in excess of those achieved therapeutically.

For example, chemiluminescence is depressed by amphotericin B at levels of 5 μg/ml (11). *In vitro*, tetracycline causes a decrease in the maximal nitroblue tetrazolium (NBT) response of human PMNs (103). The importance of these observations, however, is uncertain.

More quantitative measures of the respiratory burst of phagocytic cells have also been used. Oxygen uptake by guinea pig peritoneal exudate PMNs following phagocytosis was slightly decreased by massive amounts of polymyxin B (24). Chloramphenicol at high concentrations (6 mM, or 1,940 μg/ml) markedly inhibited postphagocytic oxygen uptake by neutrophils, although the effect was not demonstrable at 0.2 mM concentrations (62,67). Other workers have found the oxidative burst to be less sensitive to chloramphenicol suppression, with measurable effects seen only at concentrations of 10 mM (82). Tetracycline and sulfisoxazole failed to show a similar effect (82).

More detailed studies of the components of the oxidative burst have shown that iodination of *Candida* can be inhibited by sulfonamides at 50 to 500 μg/ml, and that these drugs also block the candidacidal activity of a cell-free system of myeloperoxidase (MPO), potassium iodide, and hydrogen peroxide (66). This inhibition was not demonstrable with MPO-deficient PMNs, implying a specific action of sulfonamides on MPO-mediated reactions. The candidacidal activity of PMNs is also reduced by aminoglycosides, although the mechanisms of this effect are not known (32). Activation of the hexose-monophosphate shunt appears also to be affected by certain antibiotics. Chloramphenicol in high concentrations (3.5 mM) impaired the oxidation of $1\text{-}^{14}C$-glucose in conjunction with suppression of oxygen consumption by human PMNs (67). The primary site of action of the antibiotic in the oxygen metabolic pathways was not clarified, however.

Energy metabolism may also be affected by antimicrobials. Tetracycline (300 μg/ml) was reported to increase lactate production, although no alteration of glucose uptake could be detected in human PMNs (81). Conversely, production of lactate was unaffected by massive doses of polymyxin B (in guinea pig peritoneal exudate neutrophils) or chloramphenicol (in human PMNs) (24,82). Mitochondrial synthesis of cytochrome C in fibroblast cultures has been demonstrated to be decreased by both chloramphenicol and tetracycline (91). Ascorbic acid content of leukocytes may fall in conjunction with oral tetracycline therapy, although the significance of this is uncertain (130).

Thus, the overall evidence suggests that a variety of antibiotics can modify neutrophil metabolism *in vitro*, but that these effects are not demonstrable at antibiotic concentrations usually attained *in vivo*. The relevance of these observations to neutrophil microbicidal functions *in vivo* remains uncertain at present.

ANTIBIOTIC EFFECTS ON COMPLEMENT ACTIVATION

Although not strictly an aspect of leukocyte function, complement activation is a crucial step in promoting opsonization as well as the formation of potent chemotactic factors from the complement cascade. Several antimicrobials appear capable of inhibiting activation of the complement pathways (Table 3). For instance, sulfadiazine, tetracycline, and gentamicin have all been shown to inhibit the alternate complement pathway *in vitro* (4). Such inhibition might significantly impair the ability of the host to generate chemotactic and opsonic factors in clinical situations, although this remains to be proven.

In addition, the bactericidal action of serum for *E. coli*, which requires activation of complement through the lytic steps, is inhibited by tetracycline and doxycycline (35,123). This effect is reversible when Mg^{2+} (required for alternate complement

TABLE 3. *Modification of microbial interaction with complement by antibiotics[a]*

Function	Increase	Decrease	No effect
Complement activation		Sulfonamides (4) Tetracyclines (4) Gentamicin (4)	
Susceptibility to complement-mediated lysis[b]	Ampicillin (39)	Ampicillin (70)	Ampicillin (33,118)
	Polymyxins (22,33, 95,113,118)	Chloramphenicol (123)	Penicillin[c] (131)
			Carbenicillin (33)
	Rifampin (6)	Tetracyclines (34,35,123)	Cephalothin (33)
			Aminoglycosides (33,118)

[a]Only those antibiotics that have been specifically studied are listed.
[b]Refers to lysis of gram-negative bacilli except as noted.
[c]Tested against *S. aureus*.

pathway activation) is added to the incubation medium. Similarly, following oral administration of doxycycline, human serum permitted a 55-fold greater survival of a serum-sensitive *E. coli* than was seen before antibiotic administration (34). Serum bactericidal activity against *E. coli* is also inhibited by chloramphenicol (123). Thus, antibiotics may be able to inhibit microbicidal mechanisms that supplement the PMN in eradicating infection.

ANTIBIOTIC EFFECTS ON MICROBE-LEUKOCYTE INTERACTIONS

In addition to their effects on PMNs and serum factors, antibiotics may alter bacteria so that they are made more susceptible to PMN attack (Table 4). Antibiotic treatment of bacteria may increase their sensitivity to serum bactericidal mechanisms, increase the efficiency of opsonization, alter their rate of phagocytosis, or modify intracellular survival within PMNs.

Sensitivity to Serum Bactericidal Mechanisms

Antibiotics that act on the bacterial surface have been implicated in altering bacterial susceptibility to complement (Table 3). Polymyxins, which act at the level of the bacterial membrane, have been most thoroughly investigated. Colistin and polymyxin B are synergistic with serum in killing serum-sensitive *E. coli* (22), or even serum-resistant *E. coli* (118), *S. typhimurium* (95), and *Proteus mirabilis* (113). Although this effect is attributable to increased susceptibility to serum lysozyme for some organisms (33,95), low concentrations of polymyxin also sensitize lysozyme-resistant gram-negative bacilli to complement-mediated lysis via the alternative pathway (33). No change in C3b deposition on the polymyxin-treated bacteria could be demonstrated by a hemagglutination assay, suggesting that the

TABLE 4. *Modification of specific microbe-phagocyte interactions by antibiotics*[a]

Function	Increase	Decrease	No Effect

Phagocytosis
Opsonization
	Group A streptococci
	  Lincomycin (43)
	  Clindamycin (43)
	  Erythromycin (42)
	Group B streptococci
	  Beta-lactams (56,57)
	  Vancomycin (57)
			Group A streptococci
			  Penicillin (42)
			  Chloramphenicol (42)

Ingestion	Group A streptococci, *S. pneumoniae*
	  Lincomycin (42)
	  Clindamycin (42)
	S. aureus
	  Nafcillin (38)
	E. coli
	  Gentamicin (1)
	  Streptomycin (3)
	  Polymyxin B (1)
	P. aeruginosa
	  Carbenicillin (86)
	L. monocytogenes
	  Ampicillin (2)
	  Chloramphenicol (2)
	  Tetracycline (2)
	B. recurrentis
	  Penicillin (17)
			Group A streptococci, *S. pneumoniae*
			  Penicillin (42)
			  Erythromycin (42)
			  Chloramphenicol (42)
			
			S. aureus
			  Beta-lactams (71,100)
			  Vancomycin (100)
			P. aeruginosa
			  Gentamicin (86)

Killing	*S. aureus*
	  Beta-lactams (100)
	  Vancomycin (100)
	Group A streptococci
	  Penicillin (44)
	S. pneumoniae, S. sanguis
	  Beta-lactams (58)
	
	E. coli
	  Chloramphenicol (94,96)
	  Gentamicin (96)
	B. fragilis
	  Chloramphenicol (96)
		S. aureus
		  oxacillin (71)
			S. aureus
			  Tetracycline (99)
			  Chloramphenicol (99)
			  Erythromycin (99)
			  Clindamycin (99)
			  Gentamicin (100)
			
			E. coli
			  Beta-lactams (96)

Susceptibility to lysozyme	Group A streptococci
	  Penicillin (44)
	S. pneumoniae, S. fecalis, S. aureus
	  Nafcillin (126)
	N. Catarrhalis
	  Polymyxin B (129)
	K. pneumoniae, S. typhimurium
	  Polymyxin B (33,95)
			S. aureus
			  Oxacillin (126)
			  Cephalothin (126)
			  Vancomycin (126)
			N. catarrhalis
			  Nafcillin (126)

[a]Those antibiotics which have been found to alter certain interactions of specific bacteria with leukocytes are listed next to the organism studied. References are noted in parentheses. In many cases sub-MIC concentrations of the antibiotic have been used to pretreat the bacteria. See text for details.

mechanism may be independent of a major increase in attachment of complement factors to the organisms (33).

The effect of the penicillins is less clear-cut. Ampicillin and the related compound, cyclacillin, at sub-MIC concentrations were found to increase the sensitivity of *E. coli* to lysis mediated by antibody and complement or by immunized murine spleen cells (39). However, in other work, ampicillin, carbenicillin, and cephalothin failed to increase the serum sensitivity of a variety of serum-resistant gram-negative bacilli (33,118). In fact, the filamentous or rounded forms of various gram-negative rods produced by growth in sub-MIC concentrations of ampicillin demonstrated decreased sensitivity to killing by serum or blood (70).

In contrast, sub-MIC concentrations of penicillin make some streptococci more sensitive to killing by serum, even when complement has been inactivated by heating (69). Work from our own laboratory, however, indicates that staphylococci treated with sub-MIC concentrations of penicillin are not rendered susceptible to lysis by complement even during PMN attack, and are opsonized by classical complement pathway mechanisms in the same manner as untreated bacteria (131).

Rifampin, an antibiotic not acting on the bacterial surface, has been reported to be capable of converting a serum-resistant strain of *E. coli* to a serum-susceptible form (6). Whether this is a general phenomenon with this antibiotic has not been investigated. Aminoglycoside antibiotics such as kanamycin and gentamicin appear not to confer increased serum sensitivity on gram-negative bacilli (33,118).

It should be noted that antibiotics and complement can interact in the converse manner too: complement can alter the effectiveness of antibiotics. In some cases, complement appears to render bacteria more permeable to antibiotics (26), whereas serum antagonizes the bactericidal activity of polymyxin for *Pseudomonas aeruginosa* (22).

Phagocytosis

A variety of data are available regarding the phagocytosis of antibiotic-treated organisms. Altered phagocytosis may reflect either altered opsonization or modified interaction of antibiotic-treated organisms with host phagocytic cells. Where possible, we will distinguish between these two events in reviewing the literature on this subject (Table 4).

Opsonization

Opsonization, the coating of microbes with serum factors prior to ingestion, markedly facilitates their attachment to phagocytes as the initial phase in engulfment (112). Opsonization is a crucial part of the humoral support system for phagocytic functions. Antibody and complement are the best known opsonins, although other serum factors, including fibronectin (23), are under active investigation.

Antibiotics have the potential to modulate the opsonic process at several levels. Antibiotics could alter the deposition of opsonins on the bacterial surface by direct interaction with the opsonic proteins, by modification of the reactions that lead to attachment of opsonins to the bacterial surface, or by removing (or exposing) opsonin-binding (or inhibiting) molecules associated with the bacterial surface. Alternatively, antibiotics might be able to block or otherwise alter the PMN surface receptors for C3b and for the F_c portion of IgG (51,109).

Data for the above possibilities are sparse. We have already cited information regarding some interactions of antibiotics with the complement system. We are unaware of any data which demonstrate that antibiotics modify PMN surface receptors. On the other hand recent data indicate that antiphagocytic factors may be released from the surface of certain organisms following treatment with antimicrobials.

For instance, in the case of group A streptococci bearing an antiphagocytic M protein, exposure of organisms to sub-MIC concentrations of clindamycin makes them more susceptible to phagocytosis, in association with a loss of several surface antigens, including the antiphagocytic M protein (42,43). These organisms also appear to activate complement more efficiently, suggesting indirectly the possibility of enhanced opsonization (42,43). Similarly, pneumococci treated with lincomycin show a reduction in their polysaccharide capsule (42). In extensive work with group B streptococci, Horne and Tomasz (56) have shown that penicillin pretreatment caused release of type-specific capsular material; this effect was blocked by simultaneous chloramphenicol treatment. Enhanced PMN killing could be correlated with the loss of capsular material; phagocytosis and killing were not evaluated separately in this work, however (56). This effect has also been shown with a variety of other cell-wall-active antibiotics, including cephalosporins, cefoxitin, and vancomycin (57).

Phagocytic Uptake

Although pretreatment of other organisms with antimicrobials has been shown to modify phagocytosis, the mechanisms are less clearly related to opsonization per se. Mouse peritoneal macrophage monolayers demonstrated increased ingestion and killing of *E. coli* when the organisms were pretreated with sub-MIC concentrations of polymyxin, gentamicin, or streptomycin (1,3). Pretreatment of *Pseudomonas aeruginosa* with sub-MIC concentrations of carbenicillin permitted increased uptake (measured as killing) of bacteria by rabbit PMNs; gentamicin failed to produce this effect (86).

The effect of antibiotics on staphylococci has depended on the mode of pretreatment. In one study, treatment with sub-MIC nafcillin, but not with other beta-lactam antibiotics, caused a marked enhancement of killing of staphylococci by mouse peritoneal macrophages (38). In contrast, in another study brief treatment of stationary phase *S. aureus* with erythromycin, clindamycin, or chloramphenicol permitted increased phagocytosis by rabbit alveolar macrophages, whereas no effect was seen with penicillin or cephalothin (50).

Certain staphylococci, however, which display "tolerance" to the bactericidal but not to the bacteriostatic actions of penicillins, have been noted to release excessive amounts of lipoteichoic acid into the medium during antibiotic treatment; this lipoteichoic acid has been shown to impair phagocytic uptake (97). These findings suggest that tolerant strains might be ingested less well under conditions of antibiotic treatment. This possibility has not yet been investigated.

Finally, reports from our laboratory (100) and others (71) indicate that sub-MIC penicillin treatment, although potentiating PMN-killing, fails to alter phagocytic uptake of staphylococci. Limited data are available for other organisms, as well. For instance, phagocytosis of ³H-labeled *Listeria monocytogenes* by cultured human monocytes was enhanced by pretreatment of the bacteria with sub-MIC concentrations of ampicillin, chloramphenicol, or tetracycline (2). In another investigation, *Borrellia recurrentis* was demonstrated within neutrophils with much greater frequency during treatment with penicillin, but whether this represented increased uptake of viable organisms, or simply phagocytosis of dead spirochetes was not defined (17).

The clinical significance of these *in vitro* observations of antibiotic potentiation of phagocytosis has not been investigated, but in the case of organisms for which the mechanism has been clarified, some advantage for those compounds which modify the bacterial surface is suggested.

Modified Susceptibility to Intracellular Killing

Antibiotic pretreatment can enhance killing of bacteria by phagocytes (Table 4). Certain antibiotics have been found to sensitize bacteria to the action of lysozyme present in serum as well as in the phagolysosomes of neutrophils. For instance, polymyxin at 0.5 μg/ml will sensitize serum-resistant *Klebsiella* to lysozyme (33), and both colistin and polymyxin will increase the sensitivity of *S. typhimurium* to lysozyme (95). Polymyxin also renders *Neisseria catarrhalis* sensitive to lysozyme (129) (Table 4).

Nafcillin at sub-MIC concentrations will sensitize *S. aureus* to lysozyme (124) and also to the action of trypsin (125). Concurrent suppression of bacterial protein synthesis with chloramphenicol antagonized the expression of the nafcillin effect (127). These effects are not seen following treatment with oxacillin, despite a similar MIC for staphylococci, nor with cephalothin or vancomycin (125,126). Curiously, however, oxacillin produced a decreased sensitivity to lysozyme in *S. aureus* allowed to reach stationary phase by prolonged growth in sub-MIC oxacillin (128). Among cell-wall-active antibiotics, then, nafcillin appears to have a unique effect on the staphylococcal cell surface which is dependent on continued bacterial protein synthesis. The clinical importance of this effect is not known, nor is it known if this increased susceptibility to lysozyme is important in killing of nafcillin-treated staphylococci by neutrophils.

Antibiotics can enhance bacterial killing by neutrophils in other ways, however. Brief exposure of *E. coli* to high concentrations of chloramphenicol, for instance, causes a pronounced lag period before regrowth of the culture begins, provided that antibody, complement, and neutrophils are present. In the absence of any of these factors, regrowth proceeds without a lag period (94). This suppression of regrowth may indicate enhanced killing of chloramphenicol-altered bacteria by the leukocytes during the immediate postantibiotic phase (94).

Pretreatment with high concentrations of chloramphenicol or gentamicin has also been demonstrated to enhance the killing of *E. coli* by acetate extracts of neutrophil granules; this effect was not observed following pretreatment with cell-wall-active antibiotics (96). However, neutrophil extracts kill group A streptococci pretreated with penicillin more effectively than untreated organisms (44).

Investigation of the *in vivo* consequences of antibiotic-enhanced killing of bacteria by neutrophils has been conducted with *Proteus* species (85). Despite similar sensitivities to carbenicillin, some strains of *Proteus mirabilis* are rendered more susceptible to the action of serum and neutrophils than other strains by treatment with sub-MIC concentrations of carbenicillin. Those bacteria that demonstrated increased sensitivity to serum and PMNs were cleared more rapidly from the blood in experimental bacteremia in rabbits treated with carbenicillin. This suggests the *in vitro* actions of cell-wall-active antibiotics on some gram-negative bacteria may have *in vivo* significance.

The effect of sub-MIC concentrations of antibiotics on neutrophil killing of gram-positive cocci has been investigated in depth in our laboratory. Our data indicate that treatment of gram-positive cocci with sub-MIC concentrations of cell-wall-active antibiotics enhances susceptibility to 'ntracellular killing by human neutrophils. For example, pretreatment of *S. aureus* 502A with ¼ MIC of beta-lactam antibiotics or vancomycin did not alter the rate of uptake of radiolabeled bacteria by PMNs, but did significantly increase the rate of killing (100). This enhanced susceptibility to killing was pronounced to the point that organisms were killed readily even without phagosome formation, i.e., in cytochalasin-B-treated PMNs (100). This effect has been demonstrated to require opsonization with serum, as well as binding between bacteria and neutrophils (100). Enhanced killing was not seen when bacteria were grown in sub-MIC concentrations of gentamicin, tetracycline, chloramphenicol, erythromycin, or clindamycin (99,100). Similar results have been obtained for pneumococci, as well as for autolysin-defective organisms (mutant pneumococci, *Streptococcus sanguis*) (58).

Investigation of the mechanism by which the neutrophil kills these pretreated bacteria has been undertaken. The penicillin effect on staphylococci was preserved even when oxidative killing mechanisms were blocked with azide (which inhibits MPO) or were intrinsically defective (as in patients with CGD or MPO deficiency) (101). In contrast, when streptococci (catalase-negative) were the test organisms, treatment of neutrophils with azide abolished the penicillin enhancement of killing; likewise, enhanced killing was not demonstrable with MPO deficient cells or CGD cells (58). Thus, it appears that the enhancement of bacterial killing by PMNs by penicillin pretreatment is not dependent on a cooperative interaction with bacterial autolytic enzymes. Furthermore, penicillin-treated catalase-negative organisms (i.e., streptococci) appear to be more susceptible to oxygen-dependent killing mechanisms of the PMN, whereas staphylococci (catalase-positive) are rendered more susceptible to the nonoxygen-dependent mechanisms.

The possible cooperative role of complement and neutrophils in the killing of penicillin-treated bacteria has also been investigated (131). Results indicate that enhanced killing of treated staphylococci can be demonstrated even when opsonization is impaired by heat inactivation of serum, by the use of C2-deficient or C4-deficient serum, or by the use of trypan blue to block the PMN C3b receptor, although complete omission of opsonins abolishes all PMN killing. Furthermore, serum deficient in C5 or C8 does permit penicillin-enhanced killing, indicating that penicillin treatment does not enhance complement-induced bacterial lysis during neutrophil attack (131).

These data contrast with the recently reported findings of Lorian and Atkinson (71). Using staphylococci prepared on agar-membrane surfaces with prolonged sub-MIC oxacillin treatment, they have found that neutrophil killing of treated bacteria is poorer than killing of control bacteria, although bacterial uptake by neutrophils is unaffected. The discrepancy between these results and those cited above appears to be a consequence of the method of bacterial preparation; the technique used in the work of Lorian and Atkinson (71) yields multiseptate clusters of bacteria, in which bacteria in the center of the cluster are protected from neutrophil bactericidal activity.

Overall, however, it appears that relatively brief periods of treatment of bacteria with sub-MIC concentrations of cell-wall-active antibiotics enhance susceptibility to neutrophil killing. Although it seems likely that this is a direct consequence of antibiotic alteration of the bacterial cell wall, the nature of the structural changes induced which permit this altered susceptibility remains to be defined.

CONCLUSION

The interactions of antibiotics with bacteria and host defenses are multifaceted and complex. As this review illustrates, many aspects of these interactions have only begun to be explored, and far more questions have been raised than have been answered by the data available to date. The host of possible combinations of significant factors has been met with an equally diverse array of investigative techniques and models. Although provocative observations have been made, they defy easy integration with each other.

Nevertheless, the investigation of antibiotic-neutrophil-bacteria interactions can shed light on the mechanisms of action of various antibiotics on different microbes which might have clinical relevance. Furthermore, they may provide a powerful tool with which to enhance our understanding of the normal mechanisms of chemotaxis, phagocytosis, and neutrophil bactericidal activity.

These investigations may reveal principles necessary to construct rational therapeutic strategies for infections, both in conventional situations and in situations in which host defenses are impaired. Finally, they also may stimulate the development of *in vitro* testing of antimicrobial action to more appropriately reflect the *in vivo* events. The further study of these phenomena could thus permit major advances both in understanding basic host-defense physiology as well as in devising new approaches for the management of infectious diseases.

ACKNOWLEDGMENTS

This work was funded in part by National Institutes of Health Training Grant (#5-T32-AI-7033) and United States Public Health Service Grant (#5 RO1-AI13251).

REFERENCES

1. Adam, D., Phillip, P., and Belohradsky, B. H. (1971): Studies on the influence of host defense mechanisms on the antimicrobial effect of chemotherapeutic agents. Effect of antibiotics on phagocytosis of mouse peritoneal macrophages *in vitro*. *Aerztl. Forsch.*, 25:181–184.
2. Adam, D., Schaffert, W., and Marget, W. (1974): Enhanced *in vitro* phagocytosis of *Listeria monocytogenes* by human monocytes in the presence of ampicillin, tetracycline, and chloramphenicol. *Infect. Immun.*, 9:811–814.
3. Adam, D., Staber, F., Belohradsky, B. H., and Marget, W. (1972): Effect of dihydrostreptomycin on phagocytosis of mouse peritoneal macrophages *in vitro*. *Infect. Immun.*, 5:537–541.
4. Alexander, J. W. (1975): Antibiotic agents and the immune mechanisms of defense. *Bull. N. Y. Acad. Med.*, 51:1039–1045.
5. Alexander, J. W., and Good, R. A. (1968): Effect of antibiotics on the bactericidal activity of human leukocytes. *J. Lab. Clin. Med.*, 71:971–983.
6. Alexander, J. W., Cobbs, C. G., and Curtiss, R. (1980): Modification of bacterial serum susceptibility by rifampin. *Infect. Immun.*, 28:923–926.
7. Altura, B. M., Hershey, S. G., Ali, M., and Thaw, C. (1966): Influence of tetracycline on phagocytosis, infection and resistance to experimental shock: relationship to microcirculation. *J. Reticuloendothel. Soc.*, 3:447–457.
8. Aswanikumar, S., Schiffman, E., Corcoran, B. A., Pert, C. B., Morrell, J. L., and Gross, E. (1978): Antibiotics and peptides with agonist and antagonist chemotactic activity. *Biochem. Biophys. Res. Commun.*, 80:464–471.
9. Bannatyne, R. M., Harnett, N. M., Lee, K-Y., and Biggar, W. D. (1977): Inhibition of the biologic effects of endotoxin on neutrophils by polymyxin B sulfate. *J. Infect. Dis.*, 136:469–474.
10. Belsheim, J., Gnarpe, H., and Persson, S. (1979): Tetracyclines and host defense mechanisms: interference with leukocyte chemotaxis. *Scand. J. Infect. Dis.*, 11:141–145.
11. Bjorksten, B., Ray, C., and Quie, P. G. (1976): Inhibition of human neutrophil chemotaxis and chemiluminescence by amphotericin B. *Infect. Immun.*, 14:315–317.
12. Bonventre, P. F., and Imhoff, J. G. (1970): Uptake of ³H-dihydrostreptomycin by macrophages in culture. *Infect. Immun.*, 2:89–95.
13. Brown, K. N., and Percival, A. (1978): Penetration of antimicrobials into tissue culture cells and leukocytes. *Scand. J. Infect. Dis.*, (Suppl.) 14:251–260.
14. Brumfitt, W., Glynn, A. A., and Percival, A. (1965): Factors influencing the phagocytosis of *E. coli. Br. J. Exp. Pathol.*, 40:213–226.
15. Bryant, R. E., and Hammond, D. (1974): Interactions of purulent material with antibiotics used to treat Pseudomonas infections. *Antimicrob. Agents Chemother.*, 6:702–707.
16. Bryant, R. E., Rashad, A. L., Mazza, J. A., and Hammond, D. (1980): β-lactamase activity in human pus. *J. Infect. Dis.*, 142:594–601.
17. Butler, T., Aikawa, M., Habte-Michael, A., and Wallace, C. (1980): Phagocytosis of *Borrelia recurrentis* by blood polymorphonuclear leukocytes is enhanced by antibiotic treatment. *Infect. Immun.*, 28:1009–1013.
18. Casey, S. G., Veale, D. R., and Smith, H. (1979): Demonstration of intracellular growth of gonococci in human phagocytes using spectinomycin to kill extracellular organisms. *J. Gen. Microbiol.*, 113:395–398.
19. Chan, C. K., and Balish, E. (1978): Inhibition of granulocyte phagocytosis of *Candida albicans* by amphotericin B. *Can. J. Microbiol.*, 24:363–364.
20. Chang, Y. T. (1969): Suppressive activity of streptomycin on the growth of *Mycobacterium lepraemurium* in macrophage cultures. *Appl. Microbiol.*, 17:750–754.

21. Cole, P., and Brostoff, J. (1975): Intracellular killing of *Listeria monocytogenes* by activated macrophages (Mackaness system) is due to antibiotic. *Nature (London)*, 256:515–517.
22. Davis, S. D., Iannetta, A., and Wedgwood, R. J. (1971): Paradoxical synergism and antagonism between serum and antibacterial activity of colistin. *J. Infect. Dis.*, 123:392–398.
23. Doran, J. E., Mansberger, A. R., and Reese, A. C. (1980): Cold insoluble globulin-enhanced phagocytosis of gelatinized targets by macrophage monolayers: a model system. *J. Reticuloendothel. Soc.*, 27:471–483.
24. Downey, R. J., and Pisano, J. C. (1965): Some effects of antimicrobial compounds on phagocytosis *in vitro*. *J. Reticuloendothel. Soc.*, 2:75–88.
25. DuBuy, H. G., Riley, F., and Showacre, J. L. (1964): Tetracycline fluorescence in permeability studies of membranes around parasites. *Science*, 145:163–165.
26. Dutcher, B. S., Reynard, A. M., Beck, M. E., and Cunningham, R. K. (1978): Potentiation of antibiotic bactericidal activity by normal human serum. *Antimicrob. Agents Chemother.*, 13:820–826.
27. Eagle, H. (1954): The binding of penicillin in relation to its cytotoxic action. III. The binding of penicillin by mammalian cells in tissue culture (HeLa and L strains). *J. Exp. Med.*, 100:117–124.
28. Easmon, C. S. F. (1979): The effect of antibiotics on the intracellular survival of *Staphylococcus aureus in vitro*. *Br. J. Exp. Pathol.*, 60:24–28.
29. Ekzemplyarov, O. N. (1966): Effect of tetracycline, chloramphenicol, monomycin, and streptomycin on *S. typhimurium* after phagocytosis by macrophages. *Fed. Proc.* (Transl. Suppl.), 25:T309–T312.
30. Ekzemplyarov, O. N. (1966): Penetration of tetracycline and streptomycin into macrophages cultured *in vitro*. *Fed. Proc.* (Transl. Suppl.), 25:T312–T314.
31. Esterly, N. B., Furey, N. L., and Flanagan, L. E. (1978): The effect of antimicrobial agents on leukocyte chemotaxis. *J. Invest. Dermatol.*, 70:51–55.
32. Ferrari, F. A., Pagani, A., Marconi, M., Stefanoni, R., and Siccardi, A. G. (1980): Inhibition of candidacidal activity of human neutrophil leukocytes by aminoglycoside antibiotics. *Antimicrob. Agents Chemother.*, 17:87–88.
33. Fierer, J., and Finley, F. (1979): Lethal effect of complement and lysozyme on polymyxin-treated, serum-resistant gram-negative bacteria. *J. Infect. Dis.*, 140:581–589.
34. Forsgren, A., and Gnarpe, H. (1973): Tetracycline interference with the bactericidal effect of serum. *Nature (New Biol.)*, 244:82–83.
35. Forsgren, A., and Gnarpe, H. (1973): Tetracyclines and host defense mechanisms. *Antimicrob. Agents Chemother.*, 3:711–715.
36. Forsgren, A., and Schmeling, D. (1977): Effect of antibiotics on chemotaxis of human leukocytes. *Antimicrob. Agents Chemother.*, 11:580–584.
37. Forsgren, A., Schmeling, D., and Quie, P. G. (1974): Effect of tetracycline on the phagocytic function of human leukocytes. *J. Infect. Dis.*, 130:412–418.
38. Friedman, H., and Warren, G. H. (1974): Enhanced susceptibility of penicillin-resistant staphylococci to phagocytosis after *in vitro* incubation with low doses of nafcillin. *Proc. Soc. Exp. Biol. Med.*, 146:707–711.
39. Friedman, H., and Warren, G. H. (1976): Antibody-mediated bacteriolysis: enhanced killing of cyclacillin-treated bacteria. *Proc. Soc. Exp. Biol. Med.*, 153:301–304.
40. Frost, A. J., Smith, H., Witt, K., and Keppie, J. (1972): The chemical basis of the virulence of *Brucella abortus*. X. A surface virulence factor which facilitates intracellular growth of *Brucella abortus* in bovine phagocytes. *Br. J. Exp. Pathol.*, 53:587–596.
41. Gallin, J. I., and Quie, P. G., editors (1978): *Leukocyte Chemotaxis*. Raven Press, New York.
42. Gemmell, C. G., and Abdul-Amir, M. K. (1980): Antibiotic-induced changes in streptococci with respect to their interaction with human polymorphonuclear leukocytes. In: *Current Chemotherapy and Infectious Disease*, edited by J. D. Nelson and C. Grassi, Vol. II, pp. 810–812. American Society for Microbiology, Washington, D. C.
43. Gemmell, C. G., Peterson, P. K., Schmeling, D., and Quie, P. G. (1980): *In vitro* phagocytosis of *Streptococcus pyogenes*: its potentiation by clindamycin. *Clin. Res.*, 28:369A.
44. Ginsburg, I., Neeman, N., Ephrati, C., Sela, M. N., Bierkenfeld, L., Kutani, D., and Lahav, M. (1977): Further studies on the bactericidal and bacteriolytic effects of human leukocyte extracts: modulation by antibodies, cationic proteins, lysozyme, antibiotics and by autolytic systems and the role played by some of these factors in the extraction of lipoteichoic acids from bacteria.

In: *Movement, Metabolism, and Bactericidal Mechanisms of Phagocytes,* edited by F. Rossi, P. Patriarca, and D. Romeo, pp. 323–334. Piccin Medical Books, Padua.

45. Gnarpe, H., and Belsheim, J. (1978): Tetracyclines and host defense mechanisms. Doxycycline polymethaphosphate sodium complex (DMSC) compared to doxycycline with regard to influence on some host defense mechanisms. *Microbios,* 22:45–49.

46. Gnarpe, H., and Leslie, D. (1974): Tetracyclines and host defense mechanisms. Doxcycline interference with phagocytosis of *Escherichia coli. Microbios,* 10A:127–138.

47. Goodhart, G. L. (1977): Effect of aminoglycosides on the chemotactic response of human polymorphonuclear leukocytes. *Antimicrob. Agents Chemother.,* 12:540–542.

48. Goodhart, G. L. (1979): Further evidence for the role of bivalent cations in human polymorphonuclear leukocyte locomotion: recovery from tetracycline-induced inhibition by the presence of cation ionophores. *J. Reticuloendothel. Soc.,* 25:545–554.

49. Gray, G. D., Knight, K. A., and Talley, C. A. (1980): Rifampin has paradoxical effects on leukotaxis. *Fed. Proc.,* 39:878.

50. Hand, W. L., Thompson, N. K., and Johnson, J. D. (1980): Alveolar macrophage interactions with antibiotics and bacteria. In: *Progr. Abstr. 20th Intersci. Conf. Antimicrob. Agents Chemother.,* Abstr. 725. American Society for Microbiology, Washington, D. C.

51. Henson, P. M. (1976): Membrane receptors on neutrophils. *Immunol. Commun.,* 5:757–774.

52. Hobby, G. L., Meyer, K., and Chaffee, E. (1942): Observations on the mechanism of action of penicillin. *Proc. Soc. Exp. Biol. Med.,* 50:281–285.

53. Hoeprich, P. D., and Martin, C. H. (1970): Effect of tetracycline, polymyxin B, and rifampin on phagocytosis. *Clin. Pharmacol. Ther.,* 11:418–422.

54. Holmes, B., Quie, P. G., Windhorst, D. B., Pollara, B., and Good, R. A. (1966): Protection of phagocytized bacteria from the killing action of antibiotics. *Nature (London),* 210:1131–1132.

55. Hopps, H. H., Jackson, E. B., Danauskas, J. X., and Smadel, J. E. (1959): Study on the growth of rickettsiae. IV. Effect of chloramphenicol and several metabolic inhibitors on the multiplication of *Rickettsia tsutsugamushi* in tissue culture cells. *J. Immunol.,* 82:172–181.

56. Horne, D., and Tomasz, A. (1980): Effect of penicillin on killing of group B streptococcus by human neutrophils. In: *Current Chemotherapy and Infectious Disease,* edited by J. D. Nelson and C. Grassi, Vol. II, pp. 1127–1129. American Society for Microbiology, Washington, D. C.

57. Horne, D., and Tomasz, A. (1980): Increased susceptibility of beta-lactam treated group B streptococci to the bactericidal effect of human neutrophils. In: *Progr. Abstr. 20th Intersci. Conf. Antimicrob. Agents Chemother.,* Abstr. 585. American Society for Microbiology, Washington, D. C.

58. Isturiz, R., Metcalf, J. A., and Root, R. K. (1980): Augmented killing of streptococci by human neutrophils after penicillin pretreatment. *Clin. Res.,* 28:512A.

59. Jenkins, C., and Benacerraf, B. (1960): *In vitro* studies on the interaction between mouse peritoneal macrophages and strains of *Salmonella* and *Escherichia coli. J. Exp. Med.,* 112:403–417.

60. Jensen, M. S., and Bainton, D. F. (1973): Temporal changes in pH within the phagocytic vacuole of the polymorphonuclear neutrophilic leukocyte. *J. Cell Biol.,* 56:379–388.

61. Johnson, J. D., Hand, W. L., Francis, J. B., King-Thompson, N., and Corwin, R. W. (1980): Antibiotic uptake by alveolar macrophages. *J. Lab. Clin. Med.,* 95:429–439.

62. Kaplan, S. S., Perille, P. E., and Finch, S. C. (1969): The effect of chloramphenicol on human leukocyte phagocytosis and respiration. *Proc. Soc. Exp. Biol. Med.,* 130:839–843.

63. Kapral, F. A., and Shayegani, M. G. (1959): Intracellular survival of staphylococci. *J. Exp. Med.,* 110:123–138.

64. Khan, A. J., Evans, H. E., Glass, L., Khan, P., Chang, C. T., and Nair, C. R. (1979): Abnormal neutrophil chemotaxis and random migration induced by aminoglycoside antibiotics. *J. Lab. Clin. Med.,* 93:295–300.

65. Klempner, M. S. (1980): Human neutrophils as an antibiotic delivery mechanism for clindamycin. In: *Progr. Abstr. 20th Intersci. Conf. Antimicrob. Agents Chemother.,* Abstr. 727. American Society for Microbiology, Washington, D. C.

66. Lehrer, R. I. (1971): Inhibition by sulfonamides of the candidacidal activity of human neutrophils. *J. Clin. Invest.,* 50:2498–2505.

67. Lehrer, R. I. (1973): Effects of colchicine and chloramphenicol on the oxidative metabolism and phagocytic activity of human neutrophils. *J. Infect. Dis.,* 127:40–48.

68. Lobo, M. C., and Mandell, G. L. (1973): The effect of antibiotics on *Escherichia coli* ingested by macrophages. *Proc. Soc. Exp. Biol. Med.,* 142:1048–1050.

69. Lorian, V., and Atkinson, B. (1978): Effect of serum on gram-positive cocci grown in the presence of penicillin. *J. Infect. Dis.*, 138:865–871.

70. Lorian, V., and Atkinson, B. (1979): Effect of serum and blood on Enterobacteriaceae grown in the presence of subminimal inhibitory concentrations of ampicillin and mecillinam. *Rev. Infect. Dis.*, 1:797–806.

71. Lorian, V., and Atkinson, B. (1980): Killing of oxacillin-exposed staphylococci in human polymorphonuclear leukocytes. *Antimicrob. Agents Chemother.*, 18:807–813.

72. Lowrie, D. B., Aber, V. R., and Carrol, M. E. W. (1979): Division and death rates of *Salmonella typhimurium* inside macrophages: use of penicillin as a probe. *J. Gen. Microbiol.*, 110:409–419.

73. Mackaness, G. B. (1952): The action of drugs on intracellular tubercle bacilli. *J. Pathol. Bacteriol.*, 64:429–446.

74. Magoffin, R. L., and Spink, W. W. (1951): The protection of intracellular Brucella against streptomycin alone and in combination with other antibiotics. *J. Lab. Clin. Med.*, 37:924–930.

75. Majeski, J. A., and Alexander, J. W. (1977): Evaluation of tetracycline in the neutrophil chemotactic response. *J. Lab. Clin. Med.*, 90:259–265.

76. Majeski, J. A., McClellan, M. A., and Alexander, J. W. (1976): Effect of antibiotics on the *in vitro* neutrophil chemotactic response. *Am. Surg.*, 42:785–788.

77. Majeski, J. A., Morris, M. J., and Alexander, J. W. (1978): Action of cefoxitin and cefamandole on human neutrophil function. *J. Antibiot. (Tokyo)*, 31:1059–1062.

78. Mandell, G. L. (1970): Intraphagosomal pH of human polymorphonuclear neutrophils. *Proc. Soc. Exp. Biol. Med.*, 134:447–449.

79. Mandell, G. L. (1973): Interaction of intraleukocyte bacteria and antibiotics. *J. Clin. Invest.*, 52:1673–1679.

80. Mandell, G. L., and Vest, T. K. (1972): Killing of intraleukocytic *Staphylococcus aureus* by rifampin: *in vitro* and *in vivo* studies. *J. Infect. Dis.*, 125:486–490.

81. Martin, R. R., Warr, G. A., Couch, R. B., Yeager, H., and Knight, V. (1974): Effects of tetracycline on leukotaxis. *J. Infect. Dis.*, 129:110–116.

82. McCurrach, P. H., Park, J. K., and Perry, W. L. M. (1970): The effects of some drugs which induce agranulocytosis on the metabolism of separated human polymorphonuclear leukocytes and lymphocytes. *Br. J. Pharmacol.*, 38:608–615.

83. Melby, K., and Midtvedt, T. (1977): The effect of eight antibacterial agents on the phagocytosis of ^{32}P-labeled *Escherichia coli* by rat polymorphonuclear cells. *Scand. J. Infect. Dis.*, 9:9–12.

84. Munoz, J., and Geister, R. (1950): Inhibition of phagocytosis by aureomycin. *Proc. Soc. Exp. Biol. Med.*, 75:367–370.

85. Nishida, M., Mine, Y., and Nonoyama, S. (1978): Relationship between the effect of carbenicillin on the phagocytosis and killing of *Proteus mirabilis* by polymorphonuclear leukocytes and therapeutic efficacy. *J. Antibiot. (Tokyo)*, 31:719–724.

86. Nishida, M., Mine, Y. Nonoyama, S., and Yokota, Y. (1976): Effect of antibiotics on the phagocytosis and killing of *Pseudomonas aeruginosa* by rabbit polymorphonuclear leukocytes. *Chemotherapy*, 22:203–210.

87. Nutter, J. E., and Myrvik, Q. N. (1966): *In vitro* interactions between rabbit alveolar macrophages and *Pasturella tularensis*. *J. Bacteriol.*, 92:645–651.

88. Odegaard, A., and Lamvik, J. (1976): The effect of phenylbutazone and chloramphenicol on phagocytosis of radiolabeled *Candida albicans* by human monocytes cultured *in vitro*. *Acta Pathol. Microbiol. Scand. [C]*, 84:37–44.

89. Park, J. K., and Dow, R. C. (1970): The uptake and localization of tetracycline in human blood cells. *Br. J. Exp. Pathol.*, 51:179–182.

90. Patterson, R. J., and Youmans, G. P. (1970): Multiplication of *Mycobacterium tuberculosis* within normal and "immune" mouse macrophages cultivated with and without streptomycin. *Infect. Immun.*, 1:30–40.

91. Pious, D., and Hawley, P. (1972): Effect of antibiotics on respiration in human cells. *Pediatr. Res.*, 6:687–692.

92. Plewig, G., and Schopf, E. (1975): Anti-inflammatory effects of antimicrobial agents: an *in vivo* study. *J. Invest. Dermatol.*, 65:532–536.

93. Prokesch, R. C., and Hand, W. L. (1980): Antibiotic uptake by human polymorphonuclear leukocytes. In: *Progr. Abstr. 20th Intersci. Conf. Antimicrob. Agents Chemother.*, Abstr. 726. American Society for Microbiology, Washington, D. C.

94. Pruul, H., and McDonald, P. J. (1979): Enhancement of leukocyte activity against *Escherichia coli* after brief exposure to chloramphenicol. *Antimicrob. Agents Chemother.*, 16:695–700.

95. Pruul, H., and Reynolds, B. L. (1972): Interaction of complement and polymyxin with gram-negative bacteria. *Infect. Immun.*, 6:709–717.

96. Pruul, H., Wetherall, B. L., and McDonald, P. J. (1980): Activity of human leukocyte granule extract on antibiotic-damaged bacteria. In: *Progr. Abstr. 20th Intersci. Conf. Antimicrob. Agents Chemother.*, Abstr. 732. American Society for Microbiology, Washington, D. C.

97. Raynor, R. H., Scott, D. F., and Best, G. K. (1980): Lipoteichoic acid inhibition of phagocytosis of *Staphylococcus aureus* by human polymorphonuclear leukocytes. In: *Current Chemotherapy and Infectious Disease*, edited by J. D. Nelson and C. Grassi, Vol. II, pp. 801–803. American Society for Microbiology, Washington, D. C.

98. Rhodes, M. W., and Hsu, H. S. (1974): Effect of kanamycin on the fate of *Salmonella enteritidis* within cultured macrophages of guinea pigs. *J. Reticuloendothel. Soc.*, 15:1–12.

99. Root, R. K. (1981): Antibacterial properties of polymorphonuclear leukocytes and their interactions with antibiotics. In: *Microbiology—1981*, edited by D. Schlessinger, pp. 176-180. American Society for Microbiology, Washington, D. C.

100. Root, R. K., Isturiz, R. I., Molavi, A., Metcalf, J. A., and Malech, H. L. (1981): Interactions between antibiotics and human neutrophils in the killing of staphylococci: studies with normal and cytochalasin B treated cells. *J. Clin. Invest.*, 67:247–259.

101. Root, R. K., and Metcalf, J. A. (1979): Surface binding and enhanced killing of penicillin treated *S. aureus* 502A by human neutrophils: mechanism of the effect. *Clin. Res.*, 27:480A.

102. Rous, P., and Jones, F. S. (1916): The protection of pathogenic microorganisms by living tissue cells. *J. Exp. Med.*, 23:601–612.

103. Rubenstein, A., and Pelet, B. (1973): False-negative N. B. T. tests due to transient malfunctions of neutrophils. *Lancet* 1:382.

104. Sabath, L. D., Gerstein, D. A.,Leaf, C. D., and Finland, M. (1970): Increasing the usefulness of antibiotics: treatment of infections caused by gram-negative bacilli. *Clin. Pharmacol. Ther.*, 11:161–167.

105. Seklecki, M. M., Quintiliani, R., and Maderazo, E. G. (1978): Aminoglycoside antibiotics moderately impair granulocyte function. *Antimicrob. Agents Chemother.*, 13:552–554.

106. Shaffer, J. M., Kucera, C. J., and Spink, W. W. (1953): The protection of intracellular Brucella against therapeutic agents and the bactericidal action of serum. *J. Exp. Med.*, 97:77–90.

107. Shepard, C. C. (1957): Use of HeLa cells infected with tubercle bacilli for the study of anti-tuberculous drugs. *J. Bacteriol.*, 73:494–498.

108. Showacre, J. L., Hopps, H. E., DuBuy, H. G., and Smadel, J. (1961): Effect of antibiotics on intracellular *Salmonella typhosa*. I. Demonstration by phase microscopy of prompt inhibition of intracellular multiplication. *J. Immunol.*, 87:153–161.

109. Silverstein, S. C., Steinman, R. M., and Cohen, Z. A. (1977): Endocytosis. *Annu. Rev. Biochem.*, 46:669–722.

110. Solberg, C. O. (1972): Protection of phagocytized bacteria against antibiotics: a new method for the evaluation of neutrophil granulocyte functions. *Acta Med. Scand.*, 191:383–387.

111. Solberg, C. O., and Hellum, K. B. (1978): Protection of phagocytosed bacteria against antimicrobial agents. *Scand. J. Infect. Dis.* (Suppl.), 14:246–250.

112. Stossel, T. P. (1975): Phagocytosis: recognition and ingestion. *Semin. Hematol.*, 12:83–116.

113. Sud, I. J., and Feingold, D. S. (1975): Detection of agents that alter the bacterial cell surface. *Antimicrob. Agents Chemother.*, 8:34–37.

114. Suter, E. (1952): Multiplication of tubercle bacilli within phagocytes cultivated *in vitro*, and effect of streptomycin and isonicotinic acid hydrazide. *Am. Rev. Tuberc.*, 65:775–776.

115. Suter, E. (1952): The multiplication of tubercle bacilli within normal phagocytes in tissue culture. *J. Exp. Med.*, 96:137–150.

116. Tan, J. S., Watanakunakorn, C., and Phair, J. P. (1971): A modified assay of neutrophil function: use of lysostaphin to differentiate defective phagocytosis from impaired intracellular killing. *J. Lab. Clin. Med.*, 78:316–322.

117. Thayer, J. D., Perry, M. I., Field, F. W., and Garson, W. (1957): Failure of penicillin, chloramphenicol, erythromycin, and novobiocin to kill phagocytized gonococci in tissue culture. *Antibiot. Ann. 1956-7*, pp. 513–517.

118. Traub, W. H., and Sherris, J. C. (1970): Studies on the interaction between serum bactericidal activity and antibiotics *in vitro*. *Chemotherapy*, 15:70–83.

119. Tulkens, P., and Trouet, A. (1972): Uptake and intracellular localization of streptomycin in the lysosomes of cultured fibroblasts. *Arch. Int. Physiol. Biochem.*, 80:623–624.

120. Vaudaux, P., and Waldvogel, F. A. (1979): Gentamicin antibacterial activity in the presence of human polymorphonuclear leukocytes. *Antimicrob. Agents Chemother.*, 16:743–749.

121. Vaudaux, P., and Waldvogel, F. A. (1980): Gentamicin inactivation in purulent exudates: role of cell lysis. *J. Infect. Dis.*, 142:586–593.

122. Veale, D. R., Finch, H., and Smith, H. (1976): Penetration of penicillin into human phagocytes containing *Neisseria gonorrhoeae*: intracellular survival and growth at optimum concentrations of antibiotic. *J. Gen. Microbiol.*, 95:353–363.

123. Waisbren, B. A., and Brown, I. (1964): Effect of wide-spectrum antibiotics on bactericidal activity of human serum: *in vitro* and *in vivo*. *Am. J. Med. Sci.*, 248:56–60.

124. Warren, G. H., and Gray, J. (1963): Production of a polysaccharide by *Staphylococcus aureus*. II. Effect of temperature and antibiotics. *Proc. Soc. Exp. Biol. Med.*, 114:439–444.

125. Warren, G. H., and Gray, J. (1964): Production of a polysaccharide by *Staphylococcus aureus*. III. Action of penicillins and polysaccharides on enzymic lysis. *Proc. Soc. Exp. Biol. Med.*, 116:317–323.

126. Warren, G. H., and Gray, J. (1965): Effect of sublethal concentrations of penicillins on the lysis of bacteria by lysozyme and trypsin. *Proc. Soc. Exp. Biol. Med.*, 120:504–511.

127. Warren, G. H., and Gray, J. (1967): Effect of antimicrobial drug combinations on enzymic lysis of *Staphylococcus aureus*. *Proc. Soc. Exp. Biol. Med.*, 126:15–18.

128. Warren, G. H., and Gray, J. (1967): Influence of nafcillin on the enzymic lysis of *Staphylococcus aureus*. *Can. J. Microbiol.*, 13:321–328.

129. Warren, G. H., Gray, J., and Yurchenco, J. A. (1957): Effect of polymyxin on the lysis of *Neisseria catarrhalis* by lysozyme. *J. Bacteriol.*, 74:788–793.

130. Windsor, A. C. M., Hobbs, C. B., Treby, D. A., and Cowper, R. A. (1972): Effect of tetracycline on leukocyte ascorbic acid levels. *Br. Med. J.*, 1:214–215.

131. Yourtee, E. L., Metcalf, J. A., and Root, R. K. (1980): Augmented killing of penicillin pretreated *S. aureus* by human neutrophils: role of complement. *Clin. Res.*, 28:383A.

132. Zigmond, S. H. (1978): Chemotaxis by polymorphonuclear leukocytes. *J. Cell Biol.*, 77:269–287.

Advances in Host Defense Mechanisms, Vol. 1,
edited by John I. Gallin and Anthony S. Fauci,
Raven Press, New York © 1982

Eosinophil Behavior During Host Defense Reactions

David A. Bass

*Department of Medicine, Division of Infectious Diseases and Immunology,
Bowman Gray School of Medicine, Winston-Salem, North Carolina 27103*

Eosinophil and neutrophil leukocytes share similar life cycles, morphology, many lysosomal enzymes, most chemotactic responses, phagocytic ability, and oxidative metabolic responses to membrane stimuli. This has prompted certain investigators to consider eosinophils little more than rather gaudy, and relatively ineffective neutrophils. Yet, these two granulocyte types demonstrate quite distinctive responses during specific host-defense reactions. Whereas neutrophil production and local accumulation are markedly stimulated during acute infections, eosinophils do not have a central role in defense against bacteria, and circulating eosinophils are decreased in number during host reactions involving acute inflammation. In contrast, during infestations by invasive metazoan parasites, eosinophil production is dramatically stimulated, as is the accumulation of eosinophils in the inflammatory response to the parasites. This discussion will review our current knowledge regarding the mechanisms of eosinophil responses during acute infections and parasitic infestations, and will briefly examine the nature of the inability of eosinophils to protect against bacteria and the current hypothesis that eosinophils have a central role in the host defense against metazoan parasites.

ACUTE INFECTIONS

It is generally accepted that eosinophils do not have the ability to maintain adequate host defenses against bacterial invasion. Patients with neutropenia may have a significant eosinophilia, yet recurrent bacterial infections dominate their clinical course (1,24,59). There are at least three reasons for this situation: a) Eosinophils are relatively poor phagocytic cells. b) Eosinophils appear to have an intracellular bactericidal defect. c) Acute infections are typically accompanied by an abrupt decrease in the number of circulating eosinophils and, shortly thereafter, a suppression of eosinophilopoiesis. These observations will be discussed in turn.

Phagocytosis

There is no doubt that eosinophils are able to ingest a wide variety of substances (2,3,5,39,47,64,71,81,85,98,106,113,116,131,161,164,168). However, in most studies where the phagocytic ability of eosinophils and neutrophils has been compared, phagocytosis by eosinophils has been found to be significantly less efficient than that accomplished by neutrophils (3,5,39,71,106,113). This decreased phagocytic ability by eosinophils is reflected in both smaller numbers of cells engulfing particles and fewer ingested particles per cell (39). Moreover, eosinophil phagocytosis is rarely observed *in vivo* (66), except in specific conditions in which the cells have been previously stimulated by an immunologic event and then exposed to large numbers of particles for ingestion (41,116). Phagocytosis by eosinophils appear to be an *in vitro* phenomenon of uncertain significance *in vivo*.

Intracellular Bactericidal Defect

Studies of the microbicidal ability of eosinophils, using bacteria or fungi as target organisms, have demonstrated a moderately reduced bactericidal ability of eosinophils when compared to that of neutrophils. This has generally been ascribed to the lower phagocytic rate of eosinophils. However, the eosinophils of one patient with chronic hypereosinophilia were found to have a phagocytic rate equal to that of neutrophils, yet the eosinophils had a reduced bactericidal activity against *Escherichia coli* or *Staphylococcus aureus* (Fig. 1) (47). This suggested the presence of an intracellular bactericidal defect in eosinophils.

Studies of the bactericidal mechanisms of eosinophils have been limited. Phagocytosis by eosinophils causes an oxidative metabolic burst which is qualitatively similar to that observed in neutrophils. Although the studies to date are limited, it appears that the magnitude of the oxidative bursts of normal eosinophils and neutrophils are similar (13) [eosinophils from patients with eosinophilia generate a more vigorous metabolic response (5,29,48,80,106,120,147)]. Thus, this aspect of bactericidal mechanisms is not deficient. It may be that eosinophil peroxidase (EPO) is less able than neutrophil peroxidase (NPO) to partake in the peroxidase-H_2O_2-halide bactericidal mechanism described by Klebanoff (79). Eosinophil peroxidase is potent in protein iodination and bacterial killing in the presence of H_2O_2 and iodide, but it is less able than NPO to decarboxylate amino acids or kill bacteria in the presence of H_2O_2 and chloride (74,107,108). Eosinophil peroxidase is also more readily inhibited by low concentrations of protein (74), which could be relevant to the function of this enzyme in the intact cell. Azide inhibits EPO and would presumably block the peroxidase-H_2O_2-halide bactericidal mechanism, yet Bujak and Root (29) found that azide enhanced eosinophil bactericidal activity. One possible mechanism of this azide-mediated effect could be that it enhanced phagocytosis without blocking killing (29). It should be noted that azide also increases the production of superoxide (126) and H_2O_2 (127,167) by granulocytes. The enhanced bactericidal effect of azide could be due to this increased production of oxygen derivatives with a direct bactericidal activity by these substances. These observations prompt the speculation that eosinophils have a relatively ineffective peroxidase-H_2O_2-halide mechanism, and that their bactericidal ability may rely more on direct toxicity by oxygen derivatives such as H_2O_2 and superoxide.

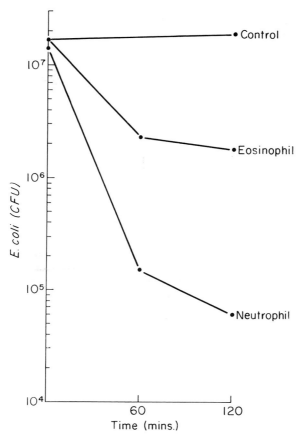

FIG. 1. Killing of *E. coli* by human neutrophils and eosinophils. These eosinophils, obtained from a patient with chronic hypereosinophilia, were shown in parallel experiments to have a phagocytic rate equal to that of the neutrophils. [Reproduced from DeChatelet et al. (47), with permission.]

The Eosinopenia of Acute Infection

The typical eosinopenia of acute infections was first described by Zappert in 1893 (166). By 1914, Schwartz (135) was able to cite over 100 references confirming the occurrence of an absolute eosinopenia as a regular event in a variety of acute bacterial and viral infections. The clinical observations were recently reviewed in detail (19) and were summarized as follows: a) Processes that elicit a significant acute inflammatory response are associated with reduction in the peripheral eosinophil count. This occurs in the great majority of acute infections but may also be seen in other inflammatory states such as systemic lupus erythematosus. b) Chronic infections cause a less predictable eosinophil reaction, but periods of active inflammation, for example in febrile patients with tuberculosis, still continue to be accompanied by eosinopenia. c) Infectious diseases causing little inflammation may cause little change in the eosinophil count. d) Once the acute process subsides, immune stimulation to eosinophilia, as in scarlet fever, may appear. In the preantibiotic era, the return of detectable circulating eosinophils was considered a harbinger of a favorable outcome in patients with acute bacterial infections (28). During the convalescent phase of infections, patients may occasionally develop a transient, usually mild eosinophilia (143).

Usually a persistent eosinophilia will be completely suppressed by a significant acute infection (111,140). However, in some patients with marked, persistent eosinophilia due to, for example, the hypereosinophilic syndrome or immune deficiency states, a partial suppression may occur, and the eosinophil count may remain in the eosinophilic range. Such a case is shown in Fig. 2. This was a patient with chronic hypereosinophilia (who has since developed acute myelomonocytic leukemia) and marked neutropenia (circulating eosinophils varying between 6,000 and 12,000 and neutrophils persistently less than 700/mm³) who developed a staphylococcal empyema following a thoracentesis procedure. With the onset of the acute infection, there was a drop in the number of circulating eosinophils, although the eosinophils remained above the normal range. It was also of interest that this patient had no history of recurrent infections in the presence of such a marked neutropenia. Once an infectious pathogen had been inadvertently introduced, the patient was able to mount an appropriate neutrophil response (Fig. 2). The mechanism of the neutropenia, which may accompany some cases of the hypereosinophilic syndrome,

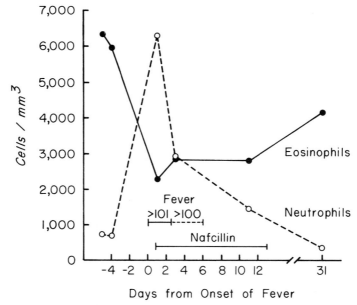

FIG. 2. Numbers of circulating eosinophils and neutrophils in a patient with hypereosinophilia with the onset and therapy of *S. aureus* empyema.

has not been elucidated. It has been reported that eosinophils may suppress neutrophil production in an *in vitro* bone marrow culture system (148); however, it appears that eosinophilic patients retain a normal neutrophil response to acute infection.

Although eosinopenia is characteristic of inflammation dominated by neutrophils, the eosinopenia occurs normally in infected patients with a variety of neutrophil defects. Eosinopenic responses to localized bacterial infections have been observed in patients with chronic granulomatous disease (CGD) (unpublished observations), the syndrome of hypergammaglobulinemia E with defective neutrophil chemotaxis (Quie, personal communication), and congenital neutropenia (1).

Several studies in animals have provided some insight into the kinetics and mechanisms of the eosinopenia of acute infection. Eosinophil kinetics during acute inflammation were examined in studies in mice (9). In order to facilitate statistical analysis of eosinopenic changes, mice were rendered predictably eosinophilic by infection with trichinosis. Then a variety of stimuli, known to elicit acute inflammatory responses, were administered. Eosinopenic reactions were observed regardless of the form of the acute inflammatory stimulant. Thus, a marked eosinopenia followed the induction of a subcutaneous pneumococcal infection (Fig. 3), unilateral pyelonephritis, coxsackie B viral pancreatitis, or subcutaneous injection of 0.1 ml of turpentine. The eosinopenia was abrupt. Even with the time required for the establishment of an infectious process, after inoculation of pneumococci, the eosinophil counts had fallen 80% to 98% of control values within 6 to 10 hr, which were the earliest time points examined. The rapidity of the response suggested that it probably involved intravascular margination of eosinophils and/or rapid mobilization of eosinophils into the tissues. Eosinopenia was not prevented by splenectomy and was not associated with an appreciable increase in eosinophils in the draining lymph nodes. Histopathologic studies of subcutaneous staphylococcal infections, 7 hr after inoculation in eosinophilic mice, revealed an accumulation of eosinophils around the area of the acute inflammatory site, suggesting this as being one site of sequestration of eosinophils during this early time period. However, these studies could not determine with certainty if this localization was sufficient to account for the entire drop in circulating eosinophils.

Studies of alterations in bone marrow eosinophils were similarly conducted in eosinophilic mice (9). A subcutaneous pneumococcal abscess was prolonged in a controlled manner by administration of the bacteriostatic agent, sulfapyridine. During the initial 36 hr there was an increase in total marrow eosinophils followed by a gradual decrease to well below control levels (Fig. 4). In order to determine if these changes were associated with changes in eosinophilopoiesis, bone marrow cells were pulse-labeled with ^{3}H-thymidine (Fig. 5). The total marrow eosinophils again increased for 36 hr then decreased. The eosinophils incorporating thymidine remained at control levels for the first 36 hr without any increased incorporation. After this period, the number of eosinophils taking up thymidine decreased abruptly, coincident with the fall in total marrow eosinophils. These data involve adrenal corticosteroids. This is supported by observations in humans and experimental

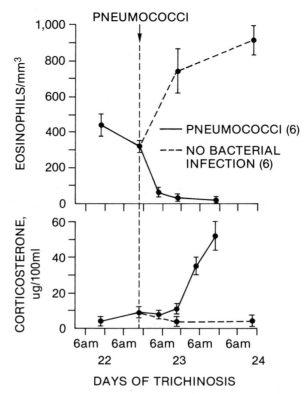

FIG. 3. Circulating eosinophils **(upper panel)** and serum corticosterone levels **(lower panel)** in eosinophilic mice following inoculation of *S. pneumoniae*, Type III, into a dorsal subcutaneous air pouch, or a sham procedure (inoculation of sterile saline). The study used mice on day 23 or day 24 of trichinosis, at the time eosinophil counts were increasing. Data are means ± SEM. [Reproduced from Bass (8), with permission.]

studies in mice. In humans, the following observations have been made. a) Infections of limited severity (with the exception of meningitis) produce only a modest stimulation of the adrenal cortex (16,20). Marked corticosteroid secretion apparently occurs only when acute infections are accompanied by a significant complication such as shock. b) Venge and co-workers (152) have suggested that serum levels of eosinophil cationic protein may reflect parallel changes in the rates of eosinophil degranulation or destruction. With the onset of an acute infection, in spite of the near absence of circulating eosinophils, serum levels of eosinophil cationic protein may be increased to nearly five times the normal level. In contrast, induction of eosinopenia by administration of corticosteroids does not cause an increase in the serum levels of eosinophil cationic proteins and β-adrenergic agonists decrease cationic protein levels (44,65). c) Patients with adrenal insufficiency, infection, and eosinopenia have been reported (165).

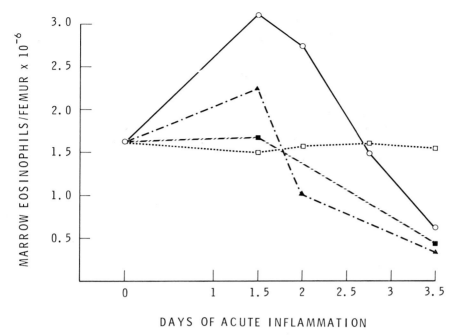

FIG. 4. Total marrow eosinophils in mice with trichinosis subjected to prolonged acute inflammation induced by pneumococcal infection *(open circles)*, *E. coli* pyelonephritis *(triangles)* or subcutaneous turpentine *(closed squares)* or, as controls, subcutaneous saline *(open squares)*. Marrows were examined on day 23 or day 24 of trichinosis. Each point is the mean of 5 to 8 mice. [Reproduced from Bass (9), with permission.]

These clinical observations were supported by direct examination of the adrenal-mediation hypothesis in the pneumococcal infected-eosinophilic mouse model described above (8). The initial studies compared serum corticosterone levels during trichinosis and pyelonephritis. It was found that during the first peak of eosinophilia of trichinosis there was an increase of serum corticosterone to four times control levels, with a gradual decrease to normal over the next week. There was a similar increase during acute pyelonephritis. However, corticosterone levels during pyelonephritis (with its eosinopenia) were actually less than those observed during the first peak of eosinophilia of trichinosis. Inoculation of pneumococci into a subcutaneous air pouch was again associated with an abrupt eosinopenia. Moreover, although the eosinopenia was marked by 6 hr after inoculation, serum corticosterone levels did not suggest that the initial increase in total eosinophils was not due to increased eosinophilopoiesis but was presumably due to an inhibition of egress of eosinophils from the bone marrow; this was then followed by a decrease in eosinophil production rates.

It was also noted that the initial increase in total marrow eosinophils varied between inflammatory stimuli. Thus, whereas pneumococcal infection caused a

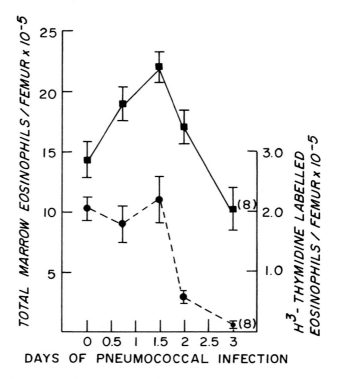

FIG. 5. Total marrow eosinophils *(squares)* and dividing marrow eosinophils, as shown by labeling with ³H-thymidine *(circles)*, in mice with pneumococcal infection prolonged by treatment with sulfapyridine (mean ± SEM). Marrows were examined on day 23 or day 24 of trichinosis. [Reproduced from Bass (9), with permission.]

doubling of bone marrow eosinophils, pyelonephritis caused only a modest increase, and turpentine injection, although causing eosinopenia for several days duration, was associated with no apparent increase in marrow eosinophils (Fig. 4). Yet all of these stimuli caused an eventual decrease in marrow eosinophils after 3½ days.

Thus, the eosinopenia of acute infection involved three separate events: An abrupt decrease in circulating eosinophils, probably due to intravascular margination and/or mobilization into tissues; an inhibition of release of mature eosinophils from the bone marrow; and a delayed suppression of eosinophilopoiesis.

Mechanisms of Eosinopenia

The mechanisms of the eosinopenia of acute infection have only been partially clarified. Adrenal corticosteroids cause similar eosinopenic responses (11), and until recently it was generally assumed that the eosinopenia of acute infection was a manifestation of adrenal stimulation by the stress of the infectious process (162). However, this hypothesis could not explain why certain stressful situations such as asthma or some parasitic infestations may be accompanied by eosinophilia, and yet localized, minimally stressful acute infections may cause eosinopenia even when superimposed on a preceding eosinophilia. It is now clear that the eosinopenia of acute infection can be mediated by mechanisms that do not significantly increase until more than 12 hr after inoculation (Fig. 3). Finally, if mice were adrenalectomized 1 to 4 days before pneumococcal inoculation, the eosinopenic response occurred normally. Thus, the eosinopenia of acute infection does not appear to be dependent on adrenal steroid mediation. The fact that it also occurs in mice 4 days after adrenalectomy without maintenance steroids suggests that it is also not due to epinephrine, since production of eosinopenia by endogenous epinephrine appears to require low or "permissive" levels of corticosteroids (67,138,149). Thus, eosinopenia occurring 4 days after adrenalectomy would strongly mitigate against epinephrine as well as corticosteroid mediation of the phenomenon.

Whether or not the alterations in eosinophilopoiesis during acute infection are also independent of adrenal stimulation, has not been so thoroughly studied but appears to be the case. Attempts to prolong the pneumococcal process in adrenalectomized mice were hampered by the fact that such mice tended to die when followed for more than 36 hr, presumably due to an Addisonian crisis. However, adrenalectomized, trichinous mice could be followed for 36 hr following pneumococcal inoculation; the bone marrow eosinophils of such mice were found to be increased significantly above that of uninfected mice (Table 1). Thus, the initial increase in marrow eosinophils occurred in these adrenalectomized animals. The delayed depression of total marrow eosinophils by acute inflammatory processes was examined following subcutaneous injection of turpentine in such eosinophilic mice (Table 1). This mild inflammatory stimulus did not cause an increase in marrow eosinophils after 24 to 36 hr in normal or adrenalectomized animals but was capable of causing the delayed suppression of eosinophil production after further prolongation of the acute inflammatory stimulus (Fig. 4, Table 1). Thus, it appears that both the initial increase in bone marrow eosinophils and the eventual suppression of eosinophilopoiesis also occur in adrenalectomized animals.

Although the eosinopenia of acute infection is thus clearly independent of adrenal corticosteroid mediation, the mechanisms of the eosinopenic response are not so well defined. At present at least two mechanisms have been discerned. The onset of eosinopenia may involve release into the circulation of small amounts of the chemotactic factors generated during acute inflammatory processes. The maintenance of the eosinopenic response, which normally persists through the period of acute inflammation, may involve other substance(s) present in acute inflammatory exudates which are first detectable 10 hr after induction of inflammatory responses in mice. The data to support these concepts are as follows.

Acute inflammation may involve the release into the circulation of chemotactic factors, in particular C5a (56,125). The possibility that such chemotactic substances might cause an eosinopenic response was examined by monitoring eosinophil counts in rabbits following intravenous injection of zymosan-activated serum, partially purified C5a, or the synthetic peptide *N*-formyl-methionyl-leucyl-phenylalanine (used by other investigators as a synthetic analog of bacterial chemotactic factor) (12).

TABLE 1. *Total marrow eosinophils in adrenalectomized mice after acute inflammatory stimuli*

Stimulus[a]	Duration	Eosinophils/femur $\times$ 10^{-6}	p
Exp. 1:			
None	—	8.6 ± 1.1 (3)	
Pneumococcal infection	36 hr	13 ± 1.2 (4)	0.02
Exp. 2:			
None	—	17.2 ± 2.9 (4)	
Subcutaneous turpentine	24 hr	18.6 ± 2.7 (4)	NS[b]
Subcutaneous turpentine	48 hr	11.7 ± 2.0 (5)	0.05

[a]Twenty-four hours following adrenalectomy, mice were given a subcutaneous pneumococcal infection, prolonged with sulfapyridine, or subcutaneous injection of 0.1 ml turpentine. Either of these stimuli markedly reduced circulating eosinophils for the duration of the experiment. Femoral bone marrow was removed and total eosinophils quantitated as in Fig. 4 and described previously (9). All marrows were examined on day 23 or day 24 of trichinosis. Means ± SEM of the indicated numbers (in parentheses) of mice.
[b]NS: Not significant.

Each of these factors caused a virtual disappearance of circulating eosinophils within 1 min, a transient return of eosinophils to approximately 50% of control levels after 10 to 90 min, and a subsequent decrease in eosinophil counts which persisted for 5 hr (Fig. 6). In contrast, the number of circulating heterophils, although dropping transiently, rapidly returned and rose to elevated levels for 6 hr after injection, as originally reported by McCall and co-workers (99). A significant eosinopenic response occurred after the injection of only 0.5 ml of ZAS or 0.2 nmoles fMLP into rabbits with blood volumes of roughly 100 ml (12). The response was not caused by adrenal mediation as it occurred normally in adrenalectomized rabbits. Also, the injection of 2 mg hydrocortisone only caused eosinopenia after 90 min and reduced eosinophil counts to 41% of control levels after 3 to 4 hr. It was also found that circulating granulocytes of humans undergoing hemodialysis, which has been reported to activate complement (43), demonstrated similar eosinopenic and neutropenic-neutrophilic responses (12). Thus, in rabbits and in man, intravascular activation or injection of chemotactic factors causes a brief, nonspecific granulocytopenia followed by a prolonged eosinopenic-neutrophilic response analogous to that seen during acute infection.

In the studies in mice described above, a rapid influx of eosinophils into the acute inflammatory site was observed (9); the question arose whether substances in the acute inflammatory exudate might mediate an eosinopenic reaction. The pneumococcal air pouch abscess provided a convenient mechanism for obtaining such exudate by merely lavaging the air pouch (10). Millipore filtration of the

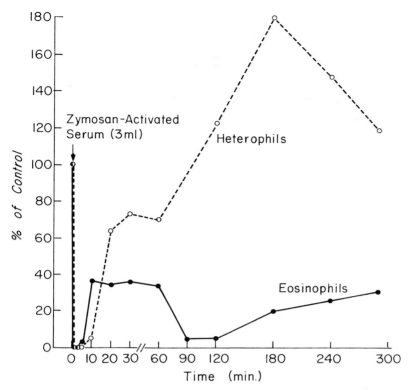

FIG. 6. Circulating eosinophils *(closed circles)* and heterophils *(open circles)* in a rabbit following intravenous injection of 3 ml of zymosan-activated rabbit serum.

exudate to remove bacteria and debris, followed by intraperitoneal inoculation of 0.1 ml of the exudate into eosinophilic mice, was associated with an eosinopenic response which was observed 15 hr later. The characterization of the eosinopenic activity included the following observations (10): The material produced an eosinopenic response which was apparent between 4 and 20 hr after intraperitoneal injection. There was no change in neutrophils during this period. The activity was destroyed by heating to 56°C for 30 min. It was retained by an ultrafiltration membrane with exclusion of molecules above 30,000 daltons. The activity was not lost after precipitation by 7% perchloric acid, which should remove the large proteins, except glycoproteins. In the pneumococcal exudate, activity was lost after 4 hr, which may have been due to pneumococcal enzymes. This loss of activity was prevented by addition of the nonspecific protease inhibitor, trasylol; this suggested, although indirectly, that the activity involved a protein. The material demonstrated a geometric dose response in its ability to suppress the eosinophilia of mice with trichinosis. The material was effective in adrenalectomized mice. The activity was detectable 10 hr after inoculation of pneumococci and reached its highest concentration 20 hr after inoculation. Thus, this activity seems to appear rather late in the inflammatory exudate and may contribute to the maintenance of the eosinopenic state.

The suppression of eosinophilopoiesis by prolonged acute inflammation may also be due, at least in part, to suppression of the lymphocyte-mediated stimulus to eosinophil production. In the eosinophilic mouse model, prolongation of acute infection was found to cause an inhibition of granulomatous responses, which was not limited to the eosinophils (19). Intravenous injection of muscle-stage *Trichinella* larvae into immune mice caused the rapid development of granulomatous inflammatory responses around the larvae within the lungs. If mice were given a pneumococcal abscess 12 hr before larval injection and the lungs examined 48 hr later, there were signs of edema around some of the larvae, but there was essentially complete suppression of the normal accumulation of mononuclear cells and eosinophils. Similarly, if the acute infection were produced 48 hr after larval injection and the lungs examined 4 days later, granulomas in infected mice were markedly reduced in size when compared with uninfected controls (19).

Thus, multiple events may contribute to the production of eosinopenia during acute inflammatory responses. The abrupt onset of eosinopenia may reflect a rapid margination of eosinophils in response to chemotactic factors released into the circulation. Part of the early eosinopenia is due to migration of eosinophils into the area of the inflammatory site, combined with inhibition of release of eosinophils from the bone marrow (the mechanism of which is unknown). Eosinopenia-producing substance(s), possibly large-molecular-weight glycoproteins, are detectable after several hours in inflammatory exudates; such activities may contribute to the maintenance of the eosinopenia. The eventual suppression of eosinophilopoiesis could be due to such activities but could also be due to an inhibition of the lymphocyte-mediated stimulus of eosinophil production.

INVASIVE METAZOAN PARASITIC INFESTATIONS

Infestations by tissue-invasive metazoa regularly cause stimulation of eosinophilopoiesis and accumulation of eosinophils around the local inflammatory response to the parasite (19). In the great majority of cases, this is associated with development of eosinophilia in the peripheral blood. The marked eosinophil response to metazoa is most pronounced during the tissue-invasive, migratory phase of their life cycles. For example, during infection in man by *Ascaris lumbricoides*, marked eosinophilia occurs during the migratory phase; once the larvae mature to adults within the gut, the eosinophilia subsides (57,58). In contrast, following infection of man by dog or cat ascarids (*Toxocara canis*), the larvae continue to migrate through the host tissues, and prolonged eosinophilia continues through the course of visceral larva migrans. Deposition of parasite eggs in tissues, as in schistosomiasis, may also cause a vigorous local inflammatory response and a marked stimulation of eosinophils. In contrast, parasites that successfully encyst and cause little inflammation within tissues, (e.g., echinococcosis or cysticercosis), cause less stimulation of eosinophils. Finally, metazoa which remain within the lumen of the gut, and similarly elicit little tissue inflammation, also cause little stimulation of eosinophils. Thus, in man, the eosinophil response to parasites correlates closely with the stimulation of a tissue inflammatory reaction.

The nature of the antigen-host interaction which leads to eosinophil stimulation remains a fundamental, and inadequately answered question. Is it a response to a specific antigenic structure? Or, is it a manifestation of the form of presentation of antigen to the immunologic apparatus? Certainly, parasites are highly antigenic (34). However, Basten and colleagues (18) and Walls and Beeson (156) found that homogenizing or solubilizing *Trichinella* antigens prior to intravenous administration to mice, aborted the subsequent eosinophilia. Administering the soluble antigen in Freund's adjuvant restored an eosinophilic response. Also, if antigens that do not usually cause eosinophilia, such as ovalbumin or human gamma globulin (133,134), dextrans (157), or toxoids (139), are administered in a particulate form (to become lodged within tissues), an eosinophilia may ensue. Thus, the eosinophilia is not merely dependent on unique antigenic structure; rather the deposition of antigen within tissues appears crucial. It is not known whether this involves a shift in the magnitude or kinetics of antigen exposure, (e.g., depot form with persistent antigen release versus bolus), subsequent antigen processing, or unusual participation by the other cells in the reaction. It is also not known why tissue-deposition of one antigen (e.g., tuberculin) causes a macrophage-lymphocyte granulomatous response, yet the analogous presentation of another (e.g., *Trichinella*) uniformly causes the recruitment of eosinophils into the reaction.

Mechanisms of Stimulation of Eosinophil Production

The eosinophil response to metazoa behaves as a part of the immunologic apparatus of the host. A major advance in our knowledge of the relationship between eosinophilia and the lymphocyte-mediated immune system was made one decade ago by Basten and Beeson (17) and their colleagues (18,26,141,142,153–158) studying rats and mice challenged with *Trichinella spiralis* and, at nearly the same time, by Speirs (137) and his colleagues (102,121) studying the response to alum precipitated tetanus toxoid in mice. Their observations have since been confirmed and extended in other experimental models, including other metazoan infestations, e.g., *Schistosoma mansoni* (mice) (54,119), *Ascaris suum* (nude mice) (114), *Nippostrongylus Braziliensis* (rats) (115), and *Fasciola hepatica* (calves) (55).

Following appropriate challenge, e.g., by intravenous administration of *Trichinella* larvae in mice, there is a delay of several days, followed by a burst of eosinophil proliferation in the bone marrow (141). Without ongoing antigenic stimulation, the eosinophil response shuts off after several days. If the animals are later rechallenged with the same antigen, an augmented eosinophil response occurs (26). This augmented response is antigen-specific (154), reminiscent of other immunologic events, such as antibody production. However, eosinophilia does not correlate with the production of hemagglutinating (18), antitoxin (137), or homocytotropic (19,145) antibody. Also, in rats (18) and guinea pigs (117), transfer of serum from stimulated animals does not cause an eosinophilia. The eosinophilia appears to be dependent on, and probably mediated by, stimulation of an intact T-lymphocyte system. Supporting data in animal models include a) a parallel suppression of T lymphocytes and eosinophilic responses, b) correlation between T lymphocyte (blastogenesis) and eosinophilic responses (134), c) transfer by sensitized lymphocytes of augmented eosinophilic responses to antigenic rechallenge, and d) direct stimulation of eosinophilia following transfer of stimulated thoracic duct lymphocytes.

In animal studies, depletion or suppression of T lymphocytes causes an equivalent suppression of the eosinophilia induced by metazoan parasites or appropriate antigenic challenge. Procedures used in these studies to cause T-lymphocyte suppression have included neonatal thymectomy (17), prolonged thoracic duct drainage (17), administration of antithymocyte sera (17,54) or immunosuppressive drugs (17,26), irradiation with lymphocyte and/or marrow reconstitution (102), neonatal thymectomy plus lethal irradiation plus bone marrow (and, as a control, thymus) reconstitution (54,155,158), and congenital T-lymphocyte deficiency (55, 114,115,119,128). In each case, depletion of T lymphocytes caused a near ablation of the normal eosinophilic responses. It should be noted that in trichinosis and schistosomiasis in T-depleted mice, a modest, transient eosinophilia occurred at the time of the onset of the normal eosinophilic response (54,158). However, studies have not examined whether this brief, T lymphocyte-independent eosinophilia reflects a stimulation of eosinophilopoiesis or a mobilization of eosinophils from storage sites such as the bone marrow or spleen.

Passive transfer of sensitized lymphocytes "primes" the recipient animals; subsequent challenge causes an augmented eosinophil response (26, 117,154,157). It is also important to note that soluble parasite antigens, which do not directly stimulate eosinophilia, also prime the animals to an augmented eosinophil response to intact parasites (156). Thus, lymphocyte-mediated antigenic "memory" can be stimulated by soluble antigens, yet the eosinophil response to the same antigens requires antigen deposition within tissues, as discussed above.

Studies indicating that lymphocytes directly mediate the stimulation of eosinophilopoiesis began with the transfer of an eosinophilic response by stimulated lymphocytes. Basten and Beeson (17) demonstrated that intraperitoneal transfer of stimulated thoracic duct lymphocytes, obtained 3 to 5 days after oral inoculation of mice with *Trichinella*, caused an eosinophilia in recipient mice. The eosinophilia also occurred when the stimulated lymphocytes were first enclosed in diffusion chambers and then implanted intraperitoneally into normal recipients. This suggested that lymphocytes release a soluble substance which causes peripheral blood eosinophilia. Evidence that this involved a stimulation of eosinophil production was obtained by McGarry and Miller (101,102), Miller et al. (109), and Miller and McGarry (110) using the peritoneal implantation of diffusion quadrachambers containing bone marrow cells and lymphocytes, separated by a Millipore membrane. It was found that antigenic stimulation of presensitized spleen cells caused an increase in the bone marrow eosinophils in the adjacent chamber.

Our knowledge of the nature of the soluble mediators of stimulation of eosino-philopoiesis is being extended by use of *in vitro* culture of bone marrow cells. At present, at least two substances appear capable of stimulating eosinophil production. Low-molecular-weight substance(s) (eosinophilopoietin, eosinophil growth-stimu-lating factor) stimulate rapid, transient growth of eosinophils *in vivo* or in liquid culture of bone marrow cells *in vitro*. A higher molecular weight substance [eosin-ophil colony-stimulating factor (ECSF)] stimulates growth of eosinophil colonies in semisolid culture of bone marrow cells after 7 to 14 days *in vitro*. Only the activity of the low-molecular-weight substance(s) has been demonstrated both *in vivo* and *in vitro*.

Eosinophilopoietin was originally described by Mahmoud and co-workers (93) as a pronase-sensitive material with a molecular weight between 613 and 1,355 daltons, which was obtained from sera of mice depleted of circulating eosinophils by pretreatment with antieosinophil serum. This substance induced increased num-bers of total and dividing marrow eosinophils and total circulating eosinophils when injected into normal mice. The production (but not the activity) of eosinophilopoietin appears dependent on an intact T-lymphocyte population (94). Similar eosinophil-opoietic activity has since been reported in sera of mice with schistosomiasis or trichinosis (94). Activity was also found in the sera of rats with trichinosis; the detectable stimulatory activity appeared in the sera 2 to 3 days before the devel-opment of peripheral blood eosinophilia in the *Trichinella*-infected rats. These investigators have also described a similar activity in sera of patients with schis-tosomiasis (94).

Eosinophil growth-stimulating factor (GSF) was defined as an activity released by antigen-stimulated mouse nonadherent spleen cells which specifically stimulated the growth of eosinophils in liquid cultures of nonadherent bone marrow cells (6,130). A recent study suggested that eosinophilopoietin and eosinophil GSF may be identical (7). Both are of low molecular weight. The kinetics of their effects in the *in vitro* liquid bone marrow culture system were remarkably parallel. Both demonstrated similar-dose response curves in the liquid culture assay. Each stim-ulant caused an increase of eosinophils which was maximal after 48 hr and was followed by a rapid decline (Fig. 7). In studies of the GSF, it appeared that the rapid cessation of eosinophilopoiesis was due to depletion of cells responsive to the stimulatory substance (6). Addition of fresh GSF to the culture after 48 hr of stimulated growth caused no further eosinophil production; conversely, the growth-stimulating activity of the culture remained essentially unchanged after 48 hr of culture, as shown by a test on fresh bone marrow cells. This could be interpreted as suggesting that this substance stimulates the terminal differentiation of eosinophil precursors but does not cause further commitment of stem cells to eosinophilo-poiesis.

Eosinophil colony-stimulating factor has been defined in studies of bone marrow culture in semisolid media. This substance induces the division and differentiation of cells at a stage before the myeloblast to form colonies of recognizable eosinophils (104–106). Antigen or mitogen-stimulated lymphocytes appear to provide the major

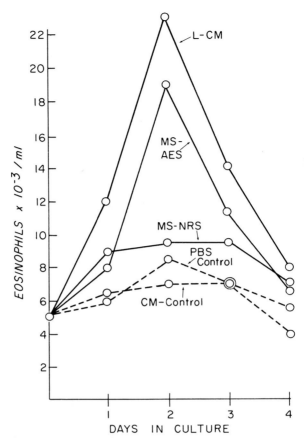

FIG. 7. Numbers of mouse bone marrow eosinophils during liquid culture *in vitro*. MS-NRS: effect of low-molecular-weight fractions of serum from mice pretreated with normal rabbit serum. MS-AES: similar fractions from mice pretreated with AES. L-CM: conditioned medium containing substances released by immune nonadherent spleen cells stimulated with excretory-secretory antigens of *T. spiralis*. CM-control: similar medium obtained by culture of immune spleen cells without antigen. PBS-control: phosphate-buffered saline. Each stimulant was tested at 10% final concentration. Each point is the mean of 2 to 4 closely agreeing determinations. [Reproduced from Bartelmez et al. (7), with permission.]

source of eosinophil CSF (38,104–106). Eosinophil CSF appears to be a glycoprotein with a molecular weight of 24,000 to 37,000 (depending on the molecular content of sialic acid) which is separable from neutrophil/macrophage CSF by isoelectric focusing, hydrophobic chromatography, and DEAE-cellulose chromatography (30).

Murine eosinophil CSF appears to be a substance quite distinct from the eosinophilopoietin/eosinophil GSF described above. Besides their differences in molecular weight, they elicit different kinetics of stimulation of eosinophilopoiesis. Whereas eosinophilopoietin/GSF cause a rapid stimulation of eosinophil production, the CSF produces eosinophil growth that is maximal after 5 to 14 days of culture. It is not unreasonable to speculate that the distinctive activity of eosinophilopoietin/eosinophil GSF and eosinophil CSF are due to different substances that act at different stages of differentiation of the eosinophil leukocyte series.

It is possible that the initiation of the eosinophilopoietic response to metazoan parasites *in vivo* involves the eosinophilopoietin/eosinophil GSF type of activity. Production of bone marrow eosinophilia by sensitized animals, challenged with the appropriate antigen, would require time for lymphocyte release of stimulatory activities and for bone marrow responses. Sensitized mice challenged intravenously with *Trichinella* larvae (141) develop bone marrow eosinophilia which is evident 2 to 4 days after challenge. The stimulation of peripheral blood eosinophilia by thoracic duct lymphocytes is detectable within 2 days after intravenous injection of the lymphocytes into normal mice (17). Thus, the onset of stimulated eosinophilopoiesis occurs with similar timing following antigen-mediated stimulation *in vivo* or following administration of eosinophilopoietin/eosinophil GSF *in vivo* or *in vitro*. If the low-molecular-weight stimulatory factors are involved in the initiation of the response, it may be that the CSF provides the necessary stimulation of very immature cells to provide the maintenance of the augmented eosinophilopoietic state.

Do Eosinophils Have a Central Role in Host Defense Against Metazoa?

The marked stimulation of eosinophils by invasive metazoa has long suggested that these cells might be a central component in host defense against such formidable pathogens. The data supporting such a role have been discussed in detail by Dessein and David in Chapter 10 of this volume. However, I include a caveat, cautioning against premature acceptance of the hypothesis that eosinophils have such a unique or crucial role in host defense.

Before an analysis of specific aspects of effective immunity can be approached, there must be some understanding, if not precise definition, of the nature of the immune defense reaction *in vivo*. Metazoan parasites are relatively huge pathogens and expose the host to a myriad of antigens (both structural and excreted or secreted by the worms). Furthermore, during its life cycle, a single parasite goes through several changes in size, structure, antigenic composition, and site (migrating or lodged within various tissues, in the blood, or relatively isolated from the host within the lumen of the gut). Thus, as the parasite progresses, it often elicits virtually every possible mechanism of immunologic stimulation. It is then necessary to determine if these immune reactions achieve any degree of immune protection of the host and at which (if any) points in the sequence such protection occurs. For example, in trichinosis, immune defense may involve reduced production of migratory larvae by the intestinal (adult) phase worms, expulsion of adult worms from the gut, and/or destruction of migratory larvae prior to their encystment in striated muscle (21–23,49–51,62,72,118,129).

Once the multiple possible sites of immune defense have been identified, then the hypothesis that eosinophils are central to specific aspects of the immune response can be examined. Data to support the hypothesis could arise by several lines of observations:

a) *In vivo* observations to determine the sites of destruction of migratory metazoa *in vivo*. This should include careful observations of the cellular accumulation and interaction in the larvicidal response, with particular emphasis on the first hours of the reaction, when the killing, rather than degradation, of the pathogen might occur, and definition of the cells interacting directly with larvae during this period.

b) Further *in vivo* observations following modification of immune responses, e.g., by antigen-specific immunization or by administration of such less specific agents as bacille Calmette Guérin (BCG). This could ascertain correlations (or the lack thereof) between enhanced eosinophil responses and effective host defense.

c) Observations regarding the effect of truly selective depletion of specific cell populations (eosinophils, neutrophils, monocytes, macrophages, basophils) on the course of the parasitic infestation. To be acceptable, the depletion of one cell population must be shown not to alter the functional integrity (not merely the numbers) of the other aspects of the host response.

d) Studies of the ability of each component (cellular and humoral) to mimic the *in vivo* defensive reaction (e.g., destruction of migratory phase larvae) during *in vitro* incubation of putative targets with purified components of the defensive system *in vitro*. Careful comparisons between the abilities of the various immunologic components, and correlation with *in vivo* events, are crucial. As discussed in the first part of this chapter, eosinophils can kill bacteria *in vitro*, but there is no doubt that eosinophils are not a central part of host defense against bacteria.

e) Definition of mechanisms of such *in vitro* reactions, hopefully to identify components possessed by specific portions of the immune armamentarium.

Each of these approaches has been used in a bewildering number of studies of host defenses, mounted by a variety of host species against diverse metazoan pathogens. Little of consistency can be discerned from the data obtained to date.

In vivo study of kinetics of development of normal cellular responses to metazoa has been limited by general inability to examine timed responses to the pathogens at the physiologic site of pathogen-host confrontation, e.g., the timed response to *Trichinella* larvae within the wall of the gut. Data have been obtained by bolus intraperitoneal, intravenous, or subcutaneous administration of parasites with subsequent peritoneal lavage or excision of lung or skin for histologic examination. Such studies, in general, reveal cellular responses similar to that in Fig. 8. There is a predominant influx of neutrophils for the initial 12 to 18 hr of the reaction. After about 12 hr, eosinophils and macrophages appear and, by 24 hr, have become the predominant cells. A qualitatively similar response to *Trichinella*, varying somewhat in timing depending on host species, has been reported by others (28,159). Also, neutrophils are the predominant cells in the early inflammatory response to schistosomula in mice (83,84). These cellular responses suggest that a pathogen

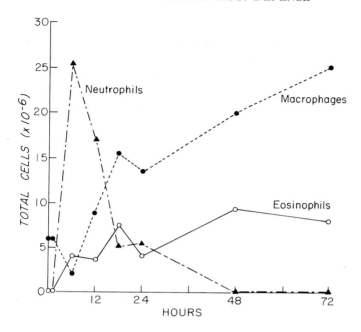

FIG. 8. Cellular response following intraperitoneal administration of 3,000 *T. spiralis* larvae to mice with trichinosis of 6 to 8 weeks duration. Peritoneal cavities were vigorously lavaged with phosphate-buffered saline (total volume, 3 ml) and eosinophil, total white cell and differential counts determined, and total cells of each type in the lavage fluid calculated. Each point is the mean of 4 mice.

would initially confront a preponderance of neutrophils, rather than eosinophils, as the front line of host defense.

Exceptions to this series of observations exist. Maddison and co-workers (87) examined skin tests in monkeys immunized by prior exposure to *S. mansoni*. Intracutaneous injection of adult worm schistosome antigens elicited an immediate (15 min) reaction which was composed predominantly of eosinophils. After 5 hr, the reaction had turned to that of an Arthus reaction with a predominance of neutrophils. Thus, this response differs from the inflammatory reactions described above by superimposition of a rapid, transient accumulation of eosinophils at the inflammatory site. Hsü and colleagues (69,70) described eosinophil-rich immediate and Arthus-like responses in monkeys which had been immunized by repeated injection of irradiated schisotosome cercariae. It is possible that this unusual response is a variant of the "retest phenomenon" described by Arnason and Waksman (4) following reinjection of tuberculin in guinea pigs and associated with an early influx of eosinophils. This retest phenomenon, although fascinating, is of limited significance for evaluating the normal sequence of inflammatory responses during host-defense reactions.

The distribution of eosinophils within granulomata varies, depending on the parasite (or other form of stimulus) studied. In immune reactions to many parasites, the eosinophils appear most concentrated in the periphery of the granulomata (27,73,135,136,146). This peripheral distribution of eosinophils at inflammatory sites has been recognized for more than 60 yr and has been demonstrated in inflammatory responses of diverse types including streptococcal pneumonia (60), subcutaneous staphylococcal infection (9), coxsackie B viral pancreatitis (9), coccidioidomycosis (78), autoimmune thyroiditis (40), and chemical injury (144). Schistosomiasis apparently again provides an exception to this series. In immune responses to schistosomula (83,84) or schistosome eggs (25), eosinophils are found scattered throughout the lesions and are occasionally found in contact with parasites. Although this could suggest that the eosinophils are involved in parasite destruction, this interpretation is limited by several other observations. A larger proportion of eosinophils appear around the penetration tracts of schistosomula than around the larvae themselves (42,83). Only a small proportion of larvae are found in contact with eosinophils. Moreover, the earliest histologic signs of parasite damage involve larval-neutrophil interactions (83,84). These observations do not, in general, support the hypothesis that the eosinophil is a primary killing cell in the host response. The delayed appearance of eosinophils and the peripheral localization of eosinophils in most inflammatory reactions would be of greater support for the concept that the eosinophil is involved in the later hypersensitivity reaction to the parasite deposited in the tissues.

Studies of effects of antigen-specific or nonspecific enhancement of immune responses *in vivo* also do not support the hypothesis that eosinophils are central to host defense. Colley and co-workers (42) attempted to immunize mice against schistosomiasis using a preparation of cercarial antigen. The "immunized" animals mounted a vigorous, eosinophil-rich inflammatory response at the dermal site of cercarial penetration, yet the cercarial-antigen pretreatment did not confer immunity. Thus, although the eosinophil response was activated, the animals were not protected. Activation of nonspecific immune mechanisms, e.g., by prior exposure to toxoplasmosis (97) or BCG (86,88), may generate a defensive response as effective as that achieved by previous exposure to (and/or chronic infestation by) a specific metazoan pathogen. Maddison et al. (86,88) examined activation of nonspecific immune responses following administration of BCG in mice or BCG plus immune serum in rhesus monkeys. Such activation caused increased host protection, monitored by decreased numbers of infective larvae surviving to adulthood in the host; however, this was associated with decreased eosinophilopoiesis and decreased eosinophils in granulomatous reactions. The available data indicate that stimulation of eosinophil responses may not confer immunity and, conversely, that enhanced protection need not involve enhanced eosinophil responses. Indeed, host protection and eosinophil responses, at least in these experimental models, appear inversely related.

Perhaps the most convincing data in support of a role for eosinophils in host defense are those from experiments using antieosinophil sera. If the hypothesis is correct, selective depletion of eosinophils (but not neutrophils, monocytes, macrophages, or basophils) should abrogate immune responses to metazoa. Characterization of the selectivity of the antisera is crucial. The antieosinophil sera of Mahmoud and co-workers (89,90,95) were probably the best characterized and were capable of blocking immunity to *S. mansoni* or *T. spiralis* in mice (Fig. 9) (63,96). This antisera did not deplete numbers of circulating neutrophils (effects on monocytes, basophils, or macrophages were not reported). However, it remains possible that such antisera could attach to neutrophils (or other effector cells), and block functional responses, without being overtly cytotoxic (36). Indeed, in preliminary experiments using Mahmoud's antihuman eosinophil serum at a 1:10 dilution [as used in *in vitro* larval killing experiments (32)], we found that the antiserum did not kill human neutrophils but that it markedly inhibited the ability to respond in the migration-under-agarose chemotaxis assay and the bactericidal activity of human neutrophils (unpublished observations). These experiments need to be repeated, as do similar experiments with the antimouse eosinophil serum. Alternatively, in the mouse model, it should be demonstrated that neutrophil-dependent host responses,

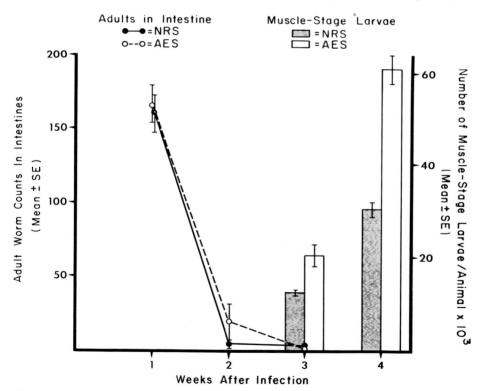

FIG. 9. Effect of antieosinophil serum (AES) and normal rabbit serum (NRS) on the natural course of *T. spiralis* infection in mice. Although AES treatment did not alter the timing of expulsion of adult worms from the gut, the number of larvae achieving muscle encystment was markedly increased. [Reproduced from Mahmoud, A.A.F. (1977): *Am. J. Trop. Med. Hyg.* 26:154, with permission.]

e.g., to a subcutaneous staphylococcal abscess, remain intact following treatment with antieosinophil serum. Finally, since the use of antineutrophil serum provided extremely valuable supporting data (it did not block immunity to parasites), it would be equally important to demonstrate that this antiserum did not alter eosinophil responses. These are not minor objections. Given the multiple possible effects of such monospecific antisera *in vivo* (e.g., what is the effect of the sudden release of the total body stores of eosinophil major basic protein (MBP) following treatment with antieosinophil serum; could lysis of the large mass of neutrophils by antineutrophil serum, with engulfment of the damaged cells by macrophages, cause activation of macrophage-mediated responses, etc.) and the demonstrated complexity of nonspecific immune activation or suppression in host defense against metazoa, a compulsive analysis of the immunologic status of animals given these antisera remains vital to the confident interpretation of the data.

Recently, several models have been devised to monitor the damage or death of migratory or tissue phases of *S. mansoni*, *T. spiralis* and *Onchocerca volvulus in vitro*. Certainly, eosinophils are capable of damaging and often killing such parasites (for detailed review, see Chapters 9 and 10). However, many investigators have found that neutrophils (14,45,46,61,68,77), monocytes (53), macrophages (35,76,92), and, with *S. mansoni*, even antibody and/or complement in the absence of cells (37,75,112,132) have a similar larvicidal ability. Comparisons of relative killing abilities have generally been limited to comparisons between eosinophils and neutrophils. We found human eosinophils and neutrophils (plus rabbit immune serum) to be equally capable of killing the migratory phase of *T. spiralis* (Fig. 10) (14). Kazura and co-workers (77) obtained similar results regarding killing of schistosomula of *S. mansoni* with human immune serum. In contrast, in the assay used by Vadas and colleagues, only eosinophils damage schistosomula; neutrophils are not even capable of continued attachment to the larval surface (150). Others have obtained data between these two extremes. The assays have differed in many respects: The immune serum used (source, heat-inactivated or not, final concentration); physical dimensions of assays [microtiter plates, which should retain an aerobic environment (14,77), or tall, thin tubes used without agitation, which could create an anaerobic environment (150)]; methods of assessing larval death (uptake of supravital dyes, chromium release, morphologic changes, infectivity), etc. Which of these best relates to events *in vivo* remains to be determined.

Regarding putative larvicidal mechanisms, eosinophils appear unusually well-endowed for the role of a killer cell. Eosinophils, at least when obtained from patients with eosinophilia, are capable of an oxidative metabolic burst which, in many ways, appears more potent than that of neutrophils. Certain migratory metazoa may be killed directly by H_2O_2 generated by granulocytes (14) or by cell-free H_2O_2-generating systems (15). Eosinophil peroxidase might contribute to certain larvicidal interactions in the peroxidase-H_2O_2-halide system (especially with iodide). The MBP is unique to eosinophils and is highly cytotoxic (33,160). If the eosinophil is not a killer cell, any alternative hypothesis of eosinophil function will have to explain why such highly toxic mechanisms exist in a pacifist cell.

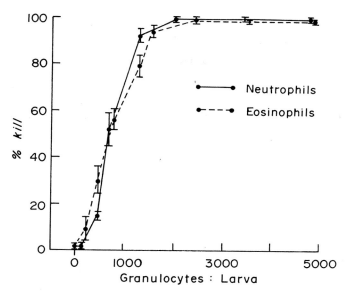

FIG. 10. Killing of newborn (migratory phase) larvae of *T. spiralis* by three preparations of purified human neutrophils (99%) or eosinophils (91% to 95%) after 18 hr incubation in medium containing 5% heat-inactivated rabbit immune serum. This immune serum promoted optimal killing by both types of granulocytes. Means ± SEM of nine determinations. [Reproduced from Bass and Szejda (14), with permission.]

In 1914, histologic study of eosinophil responses *in vivo* prompted the theory that eosinophils are not usually central components in the production of allergic or granulomatous responses but are involved in the handling of the resultant tissue reaction (135). By this view the eosinophil is seen as a scavenger, wandering around the periphery of the inflammatory process, ingesting or destroying potentially toxic by-products, and minimizing unnecessary spread of the reaction. Minor variants of this hypothesis have reappeared repeatedly during the intervening half-century (e.g., 31,122,124,151). These views have gained some further support in proposed mechanisms whereby eosinophils may counteract basophil or mast-cell-mediated reactions (19,163), and the observation that loss of eosinophils from granulomas, such as to schistosome eggs deposited in the liver, may be associated with increased damage to adjacent tissues (54,91).

With the data available at present, we have not yet proven the role(s) of the eosinophil. Perhaps it may act in immune defense in certain circumstances, and as modulator of immunologically mediated inflammatory reactions in other situations. Or perhaps, it may be that none of our currently favored hypotheses are directed with final accuracy. Forty-five years ago, Arnold Rich commented on the state of knowledge regarding the lymphocyte: "Congregated often in the more peripheral parts of the lesion, they have the appearance of phlegmatic spectators passively watching the turbulent activities of the phagocytes. Literally, nothing of importance is known regarding the potentialities of these cells other than they move and that they reproduce themselves" (123).

We have recently learned a great deal about the qualities of eosinophils and the events which control eosinophil behavior *in vivo*. If we are not lured into unwarranted acceptance of a single hypothesis, with an attendant risk of stifling new approaches, perhaps the investigation of eosinophil functions *in vivo* will now progress with the innovation, enthusiasm and success previously devoted to lymphocytes.

ACKNOWLEDGMENT

This work was supported, in part, by National Institutes of Health grants AI 14929 and HL 16769.

REFERENCES

1. Andrews, J. P., McClellan, J. T., and Scott, C. H. (1960): Lethal congenital neutropenia with eosinophilia occurring in two siblings. *Am. J. Med.*, 29:358–362.
2. Archer, G. T., and Bosworth, N. (1961): Phagocytosis by eosinophils following antigen-antibody reactions *in vivo*. *Aust. J. Exp. Biol. Med. Sci.*, 39:157–164.
3. Archer, G. T., and Hirsch, J. G. (1963): Motion picture studies on degranulation of horse eosinophils during phagocytosis. *J. Exp. Med.*, 118:287–293.
4. Arnason, B. G., and Waksman, B. H. (1963): The retest reaction in delayed sensitivity. *Lab. Invest.*, 12:737–747.
5. Baehner, R. L., and Johnston, R. B., Jr. (1971): Metabolic and bactericidal activities of human eosinophils. *Br. J. Haematol.*, 20:277–285.
6. Bartelmez, S., Dodge, W. H., and Bass, D. A. (1980): Differential regulation of spleen cell-mediated eosinophil and neutrophil-macrophage production. *Blood*, 55:489–493.
7. Bartelmez, S. H., Dodge, W. H., Mahmoud, A. A. F., and Bass, D. A. (1980): Stimulation of eosinophil production *in vitro* by eosinophilopoietin and spleen cell-derived eosinophil growth-stimulating factor. *Blood*, 56:706–711.
8. Bass, D. A. (1975): Behavior of eosinophil leukocytes in acute inflammation. I. Lack of dependence on adrenal function. *J. Clin. Invest.*, 55:1229–1236.
9. Bass, D. A. (1975): Behavior of eosinophil leukocytes in acute inflammation. II. Eosinophil dynamics during acute inflammation. *J. Clin. Invest.*, 56:870–879.
10. Bass, D. A. (1977): Reproduction of the eosinopenia of acute infection by passive transfer of a material obtained from inflammatory exudate. *Infect. Immun.*, 15:410–416.
11. Bass, D. A. (1980): Eosinopenia. In: *The Eosinophil in Health and Disease*, edited by A. A. F. Mahmoud and K. F. Austen, pp.275-289. Grune and Stratton, New York.
12. Bass, D. A., Gonwa, T. A., Szejda, P., Cousart, M. S., DeChatelet, L. R., and McCall, C. E. (1980): Eosinopenia of acute infection. Production of eosinopenia by chemotactic factors of acute inflammation. *J. Clin. Invest.*, 65:1265–1271.
13. Bass, D. A., Grover, W. H., Lewis, J., Szejda, P., DeChatelet, L. R., and McCall, C. E. (1980): Comparison of human eosinophils from normals and patients with eosinophilia. *J. Clin. Invest.*, 66:1265-1273.
14. Bass, D. A., and Szejda, P. (1979): Eosinophils versus neutrophils in host defense. Killing of newborn larvae of *Trichinella spiralis* by human granulocytes *in vitro*. *J. Clin. Invest.*, 64:1415–1422.
15. Bass, D. A., and Szejda, P. (1979): Mechanisms of killing of newborn larvae of *Trichinella spiralis* by neutrophils and eosinophils. Killing by generators of hydrogen peroxide *in vitro*. *J. Clin. Invest.*, 64:1558–1564.
16. Bassoe, H. H., Aarskog, D., Thorsen, T., and Stoa, K. F. (1965): Cortisol production rate in patients with acute bacterial infections. *Acta Med. Scand.*, 177:701–705.
17. Basten, A., and Beeson, P. B. (1970): Mechanisms of eosinophilia. II. Role of the lymphocyte. *J. Exp. Med.*, 131:1288–1305.

18. Basten, A., Boyer, M. H., and Beeson, P. B. (1970): Mechanism of eosinophilia. I. Factors affecting the eosinophil response of rats to *Trichinella spiralis*. *J. Exp. Med.*, 131:1271–1287.
19. Beeson, P. B., and Bass, D. A. (1977): *The Eosinophil*. W. B. Saunders Co., Philadelphia.
20. Beisel, W. B., and Rapoport, M. I. (1969): Interrelations between adrenocortical functions and infectious illness. *N. Engl. J. Med.*, 28:541–546.
21. Bell, R. G., and McGregor, D. D. (1980): Requirement of two discrete stimuli for induction of the intestinal rapid expulsion response against *Trichinella spiralis* in rats. *Infect. Immun.*, 29:186–193.
22. Bell, R. G., and McGregor, D. D. (1980): Rapid expulsion of *Trichinella spiralis*: Coinduction by using antigenic extracts of larvae and intestinal stimulation with an unrelated parasite. *Infect. Immun.*, 29:194–199.
23. Bell, R. G., McGregor, D. D., and Despommier, D. D. (1979): *Trichinella spiralis*: Mediation of the intestinal component of protective immunity in the rat by multiple, phase-specific, antiparasitic responses. *Exp. Parasitol.*, 47:140–157.
24. Bjorksten, B., and Lundmark, K. M. (1976): Recurrent bacterial infections in four siblings with neutropenia, eosinophilia, hyperimmunoglobulinemia A, and defective neutrophil chemotaxis. *J. Infect. Dis.*, 133:63–71.
25. Bogitsh, B. J. (1971): *Schistosoma mansoni*: Cytochemistry of eosinophils in egg-caused early hepatic granulomas of mice. *Exp. Parasitol.*, 29:493–500.
26. Boyer, M. H., Basten, A., and Beeson, P. B. (1970): Mechanism of eosinophilia. III. Suppression of eosinophilia by agents known to modify immune responses. *Blood*, 36:458–469.
27. Boyer, M. H., Spry, C. J. F., Beeson, P. B., and Sheldon, W. H. (1971): Mechanism of eosinophilia. IV. The pulmonary lesion resulting from intravenous injection of *Trichinella spiralis*. *Yale J. Biol. Med.*, 43:351–357.
28. Bracken, M. M. (1939): The prognostic significance of eosinophils in the blood in pneumonia. *Am. J. Med. Sci.*, 198:386–389.
29. Bujak, J. S., and Root, R. K. (1974): The role of peroxidase in the bactericidal activity of human blood eosinophils. *Blood*, 43:727–736.
30. Burgess, A. W., Metcalf, D., Russell, S. H. M., and Nicola, N. A. (1980): Granulocyte/macrophage, megakaryocyte-, eosinophil-, and erythroid-colony-stimulating factors produced by mouse spleen cells. *Biochem. J.*, 185:301–314.
31. Burnet, F. M. (1969): *Cellular Immunology*. Cambridge University Press, London.
32. Butterworth, A. E., Sturrock, R. F., Houba, V., Mahmoud, A. A. F., Sher, A., and Rees, P. H. (1975): Eosinophils as mediators of antibody-dependent damage to schistosomula. *Nature (London)*, 256:727–729.
33. Butterworth, A. E., Wassom, D. L., Gleich, G. J., Loegering, D. A., and David, J. R. (1979): Damage to schistosomula of *Schistosoma mansoni* induced directly by eosinophil major basic protein. *J. Immunol.*, 122:221–229.
34. Campbell, D. H. (1942): Experimental eosinophilia with keratin from *Ascaris suum* and other sources. *J. Infect. Dis.*, 71:270–276.
35. Capron, A., Dessaint, J. P., Capron, M., and Bazin, H. (1975): Specific IgE antibodies in immune adherence of normal macrophages to *Schistosoma mansoni* schistosomules. *Nature (London)*, 253:474–475.
36. Clark, R. A., Johnson, F. L., Klebanoff, S. J., and Thomas, E. D. (1976): Defective neutrophil chemotaxis in bone marrow transplant patients. *J. Clin. Invest.*, 58:22–31.
37. Clegg, J. A., and Smithers, S. R. (1972): The effects of immune rhesus monkey serum on schistosomula of *Schistosoma mansoni* during cultivation *in vitro*. *Int. J. Parasitol.*, 2:79–98.
38. Cline, M. J., and Golde, D. W. (1979): Controlling the production of blood cells. *Blood*, 53:157–165.
39. Cline, M. J., Hanifin, J., and Lehrer, R. I. (1968): Phagocytosis by human eosinophils. *Blood*, 32:922–934.
40. Cohen, S., Rose, N. R., and Brown, R. B. (1974): The appearance of eosinophils during the development of experimental autoimmune thyroiditis in the guinea pig. *Clin. Immunol. Immunopathol.*, 2:256–265.
41. Cohen, S. G., and Sapp, T. M. (1969): Phagocytosis of bacteria by eosinophils in infectious-related asthma. *J. Allergy*, 44:113–117.

42. Colley, D. G., Savage, A. M., and Lewis, F. A. (1977): Host responses induced and elicited by cercariae, schistosomula, and cercarial antigenic preparations. *Am. J. Trop. Med. Hyg.*, 26:88–95.

43. Craddock, P. R., Fehr, J., Dalmasso, A. P., Brigham, K. L., and Jacob, H. S. (1977): Pulmonary vascular leukostasis resulting from complement activation by dialyzer cellophane membranes. *J. Clin. Invest.*, 59:879–888.

44. Dahl, R., and Venge, P. (1978): Blood eosinophil leucocyte and eosinophil cationic protein. *In vivo* study of the influence of beta-2-adrenergic drugs and steroid medication. *Scand. J. Resp. Dis.*, 59:319–322.

45. Dean, D. A., Wistar, R., and Chen, P. (1975): Immune response of guinea pigs to *Schistosoma mansoni*. I. *In vitro* effects of antibody and neutrophils, eosinophils and macrophages on schistosomula. *Am. J. Trop. Med. Hyg.*, 24:74–82.

46. Dean, D. A., Wistar, R., and Murrell, K. D. (1974): Combined *in vitro* effects of rat antibody and neutrophilic leukocytes on schistosomula of *Schistosoma mansoni*. *Am. J. Trop. Med. Hyg.*, 23:420–428.

47. DeChatelet, L. R., Migler, R., Shirley, P., Muss, H., and Bass, D. A. (1978): Comparison of intracellular bactericidal abilities of human neutrophils and eosinophils. *Blood*, 52:609–617.

48. DeChatelet, L. R., Shirley, P., Muss, H., McPhail, L., and Bass, D. (1977): Oxidative metabolism of the human eosinophil. *Blood*, 50:525–535.

49. Despommier, D. (1977): Immunity to *Trichinella spiralis*. *Am. J. Trop. Med. Hyg.*, 26:68–75.

50. Despommier, D. D., Campbell, W. C., and Blair, L. S. (1977): The *in vivo* and *in vitro* analysis of immunity to *Trichinella spiralis* in mice and rats. *Parasitology*, 74:109–119.

51. Despommier, D. D., McGregor, D. D., Crum, E., and Carter, P. B. (1977): Immunity to *Trichinella spiralis*. II. Expression of immunity against adult worms. *Immunology*, 33:797–805.

52. Doenhoff, M., Musallam, R., Bain, J., and McGregor, A. (1979): *Schistosoma mansoni* infections in T-cell deprived mice, and the ameliorating effect of administering homologous chronic infection serum. I. Pathogenesis. *Am. J. Trop. Med. Hyg.*, 28:260–273.

53. Ellner, J. J., and Mahmoud, A. A. F. (1979): Killing of schistosomula of *Schistosoma mansoni* by normal human monocytes. *J. Immunol.*, 123:949–951.

54. Fine, D. P., Buchanan, R. D., and Colley, D. G. (1973): *Schistosoma mansoni* infection in mice depleted of thymus-dependent lymphocytes. I. Eosinophilia and immunologic responses to a schistosomal egg preparation. *Am. J. Pathol.*, 71:193–206.

55. Flagstad, T., Andersen, S., and Nielsen, K. (1972): The course of experimental *Fasciola hepatica* infection in calves with a deficient cellular immunity. *Res. Vet. Sci.*, 13:468–475.

56. Frank, M. M., and Atkinson, J. P. (1975): Complement in clinical medicine. *D. Month.*, 1–55.

57. Gelpi, A. P., and Mustafa, A. (1968): Ascaris pneumonia. *Am. J. Med.*, 44:377–389.

58. Gentilini, M., Pinon, J. M., Nosny, Y., and Sulahian, A. (1975): Parasitoses à nématodes: le poumon éosinophile. *Rev. Fr. Mal. Resp.*, 3:429–442.

59. Gilman, P. A., Jackson, D. P., and Guild, H. G. (1970): Congenital agranulocytosis: Prolonged survival and terminal acute leukemia. *Blood*, 36:576–585.

60. Glaser, R. J., and Wood, W. B. (1951): Pathogenesis of streptococcal pneumonia in the rat. *Arch. Pathol.*, 52:244–252.

61. Greene, B. M. (1980): Cell-mediated killing of microfilariae of *Onchocerca volvulus*. *Clin. Res.*, 28:370A (abstr.).

62. Grove, D. I., Hamburger, J., and Warren, K. S. (1978): Kinetics of immunological responses, resistance to reinfection, and pathological reactions to infection with *Trichinella spiralis*. *J. Infect. Dis.*, 136:562–570.

63. Grove, D. I., Mahmoud, A. A. F., and Warren, K. S. (1977): Eosinophils and resistance to *Trichinella spiralis*. *J. Exp. Med.*, 145: 755-759.

64. Grover, W. H., Winkler, H. H., and Normansell, D. E. (1978): Phagocytic properties of isolated human eosinophils. *J. Immunol.*, 121:718–725.

65. Hallgren, R., Venge, P., Cullhed, I., and Olsson, I. (1979): Blood eosinophils and eosinophil cationic protein after acute myocardial infarction or corticosteroid administration. *Br. J. Haematol.*, 42:147–154.

66. Harris, H. (1954): Role of chemotaxis in inflammation. *Physiol. Rev.*, 34:529–562.

67. Henry, W. L., Jr., Oliner, L., and Ramey, E. R. (1953): Relationships between actions of adrenocortical steroids and adrenomedullary hormones in the production of eosinopenia. *Am. J. Physiol.*, 174:455–458.

68. Hsü, S. Y. L., Hsü, H. F., Isacson, P., and Cheng, H. F. (1977): *In vitro* schistosomulicidal effect of immune serum and eosinophils, neutrophils and lymphocytes. *J. Reticuloendothel. Soc.*, 21:153–162.

69. Hsü, S. Y. L., Hsü, H. F., Penick, G. D., Hanson, H. O., Schiller, H. J., and Cheng, H. F. (1979): Immunoglobulin E, mast cells, and eosinophils in the skin of rhesus monkeys immunized with x-irradiated cercariae of *Schistosoma japonicum*. *Int. Arch. Allergy Appl. Immunol.*, 59:383–393.

70. Hsü, S. Y. L., Hsü, H. F., Penick, G. D., Lust, G. L., and Osborne, J. W. (1974): Dermal hypersensitivity to schistosome cercariae in rhesus monkeys during immunization and challenge. I. Complex hypersensitivity reaction of a well-immunized monkey during the challenge. *J. Allergy Clin. Immunol.*, 54:339–349.

71. Ishikawa, T., Wicher, K., and Arbesman, C. E. (1974): *In vitro* and *in vivo* studies on uptake of antigen antibody complexes by eosinophils. *Int. Arch. Allergy Appl. Immunol.*, 46:230–248.

72. James, E. R., and Denham, D. A. (1974): The stage specificity of the immune response to *Trichinella spiralis*. In: *Trichinellosis*, edited by C. Kim, pp. 345–351. Intext Publishers, New York.

73. Jones, C. E., and Rubin, R. (1974): *Nematospiroides dubius*: Mechanisms of host immunity. I. Parasite counts, histopathology and serum transfer involving orally or subcutaneously sensitized mice. *Exp. Parasitol.*, 35:434–452.

74. Jong, E. C., Henderson, W. R., and Klebanoff, S. J. (1980): Bactericidal activity of eosinophil peroxidase. *J. Immunol.*, 124:1378–1382.

75. Kassis, A. I., Warren, K. S., and Mahmoud, A. A. F. (1979): Antibody-dependent complement-mediated killing of schistosomula in intraperitoneal diffusion chambers in mice. *J. Immunol.*, 123:1659–1662.

76. Kassis, A. I., Aikawa, M., and Mahmoud, A. A. F. (1979): Mouse antibody-dependent eosinophil and macrophage adherence and damage to schistosomula of *Schistosoma mansoni*. *J. Immunol.*, 122:398–405.

77. Kazura, J. W., Fanning, M., and Mahmoud, A. A. F. (1980): Granulocyte cytotoxicity to multicellular organisms is mediated by peroxidatic mechanisms. *Clin. Res.*, 28:554A.

78. Kirshbaum, J. D. (1950): Disseminated coccidiodomycosis with severe cutaneous manifestations. *Ill. Med. J.*, 97:157–160.

79. Klebanoff, S. J. (1968): Myeloperoxidase-halide-hydrogen peroxide antibacterial system. *J. Bacteriol.*, 95:2131–2138.

80. Klebanoff, S. J., Durack, D. T., Rosen, H., and Clark, R. A. (1977): Functional studies on human peritoneal eosinophils. *Infect. Immun.*, 17:167–173.

81. Kostage, S. T., Rizzo, A. P., and Cohen, S. G. (1967): Experimental eosinophilia. XI. Cell response to particles of delineated size. *Proc. Soc. Exp. Biol. Med.*, 125:413–416.

82. Lehrer, R. I. (1971): Measurement of candidacidal activity of specific leukocyte types in mixed cell populations. II. Normal and chronic granulomatous disease eosinophils. *Infect. Immun.*, 3:800–802.

83. von Lichtenberg, F., Sher, A., Gibbons, N., and Doughty, B. L. (1976): Eosinophil-enriched inflammatory response to schistosomula in the skin of mice immune to *Schistosoma mansoni*. *Am. J. Pathol.*, 84:479–499.

84. von Lichtenberg, F., Sher, A., and McIntyre, S. (1977): A lung model of schistosome immunity in mice. *Am. J. Pathol.*, 87:105–124.

85. Litt, M. (1964): Studies in experimental eosinophilia. VI. Uptake of immune complexes by eosinophils. *J. Cell Biol.*, 23:355–361.

86. Maddison, S. E., Chandler, F. W., and Kagan, I. G. (1978): The effect of pretreatment with BCG on infection with *Schistosoma mansoni* in mice and monkeys. *J. Reticuloendothel. Soc.*, 24:615–628.

87. Maddison, S. E., Hicklin, M. D., and Kagan, I. G. (1973): Immediate, Arthus and delayed-type skin reactions in rhesus monkeys infected with *Schistosoma mansoni* or mycobacteria. *J. Allergy Clin. Immunol.*, 52:131–140.

88. Maddison, S. E., Kagan, I. G., Chandler, F. W., Gold, D., Hillyer, G. V., Slemenda, S. B., and Tsang, V. (1979): Immunization against *Schistosoma mansoni* in rhesus monkeys and the requirement of activation of both cell-mediated and humoral mechanisms. *Infect. Immun.*, 25:237–248.

89. Mahmoud, A. A. F., Kellermeyer, R. W., and Warren, K. S. (1974): Monospecific antigranulocyte sera against human neutrophils, eosinophils, basophils, and myeloblasts. *Lancet*, 2:1163–1166.

90. Mahmoud, A. A. F., Kellermeyer, R. W., and Warren, K. S. (1974): Production of monospecific rabbit antihuman eosinophil serums and demonstration of a blocking phenomenon. *N. Engl. J. Med.*, 290:417–424.

91. Mahmoud, A. A. F., and Olds, G. R. (1979): Function of the eosinophil in granulomatous hypersensitivity. *Clin. Res.*, 27:515A.

92. Mahmoud, A. A. F., Peters, P. A. S., Civil, R. H., and Remington, J. S. (1979): *In vitro* killing of schistosomula of *Schistosoma mansoni* by BCG and *C. parvum*-activated macrophages. *J. Immunol.*, 122:1655–1657.

93. Mahmoud, A. A. F., Stone, M. K., and Kellermeyer, R. W. (1977): Eosinophilopoietin. A circulating low molecular weight peptide-like substance which stimulates the production of eosinophils in mice. *J. Clin. Invest.*, 60:675–682.

94. Mahmoud, A. A. F., Stone, M. K., and Tracy, J. W. (1979): Eosinophilopoietin production: relationship to eosinophilia of infection and thymus function. *Trans. Assoc. Am. Physicians*, 92:355–359.

95. Mahmoud, A. A. F., Warren, K. S., and Boros, D. L. (1973): Production of a rabbit antimouse eosinophil serum with no cross-reactivity to neutrophils. *J. Exp. Med.*, 137:1526–1531.

96. Mahmoud, A. A. F., Warren, K. S., and Peters, P. A. (1975): A role for the eosinophil in acquired resistance to *Schistosoma mansoni* infection as determined by antieosinophil serum. *J. Exp. Med.*, 142:805–813.

97. Mahmoud, A. A. F., Warren, K. S., and Strickland, G. T. (1976): Acquired resistance to infection with *Schistosoma mansoni* induced by *Toxoplasma gondii*. *Nature (London)*, 263:56–57.

98. Mann, P. R. (1969): An electron-microscope study of the relations between mast cells and eosinophil leukocytes. *J. Pathol.*, 98:183–186.

99. McCall, C. E., DeChatelet, L. R., Brown, D., and Lachmann, P. (1974): New biologic activities following intravascular activation of the complement cascade. *Nature (London)*, 249:841–844.

100. McGarry, M. P., and Miller, A. M. (1974): Evidence for the humoral stimulation of eosinophil granulocytopoiesis in *in vivo* diffusion chambers. *Exp. Hematol.*, 2:372–379.

101. McGarry, M. P., Miller, A. M., and Colley, D. G. (1977): Humoral regulation of eosinophil granulocytopoiesis. In: *Experimental Hematology Today*, edited by S. Baum, pp. 63–70. Springer-erlag, New York.

102. McGarry, M. P., Speirs, R. S., Jenkins, V. K., and Trentin, J. J. (1971): Lymphoid cell dependence of eosinophil response to antigen. *J. Exp. Med.*, 134:801–814.

103. Metcalf, D. (1977): Eosinophil colony formation. *Rec. Results Cancer Res.*, 61:140.

104. Metcalf, D., Parker, J., Chester, H. M., and Kincade, P. W. (1974): Formation of eosinophilic-like granulocytic colonies by mouse bone marrow cells *in vitro*. *J. Cell. Physiol.*, 84:275–289.

105. Metcalf, D., Russell, S., and Burgess, A. W. (1978): Production of hemopoietic stimulating factors by pokeweed-mitogen stimulated spleen cells. *Transplant. Proc.*, 10:91–94.

106. Mickenberg, I. D., Root, R. K., and Wolff, S. M. (1972): Bactericidal and metabolic properties of human eosinophils. *Blood*, 39:67–80.

107. Migler, R., and DeChatelet, L. R. (1978): Human eosinophilic peroxidase: Biochemical characterization. *Biochem. Med.*, 19:16–26.

108. Migler, R., DeChatelet, L. R., and Bass, D. A. (1978): Human eosinophilic peroxidase: Role in bactericidal activity. *Blood*, 51:445–456.

109. Miller, A. M., Colley, D. G., and McGarry, M. P. (1976): Spleen cells from *Schistosoma mansoni*-infected mice produce diffusible stimulator of eosinophilopoiesis *in vivo*. *Nature (London)*, 262:586–587.

110. Miller, A. M., and McGarry, M. P. (1976): A diffusible stimulator of eosinophilopoiesis produced by lymphoid cells as demonstrated with diffusion chambers. *Blood*, 48:293–300.

111. Morgan, J. E., and Beeson, P. B. (1971): Experimental observations on the eosinopenia induced by acute infection. *Br. J. Exp. Pathol.*, 52:214–220.

112. Murrell, K. D., and Clay, B. (1972): *In vitro* detection of cytotoxic antibodies to *Schistosoma mansoni* schistosomules. *Am. J. Trop. Med. Hyg.*, 21:569–577.

113. Nattau-Larrier, L., and Parvu, M. (1909): Recherches sur le pouvoir phagocytaire des polynucleaires eosinophiles. *C. R. Soc. Biol.*, 66:574–576.

114. Nielson, K., Fogh, L., and Andersen, S. (1974): Eosinophil response to migrating *Ascaris suum* larvae in normal and congenitally thymus-less mice. *Acta Pathol. Microbiol. Scand. (B)*, 82:919–920.

115. Ogilvie, B. M., Askenase, P. W., and Rose, R. E. (1980): Basophils and eosinophils in three strains of rats and in athymic (nude) rats following infection with the nematodes *Nippostrongylus brasiliensis* or *Trichinella spiralis*. *Immunology*, 39:385–389.

116. Parish, W. E. (1970): Investigations on eosinophilia. The influence of histamine, antigen-antibody complexes containing γ1 or γ2 globulins, foreign bodies (phagocytosis) and disrupted mast cells. *Br. J. Dermatol.*, 82:42–64.

117. Parish, W. E., Luckhurst, E., and Cowan, S. I. (1977): Eosinophilia. V. Delayed hypersensitivity, blood and bone marrow eosinophilia, induced in normal guinea-pigs by adoptive transfer of lymphocytes from syngeneic donors. *Clin. Exp. Immunol.*, 29:75–83.

118. Perrudet-Badoux, G. R. A. (1978): Immunity against newborn *Trichinella spiralis* larvae in previously infected mice. *J. Parasitol.*, 64:187–189.

119. Phillips, S. M., DiConza, J. J., Gold, J. A., and Reid, W. A. (1977): Schistosomiasis in the congenitally athymic (nude) mouse. I. Thymic dependency of eosinophilia, granuloma formation, and host morbidity. *J. Immunol.*, 118:594–599.

120. Pincus, S. H. (1980): Peroxidase-mediated iodination by guinea pig peritoneal exudate eosinophils. *Inflammation*, 4:89–106.

121. Ponzio, N. M., and Speirs, R. S. (1975): Lymphoid cell dependence of eosinophil response to antigen. VI. The effect of selective removal of T or B lymphocytes on the capacity of primed spleen cells to adoptively transferred immunity to tetanus toxoid. *Immunology*, 28:243–251.

122. Rackemann, F. M. (1931): *Clinical Allergy*. Macmillan, New York.

123. Rich, A. R. (1936): Inflammation in resistance to infection. *Arch. Pathol.*, 22:228–254.

124. Ringoen, A. R. (1938): Eosinophil leukocytes and eosinophilia. In: *Handbood of Haematology*, Vol. 1, edited by H. Downey, p. 81. Hamish Hamilton Medical Books, London.

125. Robinson, L. D., Wooten, S. K., and Miller, M. E. (1977): Partial characterization of *in vivo* chemotactic activity: Comparison to human C5a. *J. Allergy Clin. Immunol.*, 59:353–358.

126. Roos, D., Weening, R. S., Wyss, S. R., and Aebi, H. E. (1980): Protection of human neutrophils by endogenous catalase. Studies with cells from catalase-deficient individuals. *J. Clin. Invest.*, 65:1515–1522.

127. Root, R. K., and Metcalf, J. A. (1977): H_2O_2 release from human granulocytes during phagocytosis. Relationship to superoxide anion formation and cellular catabolism of H_2O_2; studies with normal and cytochalasin B-treated cells. *J. Clin. Invest.*, 60:1266–1279.

128. Ruitenberg, E. J., Elgersma, A., Kruizinga, W., and Leenstra, F. (1977): *Trichinella spiralis* infection in congenitally athymic (nude) mice. Parasitological, serological and haematological studies with observations in intestinal pathology. *Immunology*, 33:581–587.

129. Ruitenberg, E. J., and Steerenberg, P. A. (1976): Immunogenicity of the parenteral stages of *Trichinella spiralis*. *J. Parasitol.*, 62:164–166.

130. Ruscetti, F. W., Cypess, R. H., and Chervenick, P. A. (1976): Specific release of neutrophilic and eosinophilic stimulating factors from sensitized lymphocytes. *Blood*, 475:757–765.

131. Sabesin, S. M. (1963): A function of the eosinophil: phagocytosis of antigen-antibody complexes. *Proc. Soc. Exp. Biol. Med.*, 112:667–670.

132. Santoro, F., Lachmann, P. J., Capron, A., and Capron, M. (1979): Activation of complement by *Schistosoma mansoni* schistosomula: Killing of parasites by the alternative pathway and requirement of IgG for classical pathway activation. *J. Immunol.*, 123:1551–1557.

133. Schriber, R. A., and Zucker-Franklin, D. (1974): A method for the induction of blood eosinophilia with simple protein antigens. *Cell. Immunol.*, 14:470–474.

134. Schriber, R. A., and Zucker-Franklin, D. (1975): Induction of blood eosinophilia by pulmonary embolization of antigen-coated particles: the relationship to cell-mediated immunity. *J. Immunol.*, 114:1348–1353.

135. Schwartz, E. (1914): D'e Lehre von der allgemeinen und örtlichen Eosinophilie. *Ergeb. Allgerg. Pathol. Pathol. Anat.*, 17:137–787.

136. Specht, D., and Widmer, E. A. (1972): Response of mouse liver to infection with tetrathyridia of *Mesocestoides* (Cestoda). *J. Parasitol.*, 58:431–437.

137. Speirs, R. S., Gallagher, M. T., Rauchwerger, J., Heim, L. R., and Trentin, J. J. (1973): Lymphoid cell dependence of eosinophil response to antigen. *Exp. Hematol.*, 1:150–158.

138. Speirs, R. S., and Meyer, R. K. (1949): The effects of stress, adrenal and adrenocorticotrophic hormones on the circulating eosinophils of mice. *Endocrinology*, 45:403–429.

139. Speirs, R. S., and Wenck, U. (1955): Eosinophil response to toxoids in actively and passively immunized mice. *Proc. Soc. Exp. Biol. Med.*, 90:571–574.

140. Spink, W. W. (1934): Effects of vaccines and bacterial and parasitic infections on eosinophilia in trichinous animals. *Arch. Intern. Med.*, 54:805–817.

141. Spry, C. J. F. (1971): Mechanism of eosinophilia. V. Kinetics of normal and accelerated eosinopoiesis. *Cell Tissue Kinet.*, 4:351.

142. Spry, C. J. F. (1971): Mechanism of eosinophilia. VI. Eosinophil mobilization. *Cell Tissue Kinet.*, 4:365–374.

143. Staubli, C. (1910): Die klinische Bedeutung der Eosinophilie. *Ergeb. Inn. Med.*, 6:192–220.

144. Steele, R. H., and Wilhelm, D. L. (1970): The inflammatory reaction in chemical injury. III. Leukocytosis and other histological changes induced by superficial injury. *Br. J. Exp. Pathol.*, 51:265–279.

145. Takenaka, T., Okuda, M., Kubo, K., and Uda, H. (1975): Studies on interrelations between eosinophilia, serum IgE and tissue mast cells. *Clin. Allergy*, 5:175–180.

146. Taliaferro, W. H., and Sarles, M. P. (1939): The cellular reactions in the skin, lungs, and intestine of normal and immune rats after infection with *Nippostrongylus muris*. *J. Infect. Dis.*, 65:157–192.

147. Tauber, A. I., Goetzl, E. J., and Babior, B. M. (1979): Unique characteristics of superoxide production by human eosinophils in eosinophilic states. *Inflammation*, 3:261–279.

148. Tebbi, C. K., Mahmoud, A. A. F., Polmar, S., and Gross, S. (1980): The role of eosinophils in granulopoiesis. I. Eosinophilia in neutropenic patients. *J. Pediatr.*, 96:575–81.

149. Thevathasan, O. I., and Gordon, A. S. (1958): Adrenocortical-medullary interactions on the blood eosinophils. *Acta Haematol.*, 19:162–172.

150. Vadas, M. A., Butterworth, A. E., Sherry, B., Dessein, A., Hogan, M., Bout, D., and David, J. R. (1980): Interactions between human eosinophils and schistosomula of *Schistosoma mansoni*. I. Stable and irreversible antibody-dependent adherence. *J. Immunol.*, 124:1441–1448.

151. Vaughn, J. (1953): The function of the eosinophil leukocyte. *Blood*, 8:1–15.

152. Venge, P., Stromberg, A., Braconier, J. H., Roxin, L. E., and Olsson, I. (1978): Neutrophil and eosinophil granulocytes in bacterial infection: sequential studies of cellular and serum levels of granule proteins. *Br. J. Haematol.*, 38:475–483.

153. Walls, R. S. (1976): Lymphocytes and specificity of eosinophilia. *S. Afr. Med. J.*, 50:1313–1318.

154. Walls, R. S., Bass, D. A., and Beeson, P. B. (1974): Mechanism of eosinophilia. X. Evidence for immunological specificity of the stimulus. *Proc. Soc. Exp. Biol. Med.*, 145:1240–1242.

155. Walls, R. S., Basten, A., Leuchars, E., and Davies, A. J. S. (1971): Mechanisms for eosinophilic and neutrophilic leukocytoses. *Br. Med. J.*, 3:157–159.

156. Walls, R. S., and Beeson, P. B. (1972): Mechanism of eosinophilia. VII. Importance of local cellular reactions in stimulating eosinophil production. *Clin. Exp. Immunol.*, 12:111–119.

157. Walls, R. S., and Beeson, P. B. (1972): Mechanisms of eosinophilia. IX. Induction of eosinophilia in rats by certain forms of dextran. *Proc. Soc. Exp. Biol. Med.*, 140:689–693.

158. Walls, R. S., Carter, R. L., Leuchars, E., and Davies, A. J. S. (1973): The immunopathology of trichiniasis in T-cell deficient mice. *Clin. Exp. Immunol.*, 13:231–242.

159. Walls, R. S., Hersey, P., and Quie, P. G. (1974): Macrophage-eosinophil interactions in the inflammatory response to *Trichinella spiralis*. *Blood*, 44:131–136.

160. Wassom, D. L., and Gleich, G. J. (1979): Damage to *Trichinella spiralis* newborn larvae by eosinophil major basic protein. *Am. J. Trop. Med. Hyg.*, 28:860–863.

161. Weinberg, M., and Seguin, P. (1915): Recherches biologique sur l'eosinophile, deuxieme partie, proprietes phagocytaires et absorption de produits vermineux. *Ann. Inst. Pasteur (Paris)*, 29:323–346.

162. Weiner, H. A., and Morkovin, D. (1952): Circulating blood eosinophils in acute infectious disease and the eosinopenic response. *Am. J. Med.*, 13:58–72.

163. Weller, P. F., and Goetzl, E. J. (1979): The regulatory and effector roles of eosinophils. *Adv. Immunol.*, 27:339–371.

164. Welsh, R. A., and Geer, J. C. (1959): Phagocytosis of mast cell granule by the eosinophil leukocyte in the rat. *Am. J. Pathol.*, 35:103–113.

165. West, K. M. (1953): Adrenal cortical insufficiency associated with eosinopenia: Report of a case. *J. Clin. Endocrinol. Metab.*, 13:791–794.

166. Zappert, J. (1893): Ueber das Vorkommen der Eosinophilen Zellen im menschlichen Blute. *Z. Klin. Med.*, 23:227–308.

167. Zatti, M., Rossi, F., and Patriarca, P. (1968): The H_2O_2 production by polymorphonuclear leukocytes during phagocytosis. *Experientia (Basel)*, 27:669–670.
168. Zucker-Franklin, D., Davidson, M., and Thomas, L. (1966): The interaction of mycoplasmas with mammalian cells. I. HeLa cells, neutrophils and eosinophils. *J. Exp. Med.*, 124:521–531.

Advances in Host Defense Mechanisms, Vol. 1,
edited by John I. Gallin and Anthony S. Fauci,
Raven Press, New York © 1982.

The Eosinophil in Parasitic Diseases

Alain J. Dessein and John R. David

The Department of Medicine, Harvard Medical School, and the Division of Rheumatology and Immunology, Brigham and Women's Hospital, Boston, Massachusetts 02115

The fat droplet containing leukocyte, first described by Wharton Jones in 1846 (229), was named the eosinophilic leukocyte by Ehrlich in 1879 after he noticed the affinity of its granules for aniline dyes (65). These eosinophilic granules, regarded by Ehrlich's followers as a sort of nutritive reserve, were believed to be stored by polymorphonuclear neutrophils (PMN) during a kind of ripening process. Max Schultz and Ehrlich suggested that the transition from the neutrophilic to the eosinophilic stage occurred in the bone marrow.

One hundred years later, it is known that eosinophils do differentiate in the bone marrow; they do not, however, derive from mature neutrophils, nor from any identifiable neutrophil precursors. Furthermore, the eosinophilic granules do not contain nutritive reserves but various enzymes and molecules that account for the unique biological role of this leukocyte.

In certain pathologic conditions, such as helminth infections, blood eosinophil counts reach levels 10 to 100 times higher than normal, and massive eosinophil accumulation occurs in the tissues around the invading parasite. The mechanisms underlying this impressive blood and tissue eosinophil response and the "purpose" of such a striking reaction have challenged the minds of several generations of investigators. This article as well as other recent reviews (17,39,56,85,225) are an attempt to summarize their principal findings.

PARASITIC DISEASES ASSOCIATED WITH EOSINOPHILIA

Helminthiasis

The striking association between eosinophilia and helminth infections was documented in the late 19th century, and Ehrlich named helminthiasis as a major cause of eosinophilia in his monograph *The Anemias* published in 1898 (66). In 1891, Muller and Reider (167) first described patients infected with *Uncinaria duodenalis* with an eosinophil count constituting 9.6% of the total number of leukocytes. Two years later, Zappert (232), reported a similar case with a proportion of 17% and observed Charcot Leyden crystals (CLC) in the feces. These findings were extended to *Strongyloides intestinalis*, *Ascaris lumbricoides*, *Taenia solium*, and *Taenia sa-*

ginata by Bücklers (32). In one case of ancylostomiasis, the eosinophil differential count was 53%. The impressive eosinophil accumulation occurring in the tissue around the parasite was first described by Brown in 1898 (30), in specimens of muscles removed from patients infected with *Trichinella spiralis*. A few years later *Filaria bancrofti* (43,91) and *Schistosoma haematobium* (53) were also shown to cause marked eosinophilia.

Helminths are not all equal in their ability to induce an eosinophilic response in their host (58). Penetration of host tissues and migration through the body, especially in the bloodstream, which takes parasite larvae to the lungs, is accompanied by acute eosinophilia. Larvae of metazoan parasites are retained in the lung capillary network, where they may stay a few days for further differentiation or from where they may leave the bloodstream, as do intestinal nematodes, to emerge in the alveolae and migrate to the trachea. The lung inflammatory reaction caused by larvae is often associated with a marked eosinophilia. Chronic blood and tissue eosinophilia is part of the inflammatory response against eggs (139,140), encysted parasites (30,49,122), and degenerating organisms (14,16,142,143,190,224). Leakage of fluid from a hydatid cyst, or rupture of such cysts are associated with anaphylactic reactions and eosinophilia (49,122). Abortive infections caused by the invasion of humans by parasites of animals, such as *Toxocara canis*, *Toxocara cati* (visceral larva migrans), *Ancylostoma canium*, and *Ancylostoma braziliense* (cutaneous larva migrans), trigger strong inflammatory reactions accompanied by marked tissue and blood eosinophilia (16,190).

Parasites entering an immune host induce an accelerated and enhanced eosinophil response; larval migration is often prevented in an immune host, and parasites may be found amid intense eosinophilic inflammatory infiltrates (101,102,141,207). The syndrome of tropical eosinophilia is the consequence of such an anamnestic immune response against migrating microfilariae (59,170). This disease shows a mixed clinical picture of adenopathy, eosinophilia, and pulmonary involvement, marked by cough and asthma. Its etiology remained obscure until the demonstration of the therapeutic effect of antifilarial drugs (73,231) and the discovery of microfilariae in the inflammatory infiltrates of the lung (143,224).

In summary, helminths living outside the "milieu interieur" of their host, as do most of the cestode parasites of man, induce a mild eosinophilia that is more pronounced when these worms are buried in the walls of the digestive tract. Intestinal nematodes trigger a significant eosinophilia during their migration through the body, usually coming from the skin or the intestine to the pulmonary alveolae. Schistosomes and filariae, which stay in the blood and the tissues of their vertebrate hosts, induce impressive acute and chronic eosinophilia.

Protozoan, Bacterial and Fungal Infections

Bacterial infections do not cause eosinophilia. Moreover, bacterial infections leading to an acute inflammatory reaction are often associated with eosinopenia (17). Eosinophils can hardly be detected in the blood of patients at an acute phase of a pneumococcal pneumonia. When mice are given a pneumococcal abscess 12 hr before intravenous injection of muscle-stage *Trichinella* larvae, the granulomatous response, mainly mononuclear cells and eosinophils around the larvae in the lung, is suppressed (11). This suggests that eosinopenia, due to acute pyogenic infections, involves extremely potent suppressor mechanisms. Tuberculosis is of special interest, because it produces an acute lung inflammatory response and no consistent eosinophilia.

Few protozoan infections have been shown to trigger an eosinophilic response. In 1901, Strong and Musgrave described the accumulation of a large number of eosinophils in the mucosa, the muscularis mucosae, the submucosa, and the lymph follicles of the small intestine of a patient infected with *Balantidium coli* (206). Eosinophils can also be seen in the hepatic abscess of amoebiasis, in the intestinal inflammatory reaction following *Isospora* infections (coccidosis) (17), and, possibly, in the cardiac inflammatory reaction in patients with Chagas' disease. More recently, Grimaldi and Soares (89) found a large number of eosinophils in the cutaneous lesions of mice infected with *Leishmania mexicana*. It is noteworthy that the few cases of eosinophilic tissue response to protozoans have been found in tissue where mast cells are abundant (see page 250).

Fungal infections associated with immediate hypersensitivity reactions induce blood and tissue eosinophilia. The "Valley fever" contracted 20 years ago by most of the residents of the San Joaquin Valley in California was due to coccidiomycosis. Systemic eosinophilia and allergic manifestations such as urticaria and erythema multiformis were detectable 2 to 3 wk after inhalation of the fungi. In tissues this fungus undergoes an endosporulation process leading to the liberation of multiple spores, which cause an acute inflammation; with the growth of the spores, the inflammatory response converts to a granulomatous reaction with eosinophil infiltration suggestive of the granulomatous response associated with metazoan parasites. Finally, *Aspergillus fumigatus* (aspergillosis) also invade the lungs, causing an asthmalike syndrome associated with high reaginic antibody response and marked peripheral blood eosinophilia.

MECHANISM OF THE EOSINOPHILIC RESPONSE

Production, Maturation, and Release of Eosinophils in Normal and Pathological Conditions

Eosinophils are produced in the bone marrow by multiplication of unidentified stem-cell precursors probably different from the neutrophil precursor. In the unstimulated rat, the cell cycle time is 22 to 30 hr (3,203), and the total bone marrow transit time is 5.5 days (6.5 for erythrocytes) (203). Only 10% of rat bone marrow eosinophils are nondividing (204), suggesting that eosinophil maturation occurs in other organs. When tritiated thymidine is injected into normal rats, almost no labeled eosinophils are found in the spleen after 1 hr; in contrast, 15% of the eosinophils in this organ are labeled after 40 hr, at a time when no labeled eosinophils are detected in the blood (204). This suggests that in normal rats eosinophils leave the bone marrow to lodge in the spleen where they mature before being released in the blood. This maturation probably occurs without further multiplication, because no eosinophils in mitosis were found in the spleen (204). In humans, the eosinophil emergence time in the blood (time between final division in the marrow and appearance in the blood) is 63 hr (99) versus 41 hr in the rat (203). This long postmitotic time suggests that, in humans, eosinophils mature in the marrow. This also seems to be the case in guinea pigs where 75% of the marrow eosinophils are not dividing (106). Mature eosinophils remain in the blood for only a short time. Eosinophil half-life time in the blood is 6.7 to 10.5 hr in normal rats (71,204) and 3 to 8 hr in normal humans (181). Eosinophils migrate rapidly into the connective tissue under the epithelial layer in the skin, bronchii, gastrointestinal tract, and the wall of the vagina (193).

The sequence of events following an eosinophilic stimulus has been well studied in rats given *T. spiralis* larvae intravenously. These large larvae are trapped in the lungs where they induce a granulomatous reaction. Large numbers of eosinophils accumulate in the lungs within 26 hr following larval injection (14). In rats given the larvae, the eosinophil cell cycle time was shortened from 30 hr to 9 hr, whereas the marrow transit time was reduced from 5.5 days to 3.6 days, and the emergence time was dropped from 40 hr to 17 hr. This shows that the eosinophilic stimulus may have resulted in five or six additional divisions among the youngest eosinophils (203). It followed also from Spry's study (204) that alteration in eosinophil marrow production could not influence blood or tissue levels of eosinophils, at least for the first 2 days following the larvae injection. This suggested that eosinophils, accumulating in large numbers in the lungs at this early time, were mobilized from some reserve, possibly by a soluble plasma factor—eosinophil releasing factor.

Infections causing an acute inflammatory reaction are often accompanied by an eosinopenia (17,232). This eosinopenic response is believed to be due to a rapid accumulation of eosinophils in the tissue, many of them being attracted to the inflammatory foci, and to an inhibition of the egress of mature eosinophils from the bone marrow (11). With continuation of the inflammatory process, inhibition of the bone marrow eosinophilopoiesis occurs. It is remarkable that these phenomena are the mirror image of the events triggered by an eosinophilia-producing stimulus.

Possible Mechanisms of Accelerated Eosinophilopoiesis

The first investigations on the mechanisms responsible for accelerated eosinophilopoiesis and augmented blood or peritoneal eosinophilia have been conducted in two different experimental models. Beeson and Bass (17) followed the eosinophilic response in rats given *T. spiralis* larvae orally or intravenously. Speirs (202) studied bone marrow eosinophilopoiesis and peritoneal eosinophilia induced by intraperitoneal injections of alum-precipitated tetanus toxin in mice.

It was first demonstrated that the eosinophilic response (accelerated eosinophilopoiesis and augmented blood or peritoneal eosinophilia) to larvae or tetanus toxin injections required the presence of thymus-derived lymphocytes. Neonatal thymectomy (15,70), whole-body irradiation, or injection of antilymphocyte serum prior to giving the eosinophilic stimulus abolished the eosinophilic response (15). The ability of irradiated animals to mount an eosinophilic response was restored by injection of lymphocytes and bone marrow cells (15,147). Sensitized lymphocytes obtained by thoracic-duct cannulation of rats orally infected with *T. spiralis* larvae induced elevated blood eosinophilia when injected into normal animals (15).

After considering the eosinophilic response following a second larval or tetanus toxin injection, it was demonstrated that the eosinophilic reaction has the characteristics of an immune anamnestic response; it is accelerated and augmented following homologous, but not heterologous challenge, and the anamnestic blood and bone marrow eosinophil response can be transferred to irradiated recipients with sensitized lymphocytes together with normal marrow cells (15,147,216). The nature of this immune reaction was investigated further. It was found that the eosinophilic response could not be transferred by sera from rats infected with *T. spiralis* (15). The memory cells for antitetanus toxin antibody response and for eosinophilic response were shown to appear at different times after priming (184) and to have different radiosensitivity (185). Moreover, treatment of tetanus-toxoid-primed cells with anti-IgG antiserum and complement prevented transfer of memory cells for antitetanus toxin antibody response only, whereas similar treatment with anti-θ and complement prevented transfer of memory cells for both responses (186). From these results, it was suggested that the eosinophilic response to tetanus toxin injections is a manifestation of cell-mediated immunity.

The search for factors regulating eosinophilopoiesis led to the discovery of several mediators released by lymphocytes following mitogen or antigenic stimulation able to stimulate bone marrow eosinophilopoiesis *in vitro* or *in vivo*. Metcalf and associates (162) cultured bone marrow cells in semisolid conditioned media. These culture conditions allow marrow-cell precursors to multiply and differentiate. Because of the semisolid medium, cells deriving from the same precursor remain aggregated in colonies which can be easily identified and characterized. Using this assay, Metcalf and colleagues (162) found that pokeweed mitogen stimulated mouse spleen cells to release eosinophil colony-stimulating factor(s) (EO-CSF). Spleen cells stimulated with phytohemagglutinin or concanavalin A (Con A) failed to produce such mediators. In the same experimental model, Ruscetti and Chervenick (191) demonstrated that mitogens enhanced the production of granulocyte stimulating factor(s) by thymocytes or T-derived lymphocytes. In a later study, Ruscetti and colleagues (192) reported the release of EO-CSF-like activity by *T. spiralis*-sensitized lymphocytes stimulated by *T. spiralis* antigens. Normal or bacille Calmette Guérin (BCG) sensitized lymphocytes incubated with *T. spiralis* antigens did not release detectable amount of EO-CSF. Similar results were obtained in another experimental system. Normal or stimulated spleen cells were tested for their ability to stimulate marrow eosinophilopoiesis across Millipore membranes in chambers implanted *in vivo*. In such experiments, spleen cells from mice infected with *S. mansoni* (164,165) and spleen cells from tetanus-toxoid-primed mice (148) were shown to release diffusible factors capable of enhancing marrow eosinophil-opoiesis.

Depletion of the circulating pool of eosinophils can be achieved by injection of antieosinophil serum (AES), with activity directed against determinants on mature eosinophils (160). Mice treated with AES have an enhanced marrow eosinophilo-poiesis, suggesting that AES treatment may have abolished some feedback control exerted by mature eosinophils on marrow eosinophilopoiesis. Sera of such AES-treated mice induce marrow eosinophil proliferation in normal mice. The humoral factor responsible for this activity has been named eosinophilopoietin (EPP); it is a low-molecular-weight peptidelike molecule, which is not chemotactic for eosinophilopoietic (158). A similar study has also been conducted in mice rendered eosinophilic by *T. spiralis* or *S. mansoni* infections. Eosinophilopoietin-like activity, enhancing marrow eosinophilopoiesis *in vivo* and *in vitro* (161), has been found in the sera of these parasitized animals. The EPP levels were shown to parallel marrow eosinopoietic activity. Eosinophilopoietin was not found in the sera of nude mice infected with *T. spiralis*. However, EPP obtained from heterozygote Nu/+ mice stimulated marrow eosinophilopoiesis in nude animals (161). Finally, EPP-like activity was also demonstrated in patients infected with *S. mansoni* (159).

Our present knowledge of the mechanisms leading to accelerated eosinophilo-poiesis and, possibly, to elevated blood eosinophil levels can be summarized as follows. An eosinophilic stimulus results in the antigen-specific priming of memory cells and of T-derived lymphocytes. On antigen stimulation these primed T cells release or control the release by other cells of factors capable of enhancing, in a nonantigen-specific manner, proliferation and maturation of marrow eosinophil precursors. It should be noted that these regulatory pathways may represent only some of several mechanisms controlling an eosinophilic response.

Localization of Eosinophils in Tissues

It is primarily in the tissues that eosinophils are believed to exert their functions, such as destroying invading parasites or damping hypersensitivity reactions. There-fore, the mechanisms that attract and trap eosinophils at selective sites in the tissues have received considerable attention.

The Eosinophilic Tissue Reaction

Chronic tissue response to helminth parasites varies greatly, from nil to a large inflammatory reaction, presenting the characteristics of a granuloma reaction com-posed of macrophages, lymphocytes, mast cells, and plasma cells. Eosinophils very often are part of this tissue reaction; they are more numerous at the periphery of the granuloma and may account for a large fraction of the inflammatory cells (27,30,139,140,200,207). The eosinophil granuloma is a manifestation of cell-mediated immunity (2,24,25,209,218,219); however, it has not been excluded that some cells, such as eosinophils, may be attracted to the site of a granulomatous reaction by mediators released by IgE-sensitized mast cells after triggering by parasite antigens (see page 250).

Acute eosinophilic responses having the characteristics of an immediate hypersensitivity reaction have been described in the skin of immune monkeys (102,103) and mice (141) challenged with *Schistosoma japonicum* and *S. mansoni* cercariae, respectively. In the dermis, eosinophils were found marginating in vessels surrounded by degranulated mast cells (102) and migrating from the dermis to the epidermis (102), where they formed eosinophilic aggregates around the parasite (102,141). The IgE antibodies were detected on mast cells. Mast cells migrated from the dermis to the epidermis immediately after challenge, and many of them were degranulated (103).

Finally, a third type of eosinophil-infiltrated tissue reaction against parasites is the intestinal reaction to helminths buried in the intestinal wall. This is characterized by a marked increase in the number of mucosal mast cells followed by worm expulsion (163,169,207). Eosinophils can be numerous, although not as numerous as in other tissues (92,207).

Factors that Modulate Eosinophil Migration

Several factors possibly released during parasite infections have been shown to be chemotactic and/or chemokinetic for eosinophils *in vitro*. These include activated complement components, products of the plasmin-dependent fibrinolytic cascade, lymphokines, and several mast-cell mediators. Products of complement activation, C5a (123,217) and the molecular complex C567 (137), attract eosinophils as well as neutrophils. Activation of the plasmin-dependent fibrinolytic cascade and the action of other proteolytic enzymes on fibrinogen generate fibrin fragments with chemotactic activity for eosinophils and other leukocytes (127). These activities may account for the eosinophil accumulation around fibrin deposits in parasitized tissue (207).

Sensitized lymphocytes release an antigen-containing precursor substance (ECF-P) which can be activated by specific immune complexes to yield an eosinophil chemotactic factor (52,208). Colley (54,55) and Green and Colley (87,88) described the production by phytohemagglutinin or antigen-stimulated T cells of a 25,000 to 50,000 molecular weight protein chemotactic for eosinophils. This mediator, referred to as eosinophil-stimulation promoter (ESP), was also secreted by isolated schistosome egg granulomas cultured *in vitro* (112).

The ESP-like activity has also been demonstrated in humans infected with *S. mansoni* (128) and *T. spiralis* (220). More recently, Lewis and co-workers (138) reported that culture supernatant fluid possessing ESP activity is also chemotactic for eosinophils and mononuclear cells. Since the macromolecule (ECF-L) responsible for the chemotactic activity is also a heat-stable protein with a molecular weight of 25,000 to 50;000, it was suggested that an ESP is the carrier of both activities. Recently, spleen cells from mice infected with *S. mansoni* were shown to release, on stimulation by schistosomula, some lymphokines with eosinophil-chemotactic activity. The production of this molecule(s) was specific for the early stage of development of schistosomula (116).

Lymphokines that are chemotactic and/or chemokinetic for eosinophils *in vitro* have been tested for their ability to induce an eosinophil response *in vivo*. The ESP-containing fluid injected intraperitoneally in mice enhances bone marrow eosinophil-opoiesis (146). Intradermal injection of supernatant fluids containing ESP/ECF-L into the ears of normal mice results in a cellular infiltrate composed of mononuclear cells, neutrophils, and 5% to 10% eosinophils (57).

In summary, the existence of lymphokines, which are chemotactic and chemokinetic for PMNs *in vitro*, with a preference for eosinophils, is well documented. Production of these molecules is under antigen-specific T-cell control, suggesting that they are either T-cell products or that their release is controlled by T cells. Their possible involvement in the localization of eosinophils in parasitized tissue is supported by their ability to induce eosinophil-enriched inflammatory responses when injected intradermally and by the demonstration of their release by lymphocytes obtained from helminth-infected humans and animals.

Mast-Cell Mediators Modulating Eosinophil Migration

Mediators released by IgE-sensitized mast cells after triggering by parasite antigens may be the principal factors involved in the attraction of eosinophils to invading parasites. It has been known for a long time that eosinophils accumulate at a site of an anaphylactic reaction. This was described by Schlecht and Schwenker (199) in the lungs of guinea pigs surviving systemic anaphylaxis and by Berger and Lang (21) in the local urticarial wheal induced by injection of allergens in the skin of atopic patients; these findings were confirmed by several authors (34,44,45,67,68,72,81,103,136,145,194).

Since helminth infections are characterized by high IgE antibody levels (172–174) and marked mast-cell tissue response (92,103,163,169,207,228), it is likely that mediators released during immediate hypersensitivity reactions play a major role in eosinophil accumulation in parasitized tissues. This view is supported by a recent study (61) showing that tissue eosinophil response around parasites is reduced in IgE-depleted animals. The IgE antibody response has been selectively suppressed in rats by neonatal injections of rabbit anti-rat-ϵ chain antibodies. Control and IgE-suppressed rats were infected with *T. spiralis* larvae, and the intensity of the tissue-eosinophil response around muscle-encysted larvae was evaluated 4 to 5 wk later. Many fewer eosinophils were found in the inflammatory infiltrate around encysted parasites in muscles of IgE-suppressed animals as compared to control infected animals.

Histamine and a smooth-muscle-stimulating substance, SRS-A, were the first mediators to be demonstrated in a lung diffusate after anaphylaxis (132); see also page 256. The SRS-A does not exhibit eosinophilotactic activity, and the eosinophilochemotactic effect of histamine (7) has been definitively established only recently (50,51). The first characterization of eosinophil chemotactic factor of anaphylaxis

(ECF-A) was done by Kay and co-workers (125). Molecules of ECF-A were shown to be released from actively or passively sensitized lung tissue at the time of antigen challenge by a mechanism independent of the complement system. The ECF-A molecules have an estimated molecular weight between 500 and 1,000, and therefore they differed from a previously described complement-dependent eosinophil chemotactic factor (123).

A few years before the characterization of ECF-A, the molecule in atopic sera able to sensitize lung mast cells (179,201) for the release of histamine and SRS-A was identified as immunoglobulin IgE, (108,109) which was then newly discovered. It was demonstrated that the sensitizing activity could be removed from atopic sera by anti-IgE immunoadsorbent (110). Moreover, monoclonal IgE competed with atopic sera for lung sensitization (111,124), and, finally, anti-IgE antibodies could trigger lung anaphylactic reactions (110). Kay and Austen (124) then showed that ECF-A molecules were also found in the anaphylactic diffusate recovered after antigenic challenge of human lungs passively sensitized with IgE antibodies from human atopic sera.

Two acidic tetrapeptides, Ala-Gly-Ser-Glu and Val-Gly-Ser-Glu, purified from lung diffusates or synthesized, display ECF-A-like activity (81). In addition to their direct chemotactic effects on eosinophils, ECF-A tetrapeptides enhance C5a chemotactic effect on eosinophils and at lower concentration deactivate eosinophils for further challenge (126,222). It has been suggested that ECF-A acting synergistically with other chemotactic factors may attract eosinophils to the site of an inflammatory reaction and by its low-dose effect, retain eosinophils at this site when the immediate hypersensitivity response is fading.

As well as the low-molecular-weight tetrapeptides of ECF-A, mast cells release intermediate molecular weight peptides during anaphylactic reactions that are preferentially chemotactic for eosinophils or can deactivate eosinophils to further homologous activation (26).

Mast cells are the major source of tissue histamine (188), containing about 10 μg per 10^6 mast cells for the rat (18) and 1 μg per 10^6 mast cells for the human (182). Histamine is a β-imidazolylethylamine formed in mast cells from histidine by histidine decarboxylase (198) and stored in secretory granules. Histamine exerts its effect on cells and tissues by binding to cell-surface receptors, which have been designated H1 and H2 (9). Contraction of human bronchiolar smooth muscle (64) is mediated through H1 receptors.

Although the release of histamine by the lung during anaphylaxis had been described long before the characterization of ECF-A, a definitive demonstration of the eosinophil chemotactic activity of histamine has been made only recently (50,51). Histamine at 3×10^{-7} to 10^{-6} M enhances eosinophil migration. However, at higher concentrations histamine specifically inhibits eosinophil locomotion. This inhibition is followed by a desensitization to further activation by histamine, C5a and eosinophilotactic substances released by endotoxin activated sera (50). This inactivation by a high dose may explain why histamine chemotactic activity has been controversial. The chemotactic effect of histamine is not dependent on H1 or

H2 receptors on eosinophils; however, inhibition and deactivation are mediated through H2 and H1 receptors, respectively (51).

A second group of mast-cell mediators is formed by the oxygenation of arachidonic acid. Unlike the chemotactic peptides or histamine, these mediators are not preformed mediators stored in the granules. The IgG2a-directed activation of the mast-cell-rich peritoneal cavity of rats induces the production of chemotactic and chemokinetic lipid molecules derived from arachidonic acid, which stimulate migration of eosinophils and neutrophils (213). Oxygenation of arachidonic acid by cycloxygenase from various cells generates prostaglandins such as PGD2. PGD2 is the major prostaglandin synthesized in mast cells (189) and is a potent chemokinetic factor for eosinophils (86). Oxygenation of arachidonic acid by lypoxygenase present in mast cells, eosinophils, platelets, and macrophages generates monohydroxyecosatetraenoic acids (HETEs). The 12-L-HETE produced by rat mast cells and platelets (94,171,189) is chemotactic and chemokinetic for human neutrophils and eosinophils *in vitro* (83). The HETEs are also synthesized and retained by eosinophils (86). The addition of chemotactic fragments of C5 (C5FR) to eosinophils elevates the intracellular concentration of 5-HETE and 11-HETE (86). The depletion of the endogenous eosinophil HETE pool by incubation of the cells with inhibitors of lypoxygenase activity suppresses eosinophil random migration and chemotaxis to C5Fr and to F-Met-Leu-Ala-Phe (84,86). This suggests that HETEs may be an indispensable intracellular mediator of eosinophil migration.

The involvement of mast-cell mediators in the localization of eosinophils in tissues is also supported by several experiments *in vivo*, an example being the local accumulation of eosinophils at the site of injection of purified mast-cell mediators. Injected intraperitoneally ECF-A induces local eosinophilia, just as it does if applied on abraded skin (144). In the guinea pig peritoneal cavity 12-L-HETE stimulates both a rapid accumulation of eosinophils and a later influx of neutrophils (84). Eosinophil and neutrophil responses are suppressed if 12-L-HETE is injected together with an analog, the methyl ester of 12-L-HETE.

Histamine in physiological concentrations does not usually induce eosinophilia when injected into muscle or skin of animals (45,93,202). In a few cases, local and/or systemic eosinophilia have been produced in animals after injections of physiological (7) or high doses of histamine (215). In humans, intradermal injections or topical applications of histamine to abraded skin of atopic individuals induces local eosinophilia (31,67,69,134,136,144,230). It is quite possible that individuals parasitized with helminths respond to histamine in the same manner as atopic individuals.

Since histamine is chemotactic for both neutrophils and eosinophils, the apparent selective eosinophil accumulation after histamine injections may result in a preferential retention of eosinophils at the site of the injections (180). This view is consistent with the deactivation of eosinophils demonstrated *in vitro* at high concentrations of histamine and with the ability of histamine to neutralize ECF-A chemotactic activity when a mixture of histamine and ECF-A is applied to an abraded skin of a normal individual (144).

EOSINOPHIL FUNCTIONS: DAMAGE TO HELMINTHS

In Vivo and *In Vitro* Evidence

Several lines of evidence strongly suggest that eosinophils are directly involved in the destruction of helminth parasites. In the skin of a monkey hyperimmunized with repeated injections of irradiated cercariae of *S. japonicum*, Hsü and co-workers (101,102) described eosinophils in close contact with the surface of schistosomula. One of their pictures shows eosinophils adhering to a larva. They also noticed that a large fraction of the challenge larvae were destroyed in the skin where eosinophils were the more numerous cells. Disintegrated schistosomula were seen amid eosinophil infiltrates. Eosinophil granules from disrupted eosinophils were scattered in the vicinity of the deteriorated parasite. Hsü and co-workers concluded from these observations: "As eosinophils contain a number of lysomal granules that produce several kinds of hydrolytic enzymes, it is reasonable to assume that the enzymes from eosinophils will destroy the entrapped schistosomula. It is not possible to say whether schistosomula were primarily attacked by the eosinophils or whether they were confronted first by the humoral antibodies and then attacked by eosinophils."

The demonstration that eosinophils can damage helminth larvae was provided by the work of Butterworth and co-workers (35–37). Butterworth demonstrated that eosinophils, in the presence of heat-inactivated serum from infected individuals, induce the release of isotope from ^{51}CR-labeled schistosomula. Isotope release correlated well with damage to the worm as assessed by phase-contrast microscopy (38,75,76). In a more recent study, using a technique of purification which allows the preparation of 90% to 98% pure human blood eosinophils (210), it was confirmed that eosinophils but not neutrophils can inflict serious damage to antibody-coated schistosomula *in vitro* (210). Schistosomula that have been damaged by eosinophils were not capable of maturing into adult worms when reinjected into mice (63). The link between the histological observations of Hsü and co-workers (101,102) and the demonstration of the eosinophil ability to damage schistosomula *in vitro* (36,37) was provided by the work of Mahmoud and his group (153–155). By injecting a monospecific antieosinophil serum, these authors were able to abolish the blood eosinophil response in 8- to 10-wk *S. mansoni*-infected mice (156) challenged with *S. mansoni* cercariae. Eosinophil-depleted immune mice showed a reduced ability to destroy the cercarial challenge as measured by recovering larvae from the lungs or adult worms from the liver of these mice (157).

In vivo observations of Hsü and co-workers (101–103) were confirmed and extended to other animal models and to other helminths. In describing the dermal eosinophilia in the ear pinnae of 12-wk to 16-wk infected mice challenged with cercariae, Von Lichtenberg and co-workers (141) reported the tendency of eosinophils to stream toward and around *S. mansoni* larvae, suggesting some specific interactions between these leukocytes and schistosomula. Recently, analyzing the cell response against a larval challenge in the skin of rats repeatedly infected with *Strongiloides ratti*, Moqbel (166) found numerous granuloma in which eosinophils were in intimate contact with the larval cuticle. Eosinophils may also be involved in the self-cure mechanism in *S. mansoni*-infected rats: Destruction of *S. mansoni* adult worms in the rat liver, 5 to 6 wk after infection, is preceded by a marked blood eosinophilia, and large numbers of eosinophils can be found in the inflammatory reaction around the schistosomes (135).

Butterworth's original experiments have been confirmed by a number of reports on the ability of eosinophils from humans (6), rats (149,151,152), and mice (119) to damage schistosomula *in vitro*. Concomitant with Butterworth's work, James and Colley (113,114) showed that peritoneal exudate eosinophils, obtained from *S. mansoni* infected mice, caused morphological damage to *S. mansoni* eggs. This damage was complement independent. Eosinophil-rich cell populations obtained from uninfected mice induced comparable damage when incubated with sera from 8-wk *S. mansoni*-infected mice (114). Moreover, *in vivo* eosinophil depletion with AES delays egg destruction in the liver of *S. mansoni*-infected mice (175). Eosinophils have been shown to adhere to and eventually damage several antibody-coated helminths at one stage or another of their life cycle. These include the newborn larvae of *T. spiralis* (12,129,131,150), the infective larvae of *Nippostrongylus brasiliensis* (117,151), *Wucheria bancrofti* (100), the microfilariae of *Onchocerca volvulus*, and the larvae of *Dictyocaulus viviparus* (42). Treatment of *T. spiralis*-infected mice with AES enhances the number of larvae encysted in the host muscles without affecting the expulsion of adult *T. spiralis* worms from the host intestine (90). Treatment with AES also increases the susceptibility of guinea pigs to infection by Trichostrongylus colubriformis (80). Eosinophils were also shown to kill protozoan parasites *in vitro*, such as *Trypanosoma cruzi* (1,133,195,196) in the presence of heat-activated immune sera. As yet, it is not clear if protozoan parasites have to be ingested by the eosinophil in order to be killed.

Mechanism of Eosinophil-Mediated Damage

The mechanism whereby eosinophils adhere to and kill parasites has been documented in experimental systems using schistosomula of *S. mansoni* as a target. The activity in heated immune sera that mediates eosinophil adherence and damage to the larvae is associated with IgG in man (41,211) and with IgG2a (46) in rats. Ramalho-Pinto and co-workers (187) have also shown that rat eosinophils kill schistosomula in the presence of fresh rat normal serum. Since eosinophils possess C3b receptors, and since the schistosomulum fixes C3 on its surface via the alternate complement pathway, it was suggested that C3b is the ligand in this killing reaction. In a more recent study, Anwar and colleagues (6) demonstrated that activation of the classical complement pathway enhances the antibody-dependent eosinophil-mediated damage of schistosomula. This enhancement was seen after binding of C3 to the C142-schistosomula complex and did not require additional complement components.

Butterworth and co-workers (41) and Vadas and associates (211) have shown that marked eosinophil adherence to schistosomular larvae is the result of a two-step process. The first step, which is temperature independent, is the binding of eosinophils via Fc receptors to Ab-coated schistosomula. The second step is temperature-dependent and, in contrast to the first stage, cannot be reversed by adding *Staphylococcus* protein A. Irreversibility of eosinophil adherence is achieved during the degranulation of the cell on the surface of the parasite. This was shown in experiments where Con A was used as a ligand instead of antischistosomular antibodies. Eosinophils adhere to Con A-coated schistosomula and this adherence is fully reversible by α-methylmannoside. However, Con A-dependent eosinophil adherence becomes irreversible if eosinophils are induced to degranulate on the surface of the larvae with the ionophore A28187. Eosinophils which adhere to schistosomula by Con A do not kill the larvae unless degranulation is induced by the ionophore.

Microscopic damage can be seen in the schistosomulum tegument following eosinophil degranulation (76,151,152). Major basic protein (MBP) (77,78,79) and eosinophil peroxidase (EPO) (40,151) are both released on the schistosomula tegument during degranulation and could be responsible for the damage inflicted by eosinophils to the larval tegument. The EPO-H_2O_2-halide system is toxic to schistosomula (118), and eosinophils generate H_2O_2 when incubated with schistosomula and specific antibodies (130). Purified MBP or other polycations bind avidly to the negatively charged surface of *S. mansoni* (40) and *T. spiralis* (223) larvae, and small amounts of pure MBP kill these parasites. In addition, Pincus and co-workers (183) reported that human eosinophils conserve their ability to kill schistosomula in anaerobic conditions when H_2O_2 cannot be produced. All these results taken together suggest that the death of the schistosomulum, consecutive to eosinophil degranulation on its surface, may be governed by several mechanisms, including the MBP and the EPO-H_2O_2-halide systems.

Factors Enhancing Eosinophil Damage

Several factors have been shown to enhance the ability of mouse, rat, and human eosinophils to damage parasites. First, James and Colley (115) reported that culture media conditioned with *S. mansoni* egg granuloma enhance the *in vitro* damage to *S. mansoni* eggs by mouse peritoneal eosinophils. It was suggested that ESP was responsible for the enhancement effect. More recently, Anwar and colleagues (5,6) showed that human blood eosinophils have an enhanced ability to kill complement-coated schistosomula when incubated with the tetrapeptides of ECF-A. Capron and associates (46) showed that some mediator(s), released during parasite degranulation of Ig2a-sensitized rat mast cells, enhanced the Ab-dependent killing of schistosomula by rat eosinophils. The ECF-A was found to be capable of such enhancing activity.

The mechanisms by which these mediators modulate eosinophil ability to damage schistosomula is not definitively known; Anwar and co-workers (4–6) suggested that an increase in the number of C3b receptors was responsible for this effect. Capron et al. (48) detected an increase of the number of Fc receptors on the surface of rat eosinophils incubated with tetrapeptides of ECF-A. Blood eosinophils from eosinophilic patients are more efficient in killing schistosomula (60), and they show higher levels of intracellular and intramembrane enzymatic activities (13) than eosinophils from normal individuals. A possible explanation of these results is that eosinophils are activated by factors involved in the control of marrow eosinophilopoiesis. This hypothesis was tested in this laboratory in collaboration with Vadas (Walter and Eliza Hall Institute). Semi-purified human EO-CSF preparations obtained from the laboratory of D. Metcalf (Walter and Eliza Hall Institute) were found to markedly enhance the Ab or complement-dependent killing of schistosomula by human blood eosinophils *in vitro* (62,212). Although preparations containing EO-CSF enhanced eosinophil adherence to the larvae (62), no significant increase of the number of C or Fc receptors at the surface of eosinophils was detected.

These results, taken together, suggest that the eosinophil's ability to kill parasites *in vivo* may be potentiated by lymphokines (62,115,212) or mast-cell mediators (4,5,46–48) released at the site of the inflammatory reaction triggered by the invader.

EOSINOPHIL FUNCTION: MODULATION OF PARASITE-TRIGGERED IMMEDIATE HYPERSENSITIVITY REACTIONS

Helminth infections are characterized by high IgE antibody levels (172–174). Most of these reagenic antibodies are probably not directed against parasite antigens. However, IgE antibodies with antiparasite activity are in sufficient amount to be responsible for local or systemic reactions during helminth reinvasion. As we pointed out earlier, such reactions are probably beneficial to the host in attracting different components of host immunity to the site of penetration of the invader. Anaphylactic reactions, however, can also become harmful to the host if they lead to systemic manifestations or to local tissue damage.

It has been suggested that eosinophils might have the function of dampening such reactions, and several findings support this hypothesis: a) Eosinophils tend to localize at the site of immediate hypersensitivity reactions (see localization of eosinophils in tissue, page 248); b) eosinophils may limit local accumulation of both IgE antibodies and parasite antigens by preferential phagocytosis of IgE-containing immune complexes (107); and c) eosinophils contain and release several molecules, arylsulfatase, phospholipase D, histaminase, prostaglandins, and MBP, capable of inhibiting the release of, neutralizing, or destroying some of the mast-cell mediators.

Slow-reacting substance of anaphylaxis (SRS-A) was first demonstrated in the diffusate of guinea pig lungs after anaphylactic reactions (132) and was shown to be released during immediate hypersensitivity reactions *in vivo* and *in vitro* (176,177,205). Slow-reacting substances contract smooth muscle more slowly than do histamines or acetylcholines (23). The substance was distinguished from histamine by the failure of antihistamine to inhibit its contractile activity (22). The SRS-A is an acidic polar lipid that is an oxidative product of arachidonic acid containing a thioether, and it belongs to the family of leukotrienes (168) now called LT. Because of its acidic properties (177) SRS-A might be inactivated by the MBP contained in eosinophil granules (79). Cleavage of the thioether bound by partially purified arylsulfatase (178,221) leads to the loss of biologic activity. Since eosinophil arylsulfatase is secreted during phagocytosis or when eosinophils are incubated in the presence of high concentrations of ECF-A (82), it was suggested that this enzyme was contributing, together with MBP, to inactivation of SRS-A. This hypothesis, however, should be viewed with caution since Weller and associates (227) reported recently that highly purified arylsulfatase fails to inactivate SRS-A.

Early studies suggested that eosinophils had an antihistaminic effect. Archer and Hirsch (8) reported that intact eosinophils and eosinophil extracts had the capacity to reduce the intradermal response to histamine. Broome and Archer (28) suggested that histamine was metabolically inactivated by eosinophils. Two main pathways are responsible for the catabolism of histamine in man. One is the oxidative deamination of histamine to imidazole acetic acid catalyzed by the enzyme histaminase (197), and the other is the N-methylation of histamine to methyl histamine catalyzed by histamine methyl transferase (29). Histamine activity has been demonstrated in human eosinophils and neutrophils, but not in mononuclear cells (233); conversely, histamine methyl transferase was detected in monocytes, but not in granulocytes (233). Histaminase is released by eosinophils during phagocytosis or after exposure to the calcium ionophore A21187 (234). An increase in histaminase blood level activity has been observed in several animal species immediately after anaphylactic shock (33,74). These findings raise the possibility that eosinophil histaminase together with neutrophil histaminase and monocyte methyltransferase is involved in the inactivation of histamine at a site of an inflammatory reaction.

Eosinophils may also limit the amount of histamine secreted by mast cells. Hübsher (104,105) demonstrated that immunologic stimulation of human eosinophilic leukocytes results in the synthesis and the liberation by eosinophils of an inhibitor of histamine release by leukocytes. This inhibitory factor was identified as the prostaglandins E1 and E2, which act at the target cell level by increasing the intracellular concentration of cyclic-AMP.

Histamine is also released from platelets by several mechanisms (19,20,97,98). One of those is mediated by the platelet-activating factor (PAF) released during anaphylactic reactions by IgE-sensitized basophils (19). Platelet-activating factor was thought to be inactivated by phospholipase D (120,121). This enzyme has been demonstrated in human eosinophils (121) and identified as a constituent of CLC (226). Phospholipase D was not detected in human neutrophils, mononuclear leukocytes, and platelets. It has therefore been suggested that eosinophils may also control the histamine level in immediate hypersensitivity reactions by neutralizing PAF. More recently, however, PAF has been separated from a platelet lytic activity

(PLF) by chromatography on silica gel, and it was found that phospholipase D inactivated PLF and does not affect PAF activity (214).

Thus, eosinophils may very well contribute to dampening immediate hypersensitivity reactions. The preferential localization of eosinophils at sites of such reactions and their capacity to phagocytose preferentially IgE-containing immune complexes, as well as the existence of various eosinophil products capable of destroying or inactivating mast-cell mediators, argue for such a role. It is also possible that this view oversimplifies the complex interrelationship between eosinophils and mast cells at the site of an eosinophilic reaction. It has recently been shown that EPO enhances mast-cell degranulation *in vitro* (96). Furthermore, EPO binds to mast cell granules, and bound EPO is more cytotoxic for bacteria (and possibly for mast cells) than the free enzyme (95).

SUMMARY

Eosinophils are part of the host immune response against parasites such as helminths and certain protozoa. Several lines of *in vitro* and *in vivo* evidence strongly suggest that they are directly involved in the destruction of invading larvae by antibody and/or complement-dependent cytotoxicity mechanisms. Eosinophils appear to be especially well equipped to perform this protective function, and the MBP contained in their granules probably accounts for their ability to bind irreversibly to parasite larvae, such as schistosomula of *S. mansoni*. Damage to the larvae is probably directly caused by the release of MBP and the oxidative products of the H_2O_2-EPO-halide system onto the surface of the parasite.

The mechanisms leading to the marked blood and tissue eosinophilia during helminth infections are not completely understood. It is likely, however, that eosinophils are recruited around the invader at a very early stage of the infection by mediators released by IgE-sensitized mast cells.

Finally, eosinophils are probably not only involved in the destruction of helminth larvae, but also may dampen the immediate hypersensitivity reaction induced by the parasite, thus limiting damage to the host tissues.

ACKNOWLEDGMENTS

We thank Dr. Peter Weller and Roberta David for reading the manuscript and Ramona Gonski for help in preparing it.

REFERENCES

1. Abrahamsohn, I. A., and Dias da Silva, W. (1977): Antibody-dependent cell-mediated cytotoxicity against *Trypanosoma cruzi*. *Parasitology*, 75:317–323.
2. Adams, D. O. (1976): The granulomatous inflammatory response. *Am. J. Pathol.*, 84:164–191.
3. Alexander, P., Monette, F. C., Lobue, J., Gordon, A. S., and Chan, P. C. (1969): Mechanisms of leukocyte production and release. X. Eosinophil proliferation in rats of different ages. *Scand. J. Haematol.*, 6:319–326.
4. Anwar, A. R. E., and Kay, A. B. (1977): The ECF-A tetrapeptides and histamine selectively enhanced human eosinophil complement receptors. *Nature (London)*, 269:522–524.

5. Anwar, A. R. E., and Kay, A. B. (1978): Enhancement of human eosinophil complement receptors by pharmacologic mediators. *J. Immunol.*, 121:1245–1250.
6. Anwar, A. R. E., Smithers, S. R., and Kay, A. B. (1979): Killing of schistosomula of *Schistosoma mansoni* coated with antibody and/or complement by human leukocytes in vitro: requirement for complement in preferential killing by eosinophils. *J. Immunol.*, 122:628–637.
7. Archer, R. K. (1956): The eosinophil response in the horse to intramedullary and intradermal injection of histamine, ACTH and cortisone. *J. Pathol.*, 72:87–94.
8. Archer, G. T., and Hirsch, G. F. (1963): Isolation of granules from eosinophil leukocytes and study of their enzyme content. *J. Exp. Med.*, 118:277–286.
9. Ash, A. S. F., and Schild, A. S. F. (1966): Receptors mediating some actions of histamine. *Br. J. Pharmacol. Chemother.*, 27:427–439.
10. Bainton, D. F., and Farquhar, M. G. (1970): Segregation and packaging of granules enzymes in eosinophilic leukocytes. *J. Cell Biol.*, 45:54–73.
11. Bass, D. A. (1975): Behavior of eosinophil leukocytes in acute inflammation. II. Eosinophil dynamic during acute inflammation. *J. Clin. Invest.*, 56:870–879.
12. Bass, D. A., and Szejda, P. (1979): Mechanisms of killing of newborn larvae of *Trichinella spiralis* by neutrophils and eosinophils. *J. Clin. Invest.*, 64:1558–1564.
13. Bass, D. A., Grover, W. H., Lewis, J. C., Szejda, P., DeChatelet, L. R., and McCall, C. E. (1980): Comparison of human eosinophils from normals and patients with eosinophilia. *J. Clin. Invest.*, 66:1265–1273.
14. Basten, A., Boyer, M. H., and Beeson, P. B. (1970): Mechanism of eosinophilia. I. Factors affecting the eosinophil response of rats to *Trichinella spiralis*. *J. Exp. Med.*, 131:1271–1287.
15. Basten, A., and Beeson, P. B. (1970): Mechanism of eosinophilia. II. Role of the lymphocyte. *J. Exp. Med.*, 131:1288–1305.
16. Beaver, P. C. (1956): Parasitological review. Larva migrans. *Exp. Parasitol.*, 5:587–621.
17. Beeson, P. B., and Bass, D. A. (1977): The eosinophil. In: *Major Problems in Internal Medicine*, pp. 1–269. W. B. Saunders Co., Philadelphia.
18. Benditt, E. P., Arase, M., and Roeper, M. E. (1956): Histamine and heparin isolated from mast cells. *J. Histochem. Cytochem.*, 4:419–420.
19. Benveniste, J., Henson, P. M., and Cochrane, C. G. (1972): Leukocyte-dependent histamine release from rabbit platelets. The role of IgE, basophils and a platelet-activating factor. *J. Exp. Med.*, 136:1356–1377.
20. Benveniste, J. (1974): Platelet-activating factor, a new mediator of anaphylaxis and immune complex deposition from rabbit and human basophils. *Nature (London)*, 249:581–582.
21. Berger, W., and Lang, F. J. (1931): Zur Histopathologie der idiosynkrasischen Entzündung in der menschlichen Haut. VI. Beitr. z. path. anat. u. z. allg. *Pathology*, 87:71–123.
22. Brocklehurst, W. E. (1960): The release of histamine and formation of a slow reacting substance of anaphylaxis (SRS-A) during anaphylactic shock. *J. Physiol. (London)*, 151:416–435.
23. Brocklehurst, W. E. (1962): Slow reacting substance and related compounds. *Prog. Allergy*, 6:539–552.
24. Boros, D. L., and Warren, K. S. (1970): Delayed hypersensitivity-type granuloma formation and dermal reaction induced and elicited by a soluble factor isolated from *Schistosoma mansoni* eggs. *J. Exp. Med.*, 132:488–507.
25. Boros, D. L., Schwartz, H. J., Powell, A., and Warren, K. S. (1973): Delayed hypersensitivity as manifested by granuloma formation, dermal reactivity, macrophage migration inhibition and lymphocyte transformation, induced and elicited in guinea pigs with soluble antigens of *Schistosoma mansoni* eggs. *J. Immunol.*, 110:1118–1125.
26. Boswell, R. N., Austen, K. F., and Goetzl, E. J. (1978): Intermediate molecular weight eosinophil chemotactic factors in rat peritoneal mast cells: Immunologic release, granule association, and demonstration of structural heterogeneity. *J. Immunol.*, 120:15–20.
27. Boyer, M. H.,Spry, C. J. F., Beeson, P. B., and Sheldon, W. H. (1971): Mechanism of eosinophilia. IV. The pulmonary lesion resulting from intravenous injection of *Trichinella spiralis*. *Yale J. Biol. Med.*, 43:351–357.
28. Broome, J., and Archer, R. K. (1962): Effect of equine eosinophils on histamine in vitro. *Nature (London)*, 193:446–448.
29. Brown, D. D., Tomchick, R., and Alexrod, J. (1960): The distribution and properties of histamine methylating enzyme. *J. Biol. Chem.*, 234:2948–2950.
30. Brown, T. (1898): Studies on trichinosis, with especial reference to the increase of the eosinophilic cells in the blood and muscle, the origin of these cells and their diagnostic importance. *J. Exp. Med.*, 3:315–347.

31. Bryant, D. M., and Kay, A. B. (1977): Cutaneous eosinophil accumulation in atopic and non atopic individuals: the effect of an ECF-A tetrapeptide and histamine. *Clin. Allergy*, 7:211–217.

32. Bücklers (1894): Ueber den Zusammenhang der vermehrung der eosinophilen Zellen im Blute mit dem Vorkommen der Charcotischen Krystalle in den Fäces bei Wurmkranken. *Münch. Med. Wochenschr.*, 11:21–47.

33. Buffoni, F. (1966): Histaminase and related amine oxidase. *Pharmacol. Rev.*, 18:1163–1199.

34. Bullock, J. D., Bodenbernder, J. G., Kantras, S. B., and Miller, C. E. (1968): The skin window as a diagnostic tool in pediatric allergy. *Ann. Allergy*, 26:177–184.

35. Butterworth, A. E., Sturrock, R. F., Houba, V., and Rees, P. H. (1974): Antibody-dependent cell-mediated damage to schistosomula in vitro. *Nature (London)*, 252:503–505.

36. Butterworth, A. E., Sturrock, R. F., Houba, V., Mahmoud, A. A. F., Sher, A., and Rees, P. H. (1975): Eosinophils as mediators of antibody-dependent damage to schistosomula. *Nature (London)*, 256:727–729.

37. Butterworth, A. E., Coombs, R. R. A., Gurner, B. W., and Wilson, A. B. (1976): Receptors for antibody-opsonic adherence on the eosinophils of guinea pigs. *Int. Arch. Allergy*, 51:368–377.

38. Butterworth, A. E., David, J. R., Franks, D., Mahmoud, A. A. F., David, P. H., Sturrock, R. F., and Houba, V. (1977): Antibody-dependent eosinophil-mediated damage to ^{51}Cr-labeled schistosomula of *Schistosoma mansoni*: damage by purified eosinophils. *J. Exp. Med.*, 145:136–150.

39. Butterworth, A. E. (1977): The eosinophil and its role in immunity to helminth infection. *Curr. Top. Microbiol. Immunol.*, 77:127–168.

40. Butterworth, A. E., Wassom, D. L., Gleich, G. J., Loegering, D. A., and David, J. R. (1979): Damage to schistosomula of *Schistosoma mansoni* induced directly by eosinophil major basic protein. *J. Immunol.*, 122:221–229.

41. Butterworth, A. E., Vadas, M. A., Wassom, D. L., Dessein, A., Hogan, M., Sherry, B., Gleich, G. J., and David, J. R. (1979): Interactions between human eosinophils and schistosomula of *Schistosoma mansoni*. *J. Exp. Med.*, 150:1456–1471.

42. Butterworth, A. E., personnal communication.

43. Calvert, W. J. (1902): A preliminary report on the blood in two cases of filariasis. *Bull. Johns Hopkins Hosp.*, 13:23–24.

44. Campbell, A. C. P., Drennan, A. M., and Rettie, T. (1935): The relationship of the eosinophil leukocyte to allergy and anaphylaxis. *J. Pathol. Bacteriol.*, 40:537–548.

45. Campbell, D. H. (1943): Relationship of the eosinophil response to factors involved in anaphylaxis. *J. Infect. Dis.*, 72:42–48.

46. Capron, M., Capron, A., Torpier, G., Bazin, H., Bout, D., and Joseph, M. (1978): Eosinophil-dependent cytotoxicity in rat schistosomiasis. Involvement of IgG$_{2a}$ antibody and role of mast cells. *Eur. J. Immunol.*, 8:127–133.

47. Capron, M. A., Goetl, E. J., and Austen, K. F. (1981): Tetrapeptides of the eosinophil chemotactic factor of anaphylaxis (ECF-A) enhance eosinophil F$_c$ receptor. *Nature (Lond.)* 71–73.

48. Capron, M., Goetzl, E. J., Austen, K. F., and Capron, A. (1980): Role of ECFA in IgG-dependent eosinophil cytotoxicity and enhancement of eosinophil Fc receptor. *Fourth Int. Cong. Immunol. (Paris)*, Abstr.

49. Carmalt-Jones, D. W. (1929): Hydatid disease as a clinical problem; some New Zealand experiences. *Br. Med. J.*, 1:5–9.

50. Clark, R. A. F., Gallin, J. I., and Kaplan, A. P. (1975): The selective eosinophil chemotactic activity of histamine. *J. Exp. Med.*, 142:1462–1476.

51. Clark, R. A. F., Sandler, J. A., Gallin, J. I., and Kaplan, A. R. (1977): Histamine modulation of eosinophil migration. *J. Immunol.*, 118:137–145.

52. Cohen, S., and Ward, P. A. (1971): In vitro and in vivo activity of a lymphocyte and immune complex-dependent chemotactic factor for eosinophil. *J. Exp. Med.*, 133:133–146.

53. Coles (1902): The blood in cases affected with filariasis and *Bilharzia haematobia*. *Br. Med. J.*, 1:1137–1138.

54. Colley, D. G. (1973): Eosinophils and immune mechanisms. I) Eosinophil stimulation promoter (ESP) of lymphokine induced by specific antigen or phytohemagglutinin. *J. Immunol.*, 110:1419–1423.

55. Colley, D. G. (1976): Eosinophils and immune mechanisms. IV. Culture conditions, antigen requirements, production kinetics and immunologic specificity of the lymphokine eosinophil stimulation promoter. *Cell. Immunol.*, 24:328–335.

56. Colley, D. G., and James, S. L. (1979): Participation of eosinophils in immunological systems. In: *Cell, Molecular Clinical Aspects of Allergy Disorders*, edited by S. Gupta and R. Good, pp. 55–85.

57. Colley, D. G. (1981): Lymphocyte products. In: *The Eosinophil in Health and Disease*, edited by A. A. F. Mahmoud and K. F. Austen, pp. 293–312. Grune and Stratton, New York.
58. Conrad, M. E. (1971): Hematologic manifestations of parasitic infections. *Semin. Hematol.*, 8:267–303.
59. Danaraj, T. J., Pacheco, G., Shanmugaratnam, K., and Beaver, P. C. (1966): The etiology and pathology of eosinophilic lung. *Am. J. Trop. Med.*, 15:183–189.
60. David, J. R., Vadas, M. A., Butterworth, A. E., Azevedo de Brito, P., Carvalho, E. M., David, R. A., Bina, J. C., and Andrade, Z. A. (1980): Enhanced helminthotoxic capacity of eosinophils from patients with eosinophilia. *N. Engl. J. Med.*, 303:1147–1152.
61. Dessein, A. J., Parker, W., James, S. L., and David, J. R. (1981): IgE antibody and resistance to infections. I. Selective suppression of the IgE antibody response in rats diminishes the resistance and the eosinophil response to *Trichinella spiralis. J. Exp. Med.*, 153:423–436.
62. Dessein, A. J., Vadas, M. A., Nicola, N., and David, J. R., *Submitted for publication.*
63. Dessein, A. J., Butterworth, A. E., Vadas, M. A., and David, J. R., *Submitted for publication.*
64. Dunlop, L. S., Smith, A. P., and Piper, P. J. (1977): The effect of histamine antagonists on antigen induced contractions of sensitized human bronchus in vitro. *Br. J. Pharmacol.*, 53:475P.
65. Ehrlich, P. (1880): Methodologische Beiträge zur Physiologie und Pathologie der verschiedenen Formen der Leukocyten. *Z. Klin. Med. (Berlin)*, 1:553–560.
66. Ehrlich, P., and Lazarus, A. (1898): Die Anamie. In: *Specielle Pathologie and Therapie*, edited by H. Nothnagel. Vienna, Holder. (Translated in English In *Histology of the Blood: Normal and Apathological* (1900), edited by W. Myers. Cambridge University Press, Cambridge.
67. Eidinger, D., Wilkinson, R., and Rose, B. (1964): A study of cellular responses in immune reactions utilizing the skin window technique. I. Immediate hypersensitivity reaction. *J. Allergy*, 35:77–85.
68. Feinberg, A. R., Feinberg, S. M., and Lee, F. (1967): Leucocytes and hypersensitivity reactions. Eosinophil response in skin window to ragweed extract, histamine and compound 48/80 in atopic and non-atopic individuals. *J. Allergy*, 40:73–87.
69. Fernex, M., and Fernex, S. (1966): Propriete eosinotactique de l'histamine chez l'homme. *Schweiz. Med. Wochenschr.*, 96:46–49.
70. Fine, D. P., Buchanan, R. D., and Colley, D. G. (1973): *Schistosoma mansoni* infection in mice depleted of thymus-dependent lymphocytes. I. Eosinophilia and immunologic responses to a schistosomal egg preparation. *Am. J. Pathol.*, 71:287–300.
71. Foot, E. C. (1965): Eosinophil turnover in the normal rat. *Br. J. Haematol.*, 11:439–445.
72. Fowler, J. W., and Lowell, F. C. (1966): The accumulation of eosinophils as an allergic response to allergen applied to the denuded skin surface. *J. Allergy*, 37:19–28.
73. Ganatra, R. D., and Lewis, R. A. (1955): Hetrazan in tropical eosinophilia. *Indian J. Med. Sci.*, 9:672–681.
74. Giertz, M., and Hahn, F. (1969): Mechanism of histaminase liberation in guinea pig anaphylaxis. *Int. Arch. Allergy Appl. Immunol.*, 36:41–44.
75. Glauert, A. M., and Butterworth, A. E. (1977): Morphological evidence for the ability of eosinophils to damage antibody-coated schistosomula. *Trans. Roy. Soc. Trop. Med. Hyg.*, 71:392–395.
76. Glauert, A. M., Butterworth, A. E., Sturrock, R. F., and Mouba, V. (1978): The mechanism of antibody-dependent, eosinophil-mediated damage to schistosomula of *Schistosoma mansoni* in vitro: a study by phase-contrast and electron microscopy. *J. Cell Sci.*, 34:173–192.
77. Gleich, G. J., Loegering, D. A., and Maldonado, J. (1973): Identification of a major basic protein in guinea pig eosinophil granules. *J. Exp. Med.*, 137:1459–1471.
78. Gleich, G. J., Loegering, D. A., Kueppers, F., Bajaj, S. P., and Mann, K. G. (1974): Physiochemical and biological properties of the major basic protein from guinea pig eosinophil granules. *J. Exp. Med.*, 140:313–332.
79. Gleich, G. J. (1977): The eosinophil: new aspects of structure and function. *J. Allergy Clin. Immunol.*, 60:73–82.
80. Gleich, G. J., Olson, G. M., and Merlich, H. (1979): The effect of antiserum to eosinophil on susceptibility and acquired immunity of the guinea pig to *Trichostrongylus colubriformis. Immunology*, 37:873–880.
81. Goetzl, E. J., and Austen, K. F. (1975): Purification and synthesis of eosinophilotactic tetrapeptides of human lung tissue: identification as eosinophil chemotactic factor of anaphylaxis. *Proc. Natl. Acad. Sci. U. S. A.*, 72:4123–4127.

82. Goetzl, E. J., Wasserman, S. I., and Austen, K. F. (1975): Eosinophil polymorphonuclear leukocyte function in immediate hypersensitivity. *Arch. Pathol.*, 99:1–4.
83. Goetzl, E. J., Woods, J. M., and Gorman, R. R. (1977): Stimulation of human eosinophil and neutrophil polymorphonuclear leukocyte chemotaxis and random migration by 12-L-hydroxy-5,8,10,14-eicosatetraenoic acid (HETE). *J. Clin. Invest.*, 59:170–183.
84. Goetzl, E. J., Valone, F. H., and Remold, V. N. (1979): Specific inhibition of the PMN leukocyte chemotactic response to hydroxy fatty acid metabolites of arachidonic acid by methyl ester derivatives. *J. Clin. Invest.*, 63:1181–1186.
85. Goetzl, E. J., Weller, P. F., and Valone, F. H. (1979): Biochemical and functional bases of the regulatory and protective roles of the human eosinophil. In: *Advances in Inflammation Research, Vol. 1: Proc. Int. Cong. of Inflamm.*, edited by G. Weissman, B. Samuelsson, and R. Paoletti, pp. 157–168. Raven Press, New York.
86. Goetzl, E. J. (1981): The unique role of monohydroxyeicosatetraenoic acids (HETE) in the regulation of eosinophil function. In : *The Eosinophil in Health and Disease*, edited by A. A. F. Mahmoud and K. F. Austen, pp. 167–184. Grune and Stratton, New York.
87. Green, B. M., and Colley, D. G. (1974): Eosinophils and immune mechanisms. II. Partial characterization of the lymphokine eosinophil stimulation promoter. *J. Immunol.*, 113:910–917.
88. Green, B. M., and Colley, D. G. (1976): Eosinophils and immune mechanisms. III. Production of the lymphokine eosinophil stimulation promoter by mouse T lymphocytes. *J. Immunol.*, 116:1078–1083.
89. Grimaldi, F. G., and Soares, M. J. (1980): Eosinofilia tecidual e fagocitose de *Leishmania mexicana* por eosinofilos em Leishmaniose cutanea experimental. In: *I. Jornada Cientifica*, edited by Fundação O. Cruz. Rio de Janeiro.
90. Grove, D. I., Mahmoud, A. A. F., and Warren, K. S. (1977): Eosinophils and resistance to *Trichinella spiralis. J. Exp. Med.*, 145:755–759.
91. Gulland, G. L. (1902): The condition of the blood in filariasis. *Br. Med. J.*, 1:831–832.
92. Gustowska, L., Ruitenberg, E. J. ,and Elgersma, A. (1980): Cellular reaction in tongue and gut in murine trichinellosis and their thymus dependence. *Parasite Immunol.*, 2:133–154.
93. Halpern, B. N., and Benos, S. A. (1951): Action de l'histamine sur l'eosinophilie sanguine chez l'animal et l'homme. *C. R. Soc. Biol. (Paris)*, 145:31.
94. Hamberg, M., and Samuelsson, B. (1974): Novel transformation of arachidonic acid in human platelets. *Proc. Natl. Acad. Sci. U. S. A.*, 71:3400–3404.
95. Henderson, W. R., Jong, E. C., and Klebanoff, S. J. (1980): Binding of eosinophil peroxidase to mast cell granules with retention of peroxydatic activity. *J. Immunol.*, 124:1383–1387.
96. Henderson, W. R., Chi, E. Y., and Klebanoff, S. J. (1980): Eosinophil peroxidase-induced mast cell secretion. *J. Exp. Med.*, 152:265–279.
97. Henson, P. M., and Cochrane, C. G. (1969): Immunological induction of increased vascular permeability. II. Two mechanisms of histamine release from rabbit platelets involving complement. *J. Exp. Med.*, 129:167–184.
98. Henson, P. M. (1970): Mechanisms of release of constituent from rabbit platelets by antigen-antibody complexes and complement. II. Interaction with neutrophils. *J. Immunol.*, 105:490–501.
99. Herion, J. C., Glasser, R. M., Walker, R. I., and Palmer, J. G. (1970): Eosinophil kinetics in two patients with eosinophilia. *Blood*, 36:361–370.
100. Higashi, G. I., and Chowdhury, A. B. (1970): In vitro adhesion of eosinophils to infective larvae of *Wucheria bancrofti. Immunology*, 19:65–83.
101. Hsü, S. Y. L., Lust, G. L., and Hsü, H. F. (1971): The fate of challenge schistosome cercariae in a monkey immunized by cercariae exposed to high doses of X-irradiation. *Proc. Soc. Exp. Biol. Med.*, 136:727–731.
102. Hsü, S. Y. L., Hsü, H. F., Penick, G. D., Lust, G. L., and Osborne, J. W. (1974): Dermal hypersensitivity to schistosome cercariae in rhesus monkeys during immunization and challenge. I. Complex hypersensitivity reactions of a well-immunized monkey during the challenge. *J. Allergy Clin. Immunol.*, 54:339–349.
103. Hsü, S. Y. L., Hsü, H. F., Penick, G. D., Hanson, H. O., Schiller, H. J., and Cheng, H. F. (1979): Immunoglobulin E, mast cells and eosinophils in the skin of rhesus monkeys immunized with X-irradiated cercariae of *Schistosoma japonicum. Int. Arch. Allergy Appl. Immunol.*, 59:383–393.
104. Hübscher, T. T. (1975): Role of the eosinophil in the allergic reaction. I. EDI—an eosinophil derived inhibitor of histamine release. *J. Immunol.*, 114:1379–1388.

105. Hübscher, T. T. (1975): Role of the eosinophil in the allergic reaction. II. Release of prosta-glandins from human eosinophilic leukocytes. *J. Immunol.*, 114:1389–1393.
106. Hudson, G. (1963): Changes in the marrow reserve of eosinophils following re-exposure to foreign protein. *Br. J. Haematol.*, 9:446–455.
107. Ishikawa, T., Wicher, K., and Arbeshan, C. E. (1974): In vitro and in vivo studies on uptake of antigen antibody complexes by eosinophils. *Int. Arch. Allergy*, 66:230–248.
108. Ishizaka, K., Ishizaka, T., and Hornbrock, M. M. (1966): Physicochemical properties of reaginic antibody. IV. Presence of a unique immunoglobulin as a carrier of reaginic activity. *J. Immunol.*, 97:75–85.
109. Ishizaka, K., Ishizaka, T., and Hornbrock, M. M. (1966): Physicochemical properties of reaginic antibodies. V. Correlation of reaginic activity with E globulin antibody. *J. Immunol.*, 97:840–853.
110. Ishizaka, T., Ishizaka, K., Orange, R. P., and Austen, K. F. (1970): The capacity of human immunoglobulin E to mediate the release of histamine and slow reacting substance of anaphylaxis (SRS-A) from monkey lung. *J. Immunol.*, 104:335–343.
111. Ishizaka, K., Ishizaka, T., and Lee, E. H. (1970): Biologic function of the Fc fragments of E-myeloma protein. *Immunochemistry*, 7:687–702.
112. James, S. L., and Colley, D. G. (1975): Eosinophils and immune mechanisms: production of the lymphokine eosinophil stimulation promoter (ESP) in vitro by isolated intact granulomas. *J. Reticuloendothel. Soc.*, 18:283–293.
113. James, S. L., and Colley, D. G. (1976): Eosinophil-mediated destruction of *Schistosoma mansoni* eggs. *J. Reticuloendothel. Soc.*, 20:359–374.
114. James, S. L., and Colley, D. G. (1978): Eosinophil-mediated destruction of *Schistosoma mansoni* eggs in vitro. II. The role of cytophilic antibody. *Cell. Immunol.*, 38:35–47.
115. James, S. L., and Colley, D. G. (1978): Eosinophil-mediated destruction of *Schistosoma mansoni* eggs. III. Lymphokine involvement in the induction of eosinophil functional abilities. *Cell. Immunol.*, 38:48–58.
116. James, S., and Sher, A. (1980): Immune mechanisms which stimulate mouse leukocyte migration in response to schistosomula of *Schistosoma mansoni*. *J. Immunol.*, 124:1837–1844.
117. Jarret, W. F. H., Jarrett, E. E. E., Miller, H. R. P., and Urguhart, G. M. (1968): Quantitative studies on the mechanism of self cure in *Nippostrongylus braziliensis* infection. In: *The Reaction of the Host to Parasitism*, edited by E. J. L. Soulsby, p. 191. N. G. Elwert Harburg/Lahn.
118. Jong, E. J., Mahmoud, A. A. F., and Klebanoff, S. J. (1979): Toxic effect of eosinophil peroxidase on schistosomula of *Schistosoma mansoni*. *Clin. Res.*, 27:479A.
119. Kassis, A. I., Aikawa, M., and Mahmoud, A. A. F. (1979): Mouse antibody-dependent eosinophil and macrophage adherence and damage to schistosomula of *Schistosoma mansoni*. *J. Immunol.*, 122:398–405.
120. Kater, L. A., Austen, K. F., and Goetzl, E. J. (1975): Identification and partial purification of a platelet activating factor (PAF) from rat. *Fed. Proc.*, 34:925.
121. Kater, L. A., Goetzl, E. J., and Austen, K. F. (1976): Isolation of human eosinophil phospholipase D. *J. Clin. Invest.*, 57:1173–1180.
122. Katz, A. M., and Pan, C. (1958): Echinococcus disease in the United States. *Am. J. Med.*, 25:759–770.
123. Kay, A. B. (1970): Studies on eosinophil leukocyte migration. II. Factors specifically chemotactic for eosinophils and neutrophils generated from guinea pig serum by antigen-antibody complexes. *Clin. Exp. Immunol.*, 7:723–737.
124. Kay, A. B., and Austen, K. F. (1971): The IgE-mediated release of an eosinophil leukocyte chemotactic factor from human lung. *J. Immunol.*, 107:899–902.
125. Kay, A. B., Stechschulte, D. J., and Austen, K. F. (1971): An eosinophil leukocyte chemotactic factor of anaphylaxis. *J. Exp. Med.*, 133:602–619.
126. Kay, A. B., Shin, H. S., and Austen, K. F. (1973): Selective attraction of eosinophils and syn-ergism between eosinophil chemotactic factor of anaphylaxis (ECF-A) and a fragment cleaved from the fifth component of complement (C5a). *Immunology*, 24:969–976.
127. Kay, A. B., Pepper, D. S., and McKenzie, R. (1974): The identification of fibrinogen has a chemotactic agent derived from human fibrinogen. *Br. J. Haematol.*, 27:669–677.
128. Kazura, J. W., Mahmoud, A. A. F., Karbs, K. S., and Warren, K. S. (1975): The lymphokine eosinophil stimulation promoter and human schistosomiasis mansoni. *J. Infect. Dis.*, 132:702–706.

129. Kazura, J. W., and Grove, D. I. (1978): Stage-specific antibody-dependent eosinophil-mediated destruction of *Trichinella spiralis. Nature (London)*, 274:588–590.

130. Kazura, J. W., Blumer, J., and Mahmoud, A. A. F. (1979): Parasite stimulated production of H_2O_2 from human eosinophils and neutrophils. *Clin. Res.*, 27:515A.

131. Kazura, J. W., and Aikawa, M. (1980): Host defense mechanisms against *Trichinella spiralis* infection in the mouse: eosinophil-mediated destruction of newborn larvae in vitro. *J. Immunol.*, 124:355–361.

132. Kellaway, C. H., and Trethewie, E. R. (1940): The liberation of a slow reacting smooth muscle-stimulating substance in anaphylaxis. *Q. J. Exp. Physiol.*, 30:121–145.

133. Kipnis, T. L., James, S. L., Sher, A., and David, J. R. (1981): Cell mediated cytotoxicity to *Trypanosoma cruzi*. II. Antibody dependent killing of bloodstream forms by mouse eosinophils and neutrophils. In press.

134. Kline, B. S., Cohen, M. B., and Rudolph, J. A. (1932): Histologic changes in allergic and non allergic wheals. *J. Allergy Clin. Immunol.*, 3:531–541.

135. Knopf, P. M. (1979): Peripheral and tissue eosinophilia in infected rats. *Exp. Parasitol.*, 47:232–245.

136. Knott, F. A., and Pearson, R. S. B. (1934): Eosinophilia in allergic conditions. *Guys Hosp. Rep.*, 84:230–236.

137. Lachmann, P. S., Kay, A. B., and Thompson, R. H. (1970): The chemotactic activity for neutrophil and eosinophil leukocytes of the trimolecular complex of the fifth, sixth and seventh components of human complement C567 prepared in free solution by the reactive lysis procedure. *Immunology*, 19:895–899.

138. Lewis, I. A., Carter, C. E., and Colley, D. G. (1977): Eosinophils and immune mechanisms. I. Demonstration of mouse spleen cell derived chemotactic activities for eosinophils and mononuclear cells and comparison with eosinophil stimulation promoter. *Cell. Immunol.*, 32:86–96.

139. von Lichtenberg, F. V., and Mekbel, S. (1962): Granuloma formation in the laboratory mouse. I. Reaction to *Ascaris suis* eggs in the presensitized adult and newborn. *J. Infect. Dis.*, 110:246–252.

140. von Lichtenberg, F. V. (1962): Host response to eggs of *S. mansoni*. I. Granuloma formation in the unsensitized laboratory mouse. *Am. J. Pathol.*, 41:711–731.

141. von Lichtenberg, F. V., Sher, A., Gibbons, N., and Doughty, B. L. (1976): Eosinophil-enriched inflammatory response to schistosomula in the skin of mice immune to *Schistosoma mansoni. Am. J. Pathol.*, 84:479–500.

142. von Lichtenberg, F. V., Sher, A., and McIntyre, S. (1977): A lung model of schistosome immunity in mice. *Am. J. Pathol.*, 87:105–124.

143. Lie Kian, J. (1962): Occult filariasis: its relationship with tropical pulmonary eosinophilia. *Am. J. Trop. Med. Hyg.*, 11:646–652.

144. Lindsay, W., Turnbull, D., Evans, P., and Kay, A. B. (1977): Human eosinophils, acidic tetrapeptides (ECF-A) and histamine—Interactions in vitro and in vivo. *Immunology*, 32:57–63.

145. Lowell, F. C. (1967): Clinical aspects of eosinophilia in atopic disease. *J. A. M. A.*, 202:875–878.

146. McGarry, M. P., Miller, A. M., and Colley, D. G. (1970): Humoral regulation of eosinophil granulocytopoiesis. In: *Experimental Hematology Today*, edited by S. Baum, and G. D. Ledney, pp. 63–70. Springer-Verlag, New York.

147. McGarry, M. P., Speirs, R. S., Jenkins, V. K., and Trentin, J. J. (1971): Lymphoid cell dependence of eosinophil response to antigen. *J. Exp. Med.*, 134:801–814.

148. McGarry, M. P., and Miller, A. M. (1974): Evidence for the humoral stimulation of eosinophil granulocytopoiesis in in vivo diffusion chambers. *Exp. Hematol.*, 2:372–379.

149. Mackenzie, C. D., Ramalho-Pinto, F. J., McLaren, D. J., and Smithers, S. R. (1977): Antibody-mediated adherence of rat eosinophils to schistosomula of *Schistosoma mansoni* in vitro. *Clin. Exp. Immunol.*, 30:97–104.

150. Mackenzie, C. D., Preston, P. M., and Ogilvie, B. M. (1978): Immunological properties of the surface of parasite nematodes. *Nature (London)*, 276:826–828.

151. McLaren, D. J., Mackenzie, C. D., and Ramalho-Pinto, F. J. (1977): Ultrastructural observations on the in vitro interaction between rat eosinophils and some parasitic helminths (*Schistosoma mansoni, Trichinella spiralis*, and *Nippostrongylus brasiliensis*). *Clin. Exp. Immunol.*, 30:105–118.

152. McLaren, D. J., Ramalho-Pinto, F. J., Smithers, S. R. (1978): Ultrastructural evidence for complement and antibody-dependent damage to schistosomula of *Schistosoma mansoni* by rat eosinophils in vitro. *Parasitology*, 77:313–324.

153. Mahmoud, A. A. F., Warren, K. S., and Boros, D. L. (1973): Production of a rabbit antimouse eosinophil serum with no cross-reactivity to neutrophils. *J. Exp. Med.*, 137:1526–1531.
154. Mahmoud, A. A. F., Kellermeyer, R. W., and Warren, K. S. (1974): Monospecific antigranulocyte sera against human neutrophils, eosinophils, basophils and myeloblasts. *Lancet* 2:1163–1166.
155. Mahmoud, A. A. F., Kellermeyer, R. W., and Warren, K. S. (1974): Production of monospecific rabbit antihuman eosinophil serum and demonstration of a blocking phenomenon. *N. Engl. J. Med.*, 290:417–420.
156. Mahmoud, A. A. F., Warren, K. S., and Graham, R. C. (1975): Antieosinophil serum and the kinetics of eosinophilia in *Schistosoma mansoni*. *J. Exp. Med.*, 142:560–574.
157. Mahmoud, A. A. F., Warren, K. S., and Peters, P. A. (1975): A role for the eosinophil in acquired resistance to *Schistosoma mansoni* infection as determined by antieosinophil serum. *J. Exp. Med.*, 142:805–813.
158. Mahmoud, A. A. F., Stone, M. K., and Kellermeyer, R. W. (1977): Eosinophilopoietin: a circulating low molecular weight peptide-like substance which stimulates the production of eosinophils in mice. *J. Lab. Clin. Invest.*, 60:675–682.
159. Mahmoud, A. A. F., Billings, F. T., Stone, M. K., and Kellermeyer, R. W. (1972): Human eosinophilopoietin. *Clin. Res.*, 26:555A.
160. Mahmoud, A. A. F., Warren, K. S., and Aikawa, M. A. (1978): Maturation-associated changes of eosinophil surface antigens. *Clin. Res.*, 26:506A.
161. Mahmoud, A. A. F., Stone, M. W., and Tracy, S. W. (1979): Eosinophilopoietin production: relationship to eosinophilia of infection and thymus function. *Trans. Assoc. Am. Physicians*, 92:355–359.
162. Metcalf, D., Parker, J., Chester, H. M., and Kincade, P. W. (1974): Formation of eosinophil-like granulocytic colonies by mouse bone marrow cells in vitro. *J. Cell. Physiol.*, 84:275–289.
163. Miller, H. R., and Jarret, W. F. H. (1971): Immune reactions in mucous membranes. I. Intestinal mast cell response during helminth expulsion in the rat. *Immunology*, 20:277–288.
164. Miller, A. M., and McGarry, M. P. (1976): A diffusible stimulator of eosinophilopoiesis produced by lymphoid cells as demonstrated with diffusion chambers. *Blood*, 48:293–300.
165. Miller, A. M., Colley, D. G., and McGarry, M. P. (1976): Spleen cells from *Schistosoma mansoni*-infected mice produce diffusible stimulator of eosinophilopoiesis in vivo. *Nature (London)*, 161:586–587.
166. Moqbel, R. (1980): Histopathological changes following primary, secondary and repeated infections of rats with *Strongyloides ratti* with special reference to tissue eosinophils. *Parasite Immunol.*, 2:11–27.
167. Muller, H. F., and Reider, H. (1891): Ueber Vorkommen und Klinische Bedeutung der eosinophilen Zellen. (Ehrlich) im circulirenden Blute des Menschen. *Dtsch. Arch. Klin. Med.*, 48:96–121.
168. Murphy, R. C., Hammarstrom, C., and Samuelsson, B. (1979): Leukotriene C: A slow reacting substance from mastocytoma cells. *Proc. Natl. Acad. Sci. U. S. A.*, 76:4275–4279.
169. Murray, M. (1972): Immediate-hypersensitivity effector mechanism. II. In vivo reactions. In: *Immunity to Animal Parasites*, edited by E. J. L. Soulsby, pp. 155–190. Academic Press, New York and London.
170. Neva, F. A., Kaplan, A. P., Pacheco, G., Gray, L., and Danaraj, T. J. (1975): Tropical eosinophilia—A human model of parasitic immunopathology with observation on serum IgE levels before and after treatment. *J. Allergy Clin. Immunol.*, 55:422–429.
171. Nugteren, D. H. (1975): Arachidonate lipoxygenase in blood platelets. *Biochim. Biophys. Acta*, 380:299–307.
172. Ogilvie, G. M. (1964): Reagin-like antibodies in animals immune to helminth parasites. *Nature (London)*, 4953:91–92.
173. Ogilvie, B. M., Smithers, S. R., and Terry, R. J. (1966): Reagin-like antibodies in experimental infections of *Schistosoma mansoni* and the passive transfer of resistance. *Nature (London)*, 5029:1221–1223.
174. Ogilvie, B. M., and Jones, V. E. (1970): Reaginic antibodies and helminth infection. In: *Cellular and Humoral Mechanisms of Anaphylaxy and Allergy*, edited by H. Z. Movat, p. 13. Karger, Basel.
175. Olds, G. R., and Mahmoud, A. A. F. (1980): Role of the host granulomatous response in murine *Schistosomiasis mansoni*—eosinophil-mediated destruction of eggs. *J. Clin. Invest.*, 66:1191–1199.

176. Orange, R. P., Kaliner, M. A., and Austen, K. F. (1971): The immunological release of histamine and slow reacting substance of anaphylaxis from human lung. III. Biochemical control mechanisms involved in the immunologic release of the chemical mediators. In: *Biochemistry of the Acute Allergic Reactions*, edited by K. F. Austen and E. L. Becker, pp. 189–202. F. A. Davis, Oxford, England.

177. Orange, R. P., Murphy, R. C., Karnovsky, M. L., and Austen, K. F. (1973): The physicochemical characteristics and purification of slow reacting substance of anaphylaxis. *J. Immunol.*, 110:760–770.

178. Orange, R. P., Murphy, R. C., and Austen, K. F. (1974): Inactivation of slow reacting substance of anaphylaxis (SRS-A) by arylsulfatases. *J. Immunol.*, 113:316–322.

179. Parish, W. E. (1967): Release of histamine and slow reacting substance with mast cell changes after challenge of human lung sensitized passively with reagin in vitro. *Nature (London)*, 215:738–739.

180. Parish, W. E. (1970): Investigations on eosinophilia. The influence of histamine; antigen-antibody complexes containing gamma-1 or gamma-2 globulins, foreign bodies (phagocytosis) and disrupted mast cells. *Br. J. Dermatol.*, 82:42–64.

181. Parwaresch, M. R., Walle, A. J., and Arndt, D. (1976): The peripheral kinetics of human radiolabeled eosinophils. *Virchows. Arch. (Zellpathol.)*, 21:57–66.

182. Patterson, N. A. M., Wasserman, S. I., Said, J. W., and Austen, K. F. (1976): Release of chemical mediators from partially purified human lung mast cells. *J. Immunol.*, 117:1356–1362.

183. Pincus, S. H., Butterworth, A. E., Vadas, M., Robbins, M., and David, J. R. (1981): Eosinophil specific non-oxidative killing of schistosomula. *J. Immunol.*, 126:1794–1799.

184. Ponzio, N. M., and Speirs, R. S. (1973): Lymphoid cell dependence of eosinophil response to antigen. III. Comparison of the rate of appearance of two types of memory cells in various lymphoid tissues at different times after priming. *J. Immunol.*, 110:1363–1370.

185. Ponzio, N. M., and Speirs, R. S. (1974): Lymphoid cell dependence of eosinophil response to antigen. IV. Effects of in vitro X-irradiation on adoptive transfer of amnestic cellular and humoral response. *Proc. Soc. Exp. Biol. Med.*, 145:1178–1180.

186. Ponzio, N. M., and Speirs, R. S. (1975): Lymphoid cell dependence of eosinophil response to antigen. VI. The effect of selective removal of T or B lymphocytes on the capacity of primed spleen cells to adoptively transferred immunity to tetanus toxoid. *Immunology*, 28:243–251.

187. Ramalho-Pinto, F. J., McLaren, D. J., and Smithers, S. R. (1978): Complement-mediated killing of schistosomula of *Schistosoma mansoni* by rat eosinophils in vitro. *J. Exp. Med.*, 147:147–156.

188. Riley, J. F., and West, G. B. (1953): The presence of histamine in tissue mast cells. *J. Physiol.*, 120:528–537.

189. Roberts, L. J., Lewis, R. A., and Hansbrough (1978): Biosynthesis of prostaglandins, thromboxanes, and 12-L-hydroxyl-5,8,10,14-eicosatetraenoic acid by rat mast cells. *Fed. Proc.*, 37:384A.

190. Rosen, L., Chappell, R., Laqueur, G. L., Wallace, G. D., and Weinstein, P. P. (1962): Eosinophilic meningoence-phalitis caused by a metastrongyloid lung worm of rats. *J. A. M. A.*, 179:620–624.

191. Ruscetti, F. W., and Chervenick, P. A. (1975): Release of colony-stimulating activity from thymus derived lymphocytes. *J. Clin. Invest.*, 55:520–527.

192. Ruscetti, F. W., Cypess, R. H., and Chervenick, P. A. (1976): Specific release of neutrophilic- and eosinophilic-stimulating factors from sensitized lymphocytes. *Blood*, 47:757–765.

193. Rytomma, T. (1960): Organ distribution and histochemical properties of eosinophil granulocytes in the rat. *Acta Pathol. Microbiol. Scand.*, 50 (Suppl. 140):1–118.

194. Samter, M. (1919): The response of eosinophils in the guinea pig to sensitization, anaphylaxis, and various drugs. *Blood*, 4:217–246.

195. Sanderson, C. J., Lopez, A. F., and Bunn Moreno, M. M. (1977): Eosinophils and not lymphoid K cells kill *Trypanosoma cruzi*. *Nature (London)*, 268:340–341.

196. Sanderson, C. J., Bunn Moreno, M. M., and Lopez, A. F. (1978): Antibody dependent cell-mediated cytotoxicity of *Trypanosoma cruzi*: the release of tritium-labeled RNA, DNA and protein. *Parasitology*, 76:299–307.

197. Schayer, R. S. (1959): Catabolism of physiological quantities of histamine in vivo. *Physiol. Rev.*, 39:116–126.

198. Schayer, R. W. (1963): Histidine decarboxylase in mast cells. *Ann. N. Y. Acad. Sci.*, 103:164–178.

199. Schlecht, H., and Schwenker, G. (1912): Ueber lokale Eosinophilie in den Bronchien und in der Lunge beim anaphylaktischen Meerschweinchen. *Arch. Pathol. Pharmacol.*, 68:163–170.

200. Schwartz, E. (1914): Die Lehre von der allgemeinen und ortlichen Eosinophilie. *Ergeb. Allerg. Pathol. Anat.*, 17:137–787.
201. Sheard, P., Killingback, P. G., and Blair, A. M. J. N. (1967): Antigen induced release of histamine and SRSA from human lung passively sensitized with reaginic serum. *Nature (London)*, 216:283–286.
202. Speirs, R. S. (1955): Physiological approaches to an understanding of the function of eosinophils and basophils. *Ann. N. Y. Acad. Sci.*, 59:706–731.
203. Spry, C. J. F. (1971): Mechanism of eosinophilia. V. Kinetics of normal and accelerated eosinopoiesis. *Cell Tissue Kinet.*, 4:351–364.
204. Spry, C. J. F. (1971): Mechanism of eosinophilia. VI. Eosinophil mobilization. *Cell Tissue Kinet.*, 4:365–374.
205. Stechschulte, D. J., Orange, R. P., and Austen, K. F. (1973): Detection of slow reacting substance of anaphylaxis (SRS-A) in plasma of guinea pigs during anaphylaxis. *J. Immunol.*, 111:1585–1589.
206. Strong, R. P., and Musgrave, W. E. (1901): Preliminary notes of a case of infection with *Balantidium coli. Bull. Johns Hopkins Hosp.*, 12:31–32.
207. Taliaferro, W. H., and Sarles, M. P. (1938): The cellular reactions in the skin, lungs and intestine of normal and immune rats after infection with *Nippostrongylus muris. J. Infect. Dis.*, 64:157–192.
208. Torisu, M., Yoshida, T., Ward, P. A., and Cohen, S. (1973): Lymphocyte derived eosinophil chemotactic factor. II. Studies on the mechanism of activation of the precursor substance by immune complexes. *J. Immunol.*, 111:1450–1458.
209. Unanue, E. R., and Benacerraf, B. (1973): Immunologic events in experimental hypersensitivity granulomas. *Am. J. Pathol.*, 71:349–359.
210. Vadas, M. A., David, J. R., Butterworth, A. E., Pisani, N. T., and Siongok, T. A. (1979): A new method for the purification of human eosinophils and neutrophils, and a comparison of the ability of these cells to damage schistosomula of *Schistosoma mansoni. J. Immunol.*, 122:1228–1236.
211. Vadas, M. A., Butterworth, A. E., Sherry, B., Dessein, A., Hogan, M., Bout, D., and David, J. R. (1980): Interactions between human eosinophils and schistosomula of *Schistosoma mansoni.* I. Stable and irreversible antibody-dependent adherence. *J. Immunol.*, 124:1441–1448.
212. Vadas, M. A., Dessein, A. J., Nicola, N., and David, J. R. *(in press).*
213. Valone, F. H., and Goetzl, E. J. (1978): Immunological release in the rat peritoneal cavity of lipid chemotactic and chemokinetic factors for polymorphonuclear leukocytes. *J. Immunol.*, 120:102–108.
214. Valone, F. H., Whitmer, D. I., Pichett, W. C., Austen, K. F., and Goetzl, E. J. (1979): The immunological generation of a platelet-activating factor and a platelet-lytic factor in the rat. *Immunology*, 37:841–848.
215. Vaughan, J. (1953): The function of the eosinophil leukocyte. *Blood*, 8:1–15.
216. Walls, R. S., Bass, D. A., and Beeson, P. B. (1974): Mechanisms of eosinophilia. X. Evidence for immunologic specificity of the stimulus. *Proc. Soc. Exp. Med.*, 145:1240–1242.
217. Ward, P. A. (1969): Chemotaxis of human eosinophils. *Am. J. Pathol.*, 54:121–128.
218. Warren, K. S., Domingo, E. O., and Cowan, R. B. T. (1967): Granuloma formation around schistosome eggs as a manifestation of delayed hypersensitivity. *Am. J. Pathol.*, 51:735–756.
219. Warren, K. S. (1972): Granulomatous inflammation. In: *Inflammation Mechanisms and Control*, edited by I. H. Lepow and P. A. Ward, pp. 203–217. Academic Press, New York.
220. Warren, K. S., Dard, R., Pelley, R. P., and Mahmoud, A. A. F. (1976): The eosinophil stimulation promoter test in murine and human *Trichinella spiralis* infection. *J. Infect. Dis.*, 134:277–280.
221. Wasserman, S. I., Goetzl, E. J., and Austen, K. F. (1975): Inactivation of slow reacting substance of anaphylaxis by human eosinophil arylsulfatase. *J. Immunol.*, 114:645–649.
222. Wasserman, S. I., Whitmer, D., Goetzl, E. J., and Austen, K. F. (1975): Chemotactic deactivation of human eosinophils by the eosinophil chemotactic factor of anaphylaxis. *Proc. Soc. Exp. Biol. Med.*, 148:301–306.
223. Wassom, D. L., and Gleich, G. J. (1979): Damage to *Trichinella spiralis* newborn larvae by eosinophil major basic protein. *Am. J. Trop. Med. Hyg.*, 28:860–863.
224. Webb, J. K. G., Job, C. K., and Gault, E. W. (1960): Tropical eosinophilia demonstration of microfilariae in lungs, liver and lymph nodes. *Lancet*, 1:835–842.
225. Weller, P. F., and Goetzl, E. J. (1980): The regulatory and effector roles of eosinophils. *Adv. Immunol.*, 27:339–371.

226. Weller, P. F., Goetzl, E. J., and Austen, K. F. (1980): Identification of human eosinophil lyso-phospholipase as the constituent of Charcot-Leyden crystals. *Proc. Natl. Acad. Sci. U. S. A.*, 77:7440–7443.
227. Weller, P. F., Lewis, R. A., Corey, E. J., and Austen, K. F. (1981): The interaction of purified human eosinophil arylsulfatase B with synthetic leukotrienes. *Fed. Proc.*, in press.
228. Wells, P. D. (1962): Mast cell, eosinophil and histamine levels in *Nippostrongylus brasiliensis* infected rats. *Exp. Parasitol.*, 12:82–101.
229. Wharton Jones, T. (1846): The blood corpuscle considered in its different phases of development in the animal series. *Philos. Trans. R. Soc. Lond.* [Biol. Sci.], 1:82.
230. Whited, S., and Gallin, J. I. (1980): Neutrophil chemotaxis. *Int. J. Dermatol.*, 19:130–138.
231. Wildervanck, A., Winckel, W. E. F., and Collier, W. A. (1953): Tropical eosinophilia combined with histoplasmosis. *Doc. Med. Geog. Trop.*, 5:67–71.
232. Zappert, J. (1893): Uber das Vorkommen der Eosinophilen Zellen in menschlichen Blute. *Z. Klin. Med.*, 23:227–308.
233. Zeiger, R. S., and Colten, H. R. (1977): Histamine release from human eosinophils. *J. Immunol.*, 118:540–543.
234. Zeiger, R. S., Twarog, F. J., and Colten, H. R. (1976): Histamine release from human granulo-cytes. *J. Exp. Med.*, 144:1049–1061.

Advances in Host Defense Mechanisms, Vol. 1,
edited by John I. Gallin and Anthony S. Fauci,
Raven Press, New York © 1982.

Eosinophil Effector Mechanisms in Health and Disease

*Steven J. Ackerman, **David T. Durack, and *Gerald J. Gleich

*Departments of Medicine and Immunology, Mayo Medical School,
Mayo Clinic and Mayo Foundation, Rochester, Minnesota 55905;
and **Division of Infectious Diseases, Department of Medicine,
Duke University Medical Center, Durham, North Carolina 27710*

Although the eosinophil has been recognized for over a century, its functions still remain elusive. Recent evidence indicates that the eosinophil is able to kill helminths *in vitro* (55), and experiments using anti-eosinophil serum have shown that ablation of the eosinophil abolishes or dampens immunity to the parasite (40,44,68,76). The role of the eosinophil in parasitic disease is reviewed in the two previous articles in this volume. This information strongly points to a beneficial role for the eosinophil in resistance to parasites and suggests that the eosinophil affects this resistance by directly damaging the parasite through release of its granule contents onto the surface of the parasite. The granule contents evidently disrupt the parasite's external membrane, and, in the case of schistosomula of *Schistosoma mansoni* (34,69), eosinophils actually invade the body of the parasite through the breech in the wall. The ability of the eosinophil to disrupt the external membrane of the parasite implies the existence of powerful membrane-active effector systems, many or all of which are brought into play by granule disruption. Eosinophils also possess the ability to lyse mammalian cells in the presence of a specific antibody (82). This chapter will describe the properties and activities of eosinophil proteins, their potential roles in damaging parasites and causing diseases, and a system for host resistance consisting of a homocytotropic antibody, vasoactive amine-containing cells, and eosinophils.

PROCUREMENT AND PURIFICATION OF EOSINOPHILS

Before discussing eosinophil effector mechanisms, a brief review of two key problems which confront the investigator concerned with eosinophil function is pertinent. These problems are the procurement and purification of eosinophils. Litt showed that injection of antigens into the peritoneal cavity of the guinea pig yielded exudates rich in eosinophils; cells were recovered by simple lavage of the peritoneal cavity (67). We tested his system and found that repetitive saline lavage of the peritoneal cavity of the guinea pig was sufficient to provide up to 4×10^7 eosinophils per animal; animals injected with antigen had increased mortality, and the lavage fluid contained contaminating neutrophils (36). Pincus was unable to confirm our finding, but she showed that intraperitoneal injection of polymyxin into ether-anesthetized guinea pigs stimulated up to 5.2×10^7 peritoneal eosinophils (84). We subsequently found that the choice of anesthesia for the guinea pig is critical (66). In our initial experiments with the saline lavage method, no anesthetic was used, whereas Pincus used ether. Tests of the effect of anesthesia showed that guinea pigs anesthetized with ether or halothane produced large numbers of eosinophils when injected with polymyxin. In contrast, animals anesthetized with ether did not produce eosinophils when lavaged with saline, whereas animals anesthetized with halothane did produce eosinophils. Thus, the difference in the findings evidently resides in the choice of anesthesia. We have found that guinea pigs can be lavaged weekly for up to 27 wk with little change in the recovery of eosinophils. Curiously, female guinea pigs produce significantly more eosinophils than males (66). Purification of peritoneal eosinophils is easily accomplished by means of sedimentation through a cushion of sodium diatrizoate ($d = 1.142$), or 22% sodium metrizamide.

Procurement of human cells can be accomplished by use of the cell separator. We have used both the IBM-NCI continuous-flow and the Haemonetics semicontinuous-flow-cell separator with good success, provided that hydroxyethyl starch is used in the anticoagulant. Up to 10 liters of blood can be processed, and we have recovered up to 5×10^{10} eosinophils (83). Purification of human eosinophils presents a significant problem when the starting cell preparation contains large numbers of neutrophils, and we have used adherence to nylon wool (82) and sedimentation through gradients of sodium metrizamide successfully (97).

THE GRANULE MAJOR BASIC PROTEIN

The distinctive aspect of the mature eosinophil in most mammalian species is the granule. When viewed by the electron microscope (Fig. 1) the eosinophil granule consists of an electron-dense core and an electron-radiolucent matrix (74). Presumably any particular activities of the eosinophil are mediated at least in part through molecules residing in the granule. Initial studies of horse eosinophil granules by Vercauteren and Peeters revealed arginine-rich proteins which, at high concentrations, showed antihistaminic properties (104). Later, Archer and Hirsch purified rat and horse eosinophils, isolated the granules, and found a high content of peroxidase; in contrast to neutrophil granules, lysozyme and phagocytin were not present (6). Studies from our laboratory have disclosed the presence of an eosinophil granule protein, termed the major basic protein (MBP), which comprises the core or crystalloid of the granule (37,38,63).

Physicochemical Properties of MBP

Using purified guinea pig peritoneal eosinophils we found that the cells could be readily disrupted by suspension in 0.34 M sucrose followed by mechanical agitation, such as repeated pipetting or vortexing, to yield granules (38). The

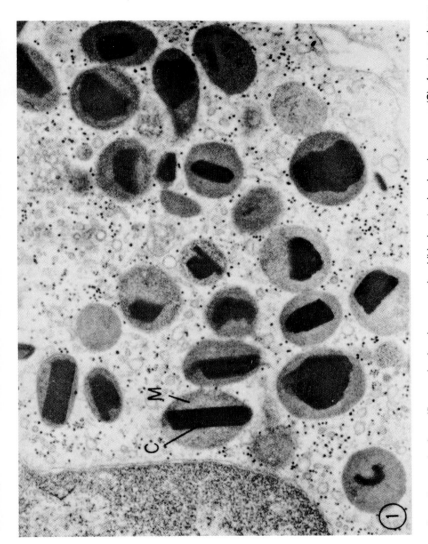

FIG. 1. Electron photomicrograph of specific granules in a human eosinophil leukocyte showing dense cores (C) of various shapes embedded in a less dense matrix (M). (× 28,000) (The regular array in the matrix is an artifact from the reproduction of the original lithograph.) [From Miller et al. (74), with permission.]

granules were readily soluble in dilute acid, and polyacrylamide gel electrophoresis (PAGE) showed the presence of a major band which stained for protein and had a molecular weight of 11,000 (37). Because this protein band accounted for over one-half of the protein staining on the gel, and because it behaved as a basic molecule, we called it the eosinophil granule MBP. Fractionation of soluble eosinophil granule proteins on Sephadex G-50 columns yielded three peaks; MBP was present in the second peak and peroxidase activity in the first peak. Analysis of the second peak by PAGE revealed a single band in the expected position of MBP, but concentration of fractions showing single bands resulted in the appearance of new bands which were multiples of the 11,000-dalton monomer (37). The aggregates were depolymerized by exposure to reducing agents, and alkylation of monomer MBP prevented polymerization.

Amino acid analysis of guinea pig MBP showed 4 moles of tryptophan; because tryptophan is not present in histones, MBP cannot be a histone (113). The basicity of the molecule is accounted for largely by the 13 residues (13%) of arginine. The molecule contains 6 moles of half-cystine; because MBP readily forms polymers and because polymer formation is related to the formation of disulfide bonds, we determined the number of sulfhydryl groups. Two sulfhydryl groups were present, indicating that these two reactive groups interacted to form disulfide-linked aggregates. Analysis of human (39) and rat eosinophil granules (65) showed the presence of a protein with properties similar to that obtained from guinea pig eosinophil granules. All these molecules contained a high content of arginine.

The MBPs from the guinea pig and human are antigenic in rabbits (64,107,108). Guinea pig MBP at concentrations greater than 50 μg/ml fixed complement in the absence of antibody (64); at lower concentrations, complement fixation was not found except in the presence of specific antibody. This study showed marked antigenic differences among guinea pig, human, and rat MBP, indicating differences in structure among these molecules. Measurement of guinea pig MBP by radioimmunoassay was achieved by using a buffer containing protamine to reduce nonspecific binding of ^{131}I-MBP (107). The MBP antigenic determinants survived reduction and alkylation in the absence of denaturing solvents; in the presence of 6 M guanidinium hydrochloride, reduction and alkylation destroyed MBP immunoreactivity. Exposure to 6 M guanidinium hydrochloride reduced immunoreactivity by approximately 50%. Polymerized MBP was only one-tenth as reactive as monomer MBP, illustrating the need for reduction and alkylation of the molecule before measurement by radioimmunoassay.

Localization of MBP in the Eosinophil Granule

The localization of MBP in the eosinophil granule was pursued by immunoelectron microscopy and by cell fractionation (63). First, by immunoperoxidase electron microscopy MBP staining was found within the crystalloid core. Specific staining of cores was seen when rabbit antiserum to MBP was used as the first-stage antibody in a double-antibody staining procedure, whereas staining was not seen when normal rabbit serum was used as the first-stage antibody. Second, by cell fractionation, crystalloids were isolated by disruption of granules and centrifugation of granule lysates. The final preparation showed numerous blunt, rod-shaped bodies similar to crystalloids. Analysis of dissolved crystalloids by PAGE revealed a band in the expected position of MBP, and 83% of the dye staining was associated with that band. Measurement of soluble core protein by radioimmunoassay showed (107) that essentially all of the protein, as measured by biuret assay, could be accounted for as MBP. Thus, these results point to the conclusion that the core of the eosinophil granule contains crystalline MBP.

Functions of MBP

Studies of MBP functions were stimulated by the presumption that any effects found would provide insights into the potential roles eosinophils themselves play in health and disease. Initial studies of MBP function did not provide many clues (37). The MBP did not increase vascular permeability and had only weak antibacterial activity. It precipitated deoxyribonucleic acid (DNA), neutralized the activity of heparin, and activated papain, presumably through the activity of the two sulfhydryl groups; all of these activities are predictable based on the physicochemical properties of MBP.

Insight into the potential function of MBP came about as a consequence of analysis of the effect of MBP on schistosomules of *S. mansoni* (16). These results showed that MBP as well as certain basic proteins, including protamine, damaged the schistosomules. The MBP bound to the membrane of the schistosomules and caused disruption of the membrane. When eosinophils in the presence of antibody attacked the schistosomule, they deposited MBP on the surface of the parasite, and increased concentrations of MBP could be detected in culture supernatants. Subsequently, eosinophils but not neutrophils were shown to adhere irreversibly to schistosomules in the presence of antibody (96). The MBP and protamine enhanced both eosinophil and neutrophil adherence to the schistosomules (15). Concanavalin A also caused adherence of eosinophils to schistosomules, and this adherence could be made irreversible and converted into an attack on the parasite by addition of the calcium ionophore, A23187. Under these conditions, MBP was released into the culture supernatants. These studies indicate that the irreversible adherence of eosinophils to schistosomules is associated with degranulation and release of MBP. In an extension of this work the effect of MBP on newborn larvae of *Trichinella spiralis* was tested (106). When these larvae were cultured with MBP at concentrations of 5×10^{-5} M or higher, all of the larvae were rendered immobile. The effect of MBP was detected as early as 2 hr after treatment when the larvae became progressively stiff and sluggish. Controls consisting of other basic proteins were negative except for polyarginine, which killed 20% of larvae in 24 hr. Recently, MBP was found to kill *Trypanosoma cruzi* in the bloodstream trypomastigote stage; this effect was inhibited by heparin, by antibody to MBP, but not by normal rabbit serum, and the toxic effect of MBP was destroyed by heating at 56° C for 30 min

(57). Interestingly, the antigenic activity of MBP is also abolished by heating at 56° C for 30 min (107,108).

Because MBP was toxic to schistosomules, its capacity to damage mammalian cells was tested. In the first experiments, Butterworth and co-workers found that MBP damaged two varieties of murine ascites tumor cells (16). This observation raised the possibility that MBP might damage other cells, including cells from organs which are infiltrated by eosinophils in certain disease states. Tests of this hypothesis showed that MBP damaged intestinal, splenic, cutaneous, and peripheral blood mononuclear cells in a dose-related manner (35). The MBP also damaged guinea pig tracheal rings as judged by total absence of ciliary beating at high concentrations and reduced ciliary beating at lower concentrations. Therefore, MBP can damage many types of mammalian cells, including those in the respiratory tract.

Further studies of MBP damage to respiratory tissue were conducted using guinea pig tracheal rings as a model (32). Guinea pig MBP concentrations as low as 10 μg/ml (9×10^{-7} M) produced exfoliation of epithelial cells and impairment of ciliary beating in circumscribed areas at 48 hr, whereas another basic protein, protamine, 1×10^{-4} M, produced neither exfoliation nor alteration of ciliary beating when incubated with tracheal rings for 72 hr. Microscopic examination of fixed tissue showed varying degrees of epithelial damage. With the lowest concentration of MBP tested (9×10^{-7} M), the epithelium was disrupted, and damaged cells were free in the lumen. With MBP levels of 50 μg/ml (4.5×10^{-6} M) and 100 μg/ml (9×10^{-6} M), the epithelium was damaged extensively, showing detachment of ciliated and brush cells and destruction of individual cells leaving only basal cells. Exfoliated cells were severely damaged, with lysis of the cellular membrane and liberation of cell contents. Cilia were stripped from cells, and exhibited a distinctive beaded appearance. The normal microtubular structure of the axonemes was lost. The lamina propria appeared edematous, with separation of collagen fibrils. These effects of MBP on bronchial epithelium are remarkably similar to the pathologic changes in human bronchial asthma. Specifically, excessive shedding and desquamation of the bronchial epithelium down to the level of the lamina propria are reported as constant findings in bronchial asthma (17,20,27,48,75). The superficial columnar cells undergo detachment, leaving behind them a layer of basal cells; regeneration of the mucosa occurs from these cells. Finally, mucociliary clearance is impaired in asthma (71,87).

Relationship to Human Disease

The findings that MBP damaged guinea pig respiratory tissue and that the damage mimicked in part the pathology of asthma pointed to the hypothesis that eosinophils, known to be a hallmark of bronchial asthma (79), damage bronchial epithelium in asthma. The MBP of both humans and guinea pigs damaged respiratory epithelium of both species, indicating that the MBP was not preferentially active on one or the other tissue (32,33). Furthermore, human MBP was similar to that of the guinea pig in its effect on the bronchial epithelium (33). To determine whether MBP is present in sputum, MBP was measured in the sera and sputa of patients with respiratory disease in general and in asthma in particular (33,108). First, the sputa of 100 patients with various respiratory diseases were examined for MBP content by radioimmunoassay. Sputa of 13 patients contained MBP levels greater than 0.1 μg/ml, and 11 of these patients had asthma. Second, sputa of 15 patients hospitalized for asthma were analyzed sequentially for MBP content. During hospitalization, all patients were treated with intravenous aminophylline, adrenergic agonists, and all but one received glucocorticoids. With this therapy, peak expiratory flow rates increased linearly from day 1 to day 4 and continued to rise until day 6, when the values approached a plateau (Fig. 2). Conversely, blood eosinophils dropped linearly from day 1 to day 4, after which they increased before dropping again. Serum MBP levels dropped from day 1 to a low point on day 7; the changes from admission on day 1 to discharge were significant ($p < 0.01$; paired t-test). Sputum MBP levels were elevated in all patients and rose from admission to day 3 before falling on day 8. The peak levels of sputum MBP in the 15 patients ranged from 0.3 μg/ml to 92.9 μg/ml, with a geometric mean of 7.1 μg/ml. These results indicated that an elevated sputum MBP was a good marker for bronchial asthma and that high concentrations of MBP are present in sputa of some patients with asthma. Certain sputa processed within a few minutes after expectoration contained high MBP levels, suggesting that the elevation of MBP in the sputa is not merely a consequence of *in vitro* cell death and liberation of granule contents.

In a second set of experiments to test the hypothesis that eosinophils mediate tissue damage through MBP, lung tissues from autopsies of patients who had died of asthma were examined for intracellular and extracellular MBP by immunofluorescence (31). The results, although preliminary, clearly show that eosinophils in the lung tissues fluoresce brightly; the immunofluorescence is specific in that normal rabbit serum does not cause it, and the ability of antiserum to MBP to stain eosinophils can be removed by immunosorption with MBP and not by other basic proteins. Eosinophils staining for MBP are distributed throughout the lamina propria, epithelium, and mucous plugs of lung tissues from patients with asthma. In addition, MBP is present outside of the eosinophil, in mucous plugs, and in areas of damaged bronchial epithelium. The detection of extracellular MBP suggests that the eosinophil releases its granule contents into the bronchial lumen in asthma.

We have also tested sera from patients with a variety of human diseases associated with blood eosinophilia and found that patients with the hypereosinophilic syndrome had high concentrations of MBP, up to 14 μg/ml (108). Overall there was a correlation between the levels of serum MBP and blood eosinophilia ($r = +0.71$; $p < 0.001$). Interestingly, patients with skin diseases frequently showed elevated serum MBP levels in the absence of blood eosinophilia. Analyses of other biological fluids indicate that MBP is elevated (above serum concentrations) in blister fluid from patients with bullous pemphigoid (114) and that markedly elevated concentrations of MBP and Charcot-Leyden crystal protein (CLC) are present in the tears of patients with vernal conjunctivitis (94). In addition, the pleural fluid

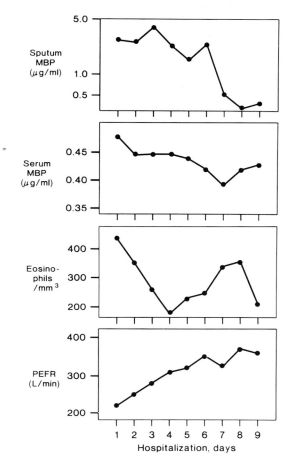

FIG. 2. Changes in peak expiratory flow rates (PEFR), blood eosinophil levels, and serum and sputum MBP levels in 15 patients hospitalized with asthma. The points for the peak expiratory flow rates, blood eosinophils, and serum MBP levels are arithmetic means of the daily observations. Sputum MBP levels are geometric means of the values shown in Table 1 of reference 33. [From Frigas et al. (33), with permission.]

of a patient with eosinophilic pneumonia contained 30 μg MBP/ml, the upper limit of normal in serum from normal patients being 0.6 μg/ml (35).

Thus, the present results encourage belief that eosinophils degranulate in tissues and release granule constituents, including MBP. However, MBP present in serum and sputum is bound to serum proteins and has molecular weights greater than 50,000 (33,108). Monomer human MBP, 9,300 daltons, can be recovered from sera and secretions by reduction with dithiothreitol and alkylation with iodoacetamide and by gel filtration on Sephadex G-50 equilibrated with HCl. The *in vitro* studies showing that MBP damages parasites and cells (16,32,33,35,57,106) used alkylated monomer MBP because nonalkylated MBP readily oxidizes to form di-sulfide-linked polymers which may precipitate from solution. The MBP in the eosinophil granule is present as monomer with two sulfhydryl groups. We do not know if the monomer MBP as it is released from the cell is toxic. Experiments to test the toxicity of nonalkylated monomer MBP are fraught with difficulty in that the molecule undergoes self-polymerization and also reacts with other proteins to form disulfide-linked polymers. Indeed this very tendency, although a curse from the experimental point of view, could enhance the toxicity of MBP by permitting it to react with membrane proteins. Further experiments must compare the toxicity of alkylated MBP, nonalkylated monomer MBP, and the polymerized MBP.

THE EOSINOPHIL PEROXIDASE

The suggestion that eosinophils possess peroxidase activity was made by the work of Vercauteren and Blonde (103) and of Rytomaa and Teir (86). Subsequently, peroxidase activity was demonstrated in the eosinophils of numerous species, in-cluding laboratory animals (8,56,115) and humans (30). The intensity of peroxidase staining is so great that it can be used for enumeration of eosinophils, as in the automated continuous-flow cytochemistry devices now used to perform differential counts. Interestingly, the eosinophils of many members of the cat family, including the lion, the tiger, and the domestic cat (*Felis domestica*), do not contain peroxidase (95). Peroxidase activity is localized to the matrix of the eosinophil granule (8,30,56,115), is released into the phagocytic vacuole following ingestion of zymo-san or *Escherichia coli* (19), and is deposited onto the surface of parasites (34).

Physicochemical Properties of Eosinophil Peroxidase

Studies of partially purified rat eosinophil peroxidase (EPO) showed spectral differences from neutrophil myeloperoxidase (MPO) and a Soret maximum of 403 nm for oxidized peroxidase and 437 nm for reduced peroxidase (4). Guinea pig EPO has been purified from marrow cells by detergent extraction and by ion exchange and gel filtration chromatography (26). The purified molecule was ho-mogeneous by immunodiffusion and existed as a monomer of 75,000 daltons and a dimer of 150,000 daltons as measured by gel filtration. Both monomer and dimer had the same specific activity, the same absorption spectrum, with a Soret maximum at 425 nm, and the same ratio of absorbance at 415 nm and 280 nm. Eosinophil peroxidase evidently consists of a single polypeptide chain as indicated by a single band in PAGE in sodium dodecyl sulfate (SDS-PAGE). The EPO and MPO differed in their antigenicity, subunit structure, and electrophoretic behavior. A study of human EPO showed spectral properties similar to those of lactoperoxidase (LPO) and a Soret band at 448 nm (112).

Functions of EPO

Eosinophil peroxidase catalyzes the oxidation of many substances by hydrogen peroxide. However, in spite of the high concentrations of EPO in eosinophils, its function is unknown. Klebanoff showed that MPO plus hydrogen peroxide and free iodide can function to iodate and kill bacteria and that the activity of this system is increased in phagocytizing neutrophils (59). The combination of MPO, H_2O_2, and halide also will kill viruses (11), mycoplasma (50), and fungi (62). Because eosinophils generate considerable H_2O_2 (7,60,61,72), the activities of the EPO + H_2O_2 + halide system in the killing of microorganisms has been explored. Studies by Bujak and Root showed that eosinophils killed *Staphylococcus aureus* in the presence of sodium azide added as a peroxidase inhibitor (14). Migler and co-workers found that eosinophil extracts killed *S. aureus* and *E. coli* only in the presence of iodide, not chloride (73). Using purified EPO, Jong and colleagues showed that EPO could kill *E. coli* in the presence of H_2O_2 and iodide as well as chloride and bromide (52). They attributed the difference between their results and that of Migler and co-workers to the presence of gelatin in the reaction mixture in the latter experiments; Jong et al. showed that gelatin and albumin inhibit killing of *E. coli* by the EPO system. Subsequently, Henderson et al. showed that EPO could bind to mast cells and that the EPO-mast cell complex retained the ability to catalyze iodination of proteins and killing of microorganisms (47). They suggested that such complexes could form extracellularly and affect the inflammatory response. In an interesting extension of this line of work, Henderson et al. showed that EPO supplemented by H_2O_2 and a halide induced mast-cell degranulation and histamine release (46). At low EPO concentrations this reaction was noncytotoxic, but at higher concentrations there was ultrastructural evidence of mast-cell damage. The EPO–mast-cell-granule complex was more effective than free EPO in stimulation of mast-cell secretion. Henderson and co-workers proposed that eosinophils, either by secretion or by cell lysis, could release EPO; EPO in the presence of H_2O_2 (generated by eosinophils or other phagocytes in the area), chloride, and iodide initiates mast-cell secretion. At pH 7.4, EPO was active in the presence of physiological concentrations of chloride plus iodide at 10^{-6} M; the iodide concentration is above that present in extracellular fluid. Thus, these findings suggest a role for the EPO + H_2O_2 + halide system in the inflammatory response. Whether or not the proposed reactions occur *in vivo* will require further study. The possibility that EPO might play a role in hypersensitivity reactions is strengthened by observations showing leakage of EPO from granules into cytoplasm and apparent extracellular release following allergen provocation of human nasal mucous membranes (109). Finally, Jong et al. have shown that the EPO + H_2O_2 + halide system is toxic to schistosomules of *S. mansoni* as judged by loss of motility and by ^{51}Cr-release (53).

EOSINOPHIL CATIONIC PROTEINS

Analyses by Olsson and Venge of cationic proteins of human leukemic myeloid cells showed seven cationic protein components (77). In these experiments leukocytes obtained from patients with myeloid leukemia were disrupted; the granule fraction was obtained by centrifugation, and granules were extracted at pH 4. Granule proteins were separated by gel filtration, preparative electrophoresis, and ion exchange chromatography, and their physicochemical and immunological properties were compared. Four of the components formed a group with molecular weights of 25,500 to 28,500 and similar amino acid compositions. The remaining three components had molecular weights from 21,000 to 29,000 and showed immunologic identity; the amino acid composition of component 5 differed greatly from components 1, 2, and 3. Subsequent investigations showed that components 5, 6, and 7 were derived from eosinophils (78), and they have been termed eosinophil cationic proteins (ECP) (100).

Physicochemical Properties of ECP

The isoelectric points of ECP are greater than pH 11; they contain 11% arginine and 10 half-cystines. Component 5 has a molecular weight of 21,000 and is composed of a single polypeptide chain as determined by SDS-PAGE (100). Of interest is the presence of 2.5 moles of zinc per mole of protein (78). Although ECP forms aggregates, these are depolymerized by detergents, indicating that they are not formed by covalent bonds as is the case with MBP. Finally, ECP accounts for approximately 30% of the weight of the granule's proteins.

The physicochemical properties described above seem to differentiate MBP from ECP, and, recently, in an exchange of reagents with Venge and Olsson we have found that the proteins are immunologically distinct. The ECP has not been localized within the eosinophil granule; the finding that MBP constitutes the crystalline core points to the granule matrix as the likely source of ECP. Although the term ECP was initially used to refer to the family of proteins, components 5 to 7, evidently component 5 is the most abundant of these, and ECP, as used hereinafter, refers to that component.

Functions of ECP

The ECP did not possess bactericidal or esterolytic activity; it did not contract the guinea pig ileum, nor did it have any inhibitory effect on histamine-induced or guinea pig anaphylotoxin-induced contractions of the ileum (78). The ECP bound to heparin and neutralized its anticoagulant activity (100). The ECP shortened the coagulation time of normal plasma in a dose-dependent manner when incubated for 30 sec; when the incubation with normal plasma was prolonged beyond 10 min, there was a marked lengthening of the clotting time (99). The ECP shortened the recalcification time of plasmas deficient in Factors V, VII, VIII, IX, X, and XI but prolonged the recalcification time of Factor XII-deficient plasma, suggesting that Factor XII was the target of ECP interaction. Kallikrein activation, which is dependent on Factor XII, was also enhanced by ECP (99).

An effect of ECP on fibrinolysis is suggested by experiments showing that ECP enhances hydrolysis of a plasmin-specific substrate by plasmin in a dose-related fashion (22). In contrast, plasminogen activation by streptokinase was abolished by ECP; this effect was presumably due to the formation of a precipitate between streptokinase and ECP. The enhancement of plasminogen activation by ECP was not associated with the formation of a complex between ECP and fibrinogen.

Relationship to Human Disease

Venge and co-workers developed a radioimmunoassay for measurement of ECP in human biological fluids (101). The major portion of serum ECP, unlike MBP, is not complexed to proteins, so that samples can be assayed without prior chemical treatment. The normal range of serum ECP is 5 to 55 μg/liter; in normal persons there is a good correlation between the number of blood eosinophils and serum ECP (100). A study of 11 patients with myocardial infarction showed no apparent relationship between serum ECP levels and levels of myoglobin; in addition, administration of glucocorticoids did not depress serum ECP levels (45).

Following bronchial challenge of asthmatic patients with specific antigen, Dahl and co-workers found that the initial symptoms were associated with a decrease in blood eosinophils and an increase in serum ECP 30 to 60 min after challenge (24). After reaching a peak, ECP levels rapidly decreased. In patients with late allergic reactions an increase in blood eosinophils was seen, but there was not a corresponding increase of serum ECP. Serum ECP was lower than expected in asthmatic patients (102). In a study of the effect of medications on ECP levels in patients with asthma, salbutamol administration caused a significant decrease in serum ECP (21). The authors state that the low ECP levels found in patients with asthma (102) cannot be explained by administration of beta-adrenergic agonists (21). However, the duration of the beta-adrenergic effect on ECP levels is not reported. Finally, Dahl and colleagues reported that normal patients and patients with asthma showed a similar diurnal variation in blood eosinophil count (23); eosinophils showed the highest values at 4:00 a.m. and a fall by 8:00 a.m., whereas ECP levels were highest at 8:00 p.m. Although the changes in ECP levels are statistically significant, they are not marked.

THE CHARCOT-LEYDEN CRYSTAL PROTEIN

The Charcot-Leyden crystal was initially described in 1853 in a patient with leukemia and later in 1872 in the sputa of patients with asthma (9). Since then the appearance in tissues and body fluids of these hexagonal bipyramidal crystals have been a hallmark of the eosinophil.

Physicochemical Properties of CLC Protein

Initial studies of CLC indicated the presence of a low-molecular-weight protein (13,49) and suggested that they formed from cytoplasm (5). In subsequent studies purified CLC dissolved in acid or detergent and, analyzed by SDS-PAGE, gave a single band which stained for protein (39). Similarly, CLC gave a single symmetrical peak when analyzed by gel filtration in 6 M guanidinum hydrochloride after reduction and carboxymethylation of CLC protein. The molecular weight of CLC was

$12{,}977 \pm 233$ ($\bar{X} \pm$ SD; $N = 5$). The presence of a single band by SDS-PAGE and a single peak by gel filtration in the presence of denaturing solvents indicates a single polypeptide chain. The CLC protein contained only 1.2% carbohydrate and had a 280 nm E $^{1\%}_{1\,cm}$ = 12.0. Amino acid analyses showed 117 to 119 amino acids, in keeping with the molecular weight, with 6 residues of arginine, 18 to 19 of glutamic acid, and 12 of valine (39).

A subsequent study of the immunochemical properties of CLC was aided by the finding that slow freezing of eosinophil extracts markedly increased the yield of crystals (2). The CLC were solubilized by lyophilization and exposure of the dry powder to slightly basic solutions; at a pH 9 in borate-HCl such solutions contained up to 868 μg/ml. The SDS-PAGE analyses of these solutions showed a single band with a molecular weight of 13,000 when CLC protein was reduced prior to electrophoresis, whereas nonreduced samples showed a minor band at 26,000 daltons, presumably a dimer; this explanation is strengthened by the finding that CLC protein had one sulfhydryl group. Electrophoresis of CLC protein in PAGE at pH 8.9 showed multiple bands; reduction prior to analysis failed to eliminate this heterogeneity. Similarly, electrofocusing of CLC protein showed two major and four minor bands with isoelectric points between 5.7 and 5.1. Immunodiffusion analyses of CLC protein showed a single precipitin band. An explanation of the heterogeneity of CLC protein in PAGE was provided by the observation that the materials in the major bands were immunochemically identical (2) when analyzed by agar gel diffusion and by radioimmunoassay. This result indicated that the presence of multiple bands was due to aggregation, carbohydrate heterogeneity, or possibly small variations in amino acid sequence rather than contaminating proteins or markedly different types of CLC protein.

Functions of CLC Protein

We found CLC protein did not increase vascular permeability in blued guinea pigs; it did not contract the isolated guinea pig ileum, nor did it antagonize the effect of bradykinin or histamine (39). In another approach to the proteins associated with eosinophils, Weller and co-workers have analyzed the properties of enzymes preferentially present in the eosinophil (111). Histochemical analyses of eosinophils by Ottolenghi and colleagues showed the presence of prominent lysophospholipase activity in rat eosinophils by histochemistry (81) and by biochemical titration of liberated fatty acid from lysolecithin (80). Weller and colleagues (111) later confirmed the increased concentrations of lysophospholipase activity in eosinophils by showing a mean activity of 79 units per 5×10^6 cells as compared to 10 units per 5×10^6 neutrophils, 28 units per 5×10^6 mononuclear cells, and 0.4 units per 5×10^6 platelets. Subsequent studies showed that lysophospholipase could be purified by sonication of eosinophils followed by gel filtration on Sephadex G-100, organomercurial agarose chromatography, and heparin-Sepharose chromatography (110). The fall-through fractions from the heparin-Sepharose column were homogeneous by SDS-PAGE and by PAGE at pH 8.9. In these experiments the molecular weight of lysophospholipase activity was $17,220 \pm 260$ ($\bar{X} \pm$ SGM; $N = 9$). When purified lysophospholipase activity was concentrated, crystals with a morphology identical to CLC formed (110). The difference between the molecular weight of CLC protein found earlier [13,000 (2,39)] and that found by Weller et al. [17,220 (110)] has been shown to be due to differences in the percentage of SDS used in SDS-PAGE gels (*unpublished communications*); Gleich et al. (39) and Ackerman et al. (2) used gels containing 1% SDS as compared to 0.1% SDS used by Weller et al. (110). The 13,000 molecular weight of CLC protein (2) is consistent with the molecular weight determined by agarose column chromatography under highly denaturing conditions using 6 M guanidinum hydrochloride (39).

Lysophospholipase (EC 3.1.1.5) (110) catalyzes the removal of a single fatty acid from lysophospholipids. Lysophospholipids are formed by the action of phospholipase A_2 which catalyzes the hydrolysis of fatty acid from the 2-position of phospholipids. Because arachidonic acid is esterified to phospholipids at the 2-position, phospholipase A_2 liberates arachidonic acid and thus provides substrate for the formation of cyclooxygenase and lysooxygenase products. Lysophospholipids formed as a consequence of phospholipase A_2 activity are potentially cytotoxic and can be neutralized among other mechanisms by lysophospholipase which deacylates at the 1-position.

Localization of CLC Protein

As Weller and co-workers point out, several lines of evidence suggest that lysophospholipase (CLC protein) is localized in the plasma membrane of the eosinophil (111). In their experiments, granule fractions showed no lysophospholipase activity, whereas activity was found in fractions containing magnesium-dependent adenosine triphosphatase (ATP) activity, a membrane marker. That lysophospholipase activity was not free was shown by the observation that it could be sedimented at $100,000 \times g$. Finally, lysophospholipase activity of intact eosinophils was inhibited by cell impermeant probes such as *p*-chloromercuribenzene sulfanate.

Relationship to Human Disease

Charcot-Leyden crystal protein can be measured by radioimmunoassay; in patients with eosinophilia, CLC levels are increased above normal serum levels (2). The level of CLC protein in normal serum was 37.0 ± 4.7 ng/ml ($\bar{X} \pm$ SEM; $N = 10$) with a range of 15 to 67 ng/ml, whereas 10 patients with eosinophilia had markedly elevated levels with a mean of 8,507 ng/ml and a range of 340 to 25,500 ng/ml. Analyses of serum CLC protein in 103 normal patients provided a normal level of 41.0 ± 4.0 ng CLC/ml with a range of 8 to 199 ng/ml, with 95% of patients below 114 ng/ml (3). Subsequent analyses of serum CLC protein showed that the antigen was stable when serum was frozen and that freezing and thawing serum up to six times did not destroy activity (3). In contrast, freezing and thawing purified CLC protein from crystals reduced activity by 20 to 40%. Both purified CLC protein and serum CLC protein were destroyed (99% loss of activity) by heating at 56° C for 4 hr, whereas CLC protein was stable at 4°, 22°, and 37° C. The CLC protein and serum CLC protein lost antigenic activity when exposed to pH 6; at pH 2, up to 99% of activity was lost. When serum was fractionated by gel filtration, CLC protein as measured by radioimmunoassay emerged as a distinct peak, but CLC protein in various sera differed in its elution volume, suggesting that it is heterogeneous. The CLC protein level was elevated in the sera of many patients with diseases associated with eosinophilia, including asthma, rheumatoid arthritis, and malignancy; 94% of patients with the hypereosinophilic syndrome had an elevated CLC protein level (3).

We have also investigated the dynamic relationships between developing eosinophilia and changes in serum levels of CLC protein (lysophospholipase) and the granule MBP in 37 patients with Bancroftian filariasis who were treated with diethylcarbamazine (DEC) (1). Prior to treatment of microfilaremic patients with DEC, peripheral blood eosinophil levels, serum concentrations of CLC protein and of MBP were unrelated to the microfilarial worm burdens of the host. Treatment with DEC resulted in significant blood eosinophilia, and the degree of eosinophilia and the elevations in serum levels of CLC protein and MBP during treatment were significantly correlated with the patients' microfilarial worm burdens before treatment. In microfilaremic patients treated with DEC, a statistically significant increase in serum MBP levels was observed concomitant with an initial eosinopenia observed on day 1 of therapy in these patients. The alterations in CLC protein levels during DEC therapy were the most striking. The CLC protein levels did not increase significantly on day 1 of therapy but rose to greater than 1,200% of pretreatment levels by day 14 of therapy in filariasis patients with >1,000 microfilaria per ml of blood. Patients with filariasis (elephantiasis, hydrocoeles, or filarial fevers) but without microfilaremia, as well as an uninfected but exposed endemic control population, showed no changes in eosinophil levels or serum CLC protein or MBP levels during an identical course of DEC therapy. Although this study also showed excellent correlations between serum concentrations of CLC protein and of MBP and peripheral blood eosinophil levels following DEC treatment. While these results are compatible with the notion of release of these proteins from circulating eosinophils, the source(s) of serum CLC protein and MBP are not known. The CLC protein and MBP in serum may be derived from eosinophils in tissues, blood, or in bone marrow.

THE EOSINOPHIL-DERIVED NEUROTOXIN

Eosinophils contain a powerful neurotoxin that can severely damage myelinated neurons in experimental animals (43,58,70,88,93). M. H. Gordon first described this neurotoxic reaction in 1932 and is now known as the "Gordon phenomenon" in his honor. The biological and clinical significance of the Gordon phenomenon remains uncertain, and the eosinophil-derived neurotoxin (EDN) has not been characterized. Because patients with idiopathic hypereosinophilic syndrome and cerebrospinal fluid eosinophilia exhibit varied neurologic abnormalities (10,18,90,92,116), the EDN may play an important role in central nervous system disease in humans.

Physicochemical Properties of EDN

Using the production of the Gordon phenomenon as an assay, Durack et al. analyzed certain of the properties of EDN (29). The EDN was partially purified by ultracentrifugation of sonicated human eosinophils followed by fractionation of the supernatant on Sephadex G-50 columns at neutral pH. Fractions with neurotoxic activity eluted at an apparent molecular weight of approximately 15,000. The partially purified material withstood lyophilization and dialysis, but its neurotoxic activity was destroyed by heating at 90° C. In a subsequent study, extracts of whole human eosinophils and purified eosinophil granules were sequentially fractionated by gel filtration at acid and alkaline pH. Fractions were analyzed by SDS-PAGE and for their ability to produce the Gordon phenomenon by intrathecal injection into rabbits (28). In confirmation of prior studies, extracts of whole eosinophils possessed potent neurotoxic activity. Similarly, extracts of highly purified eosinophil granules were also active. Fractionation of eosinophil granule extracts on Sephadex G-50 at pH 4.3 yielded three major peaks as shown in Fig. 3a. Eosinophil enzymes including peroxidase are included in peak 1, whereas MBP constitutes the protein in peak 3. Neither peak 1 nor peak 3 protein produced the Gordon phenomenon. Fractions comprising peak 2 were concentrated and fractionated on Sephadex G-50 at pH 7.4. As shown in Fig. 3b a single peak resulted, and injection of 50 μg (assuming $E\,{}^{1\%}_{1\,cm} = 10.0$ at 277 nm) caused the Gordon phenomenon. By SDS-PAGE the active material gave a single band with a molecular weight of

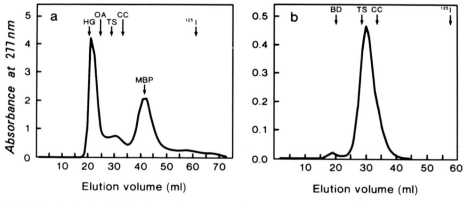

FIG. 3. Sephadex G-50 column chromatography of acid-solubilized eosinophil granules. a) Two milliliters of an acid-solubilized eosinophil granule extract were chromatographed on a Sephadex G-50 column equilibrated with 0.025 M acetate buffer, pH 4.2, 0.15 M NaCl. Fractions eluting between 27 and 33 ml (second protein peak) were pooled, dialyzed overnight against phosphate-buffered saline (PBS), and centrifuged at 12,000 x g for 10 min. b) This sample (1.2 ml; 0.323 absorbance units/ml) was chromatographed on a second G-50 column equilibrated with PBS. Fractions eluting between 27 and 33 ml were pooled and concentrated to 0.6 ml (0.129 absorbance units at 277 nm) on an Amicon UM-2 membrane. Molecular-weight markers for the columns included blue dextran (BD, > 2 × 10^6), human gamma globulin (HG; 150,000), ovalbumin (OA; 49,000), trypsinogen (TS; 24,000), cytochrome C (CC; 12,400), and ^{125}I. [From Durack et al. (28) with permission.]

17,913. Likewise, EDN was purified from whole eosinophil extracts of two other patients and showed a single band by SDS-PAGE, and both produced the Gordon phenomenon; EDN from these patients had molecular weights of 19,219 and 17,733, respectively. In these same studies purified CLC protein (lysophospholipase) and MBP did not produce the Gordon phenomenon. Finally, the relationship between EDN and ECP is obscure. The lower molecular weight of EDN compared to those reported for ECP discourages belief that the two are the same. In addition, purified EDN contained less than 0.1% ECP as determined by radioimmunoassay (*unpublished data*).

Localization of EDN

Seiler et al. reported that EDN activity was possessed by eosinophil granule extracts, but inspection of the electron photomicrographs indicates that a mixture of mitochondria, eosinophil granules, and mast-cell granules was present (89). As noted above, extracts of highly purified eosinophil granules produced the Gordon phenomenon (28); this result points to the eosinophil granule as the source of EDN. Because MBP forms the crystalloid, it seems likely that EDN is present in the granule matrix.

Functions of EDN

The only function presently associated with EDN is its ability to provoke the Gordon phenomenon. When injected intrathecally into experimental animals (usually rabbits and guinea pigs), EDN produces a predictable syndrome which begins with stiffness, most pronounced in the forelimbs, and mild ataxia, followed by incoordination and severe ataxia such that animals have difficulty in remaining upright. The final phase of the Gordon phenomenon is characterized by severe weakness and muscle wasting (29). Some animals develop nystagmus and jerky, repetitive head movements. No evidence of neurologic abnormalities of higher level functions is observed; animals remain alert and eat and drink in a normal fashion, provided food and water are placed within reach. The latent period between injection of purified EDN and the onset of neurologic manifestations ranged from 3 to 11 days (28).

Histopathologic changes produced in rabbits have been thoroughly described by Durack et al. (29). On light microscopy, the histologic abnormalities are concentrated in the cerebellum, pons, and spinal cord. A hallmark of the Gordon phenomenon is the disappearance of Purkinje cells from the cerebellum. In addition, the white matter of cerebellum, pons, and spinal cord shows a gross spongiform change; the gray matter remains essentially normal (29).

Relationship to Disease

The observation that patients with hypereosinophilic syndrome (18) and some patients with parasitic infections (92,116) display a variety of neurologic abnormalities points to the possibility that eosinophils may cause abnormalities of the central nervous system. To date this possibility has not been tested.

ENZYMES PREFERENTIALLY PRESENT IN THE EOSINOPHIL

This subject has been thoroughly reviewed by Weller et al. (111). Among these enzymes are arylsulfatase B, phospholipase D, and the phospholipid exchange protein. The activities and possible biological functions of certain of these proteins will be discussed below.

THE FUNCTIONS OF THE EOSINOPHIL

Present evidence suggests that eosinophils, like the immune response in general, may act for the benefit and for the detriment of the host. Information reviewed in detail elsewhere in this volume suggests that the eosinophil acts to damage certain forms of parasites *in vitro* and presumably *in vivo*. This view would provide a rationale for the known occurrence of eosinophils in and around the sites of parasite infestation. Additional evidence is needed, however, to support the view that the eosinophil actually damages parasites *in vivo*. The present information derived mainly from experiments testing antisera to eosinophils (40,44,68,76), although persuasive, is not conclusive. Furthermore, in man there is a paucity of information pointing to a role for the eosinophil as an *in vivo* parasite killer cell.

Another possible beneficial role for the eosinophil is the detoxification of the mediators of anaphylaxis. Goetzl et al. proposed that eosinophils dampen the inflammatory response induced by mast-cell degranulation (42). The proposal is suggested by the activities of the enzymes possessed by the eosinophil which endow the cell with the capability to degrade the mediators of anaphylaxis (111). For example, arylsulfatase B inactivates the slow-reacting substance of anaphylaxis (leukotriene C) (105); phospholipase D mediates the destruction of platelet lytic factor (54); eosinophil histaminase enzymatically destroys histamine activity (117); and lysophospholipase permits the eosinophil to inactivate membrane-active lysophosphatides (110). Again, evidence is needed to determine if this proposed activity of the eosinophil actually occurs *in vivo*. One experiment testing the effect of eosinophils on the levels of histamine released *in vivo* did not find any increase in the quantity of histamine released in the absence of the eosinophil, as predicted by this hypothesis; in fact, in the absence of eosinophils a reduction in the quantity of histamine released was observed, suggesting that the eosinophil and mast cell might interact in some manner (41). Clearly, further experiments are needed to determine if eosinophils function to dampen inflammation and to support the concept that the eosinophil serves a protective detoxifying role.

Finally, the MBP results discussed earlier point to the possibility that the eosinophil may serve to damage tissues during hypersensitivity reactions. The finding that MBP is a cytotoxic molecule, that it is present in high concentrations in fluids bathing diseased organs, as in the sputum of patients with asthma, and that the effect of MBP on the respiratory epithelium mimicks the pathologic changes seen in asthma points to the possibility that the eosinophil damages tissues. The demonstration of the ability of EPO to damage membranes suggests another mechanism by which eosinophils might mediate cell damage. In the final analysis it seems intuitively obvious that any destructive capabilities of the eosinophil, useful in a protective role, could be turned against the host during hypersensitivity reactions.

A SYSTEM FOR HOST RESISTANCE COMPRISING HOMOCYTOTROPIC ANTIBODY, VASOACTIVE AMINE-CONTAINING CELLS AND EOSINOPHILS

A series of recent observations, taken together, points to the existence of an interactive system composed of homocytotropic antibodies, such as IgE and IgG, mediator-containing cells, such as mast cells and basophils, and eosinophils in host defense against parasites. It has long been known that certain organs such as the skin, the respiratory tract, and the gastrointestinal tract display a parallelism in their content of mediators and cells. Rytomaa showed that eosinophils are concentrated in the skin, gastrointestinal tract, and respiratory tract (85). Van Arsdel and Beall (98) showed that the content of extractable histamine, presumably reflecting the resident mast cell and basophils, is increased in these same organs. Tada and Ishizaka have found that IgE is localized in cells in the respiratory and gastrointestinal tracts (91). Among human diseases the most marked elevations of serum IgE occur among patients with skin disease followed by patients with diseases of the respiratory tract, especially allergic asthma, and by patients with allergic diseases of the gastrointestinal tract (51). Finally, peripheral blood eosinophilia is commonly seen in diseases affecting the same organ systems. Although this view could be regarded as arbitrary, the parallelisms among IgE, histamine, and eosinophils point to the possibility that in some manner they comprise a system.

Recent observations support the existence of this system. Dessein et al. (25) found that repeated injection of rats with antiserum to IgE suppressed the production of IgE antibody to ovalbumin and, of greater interest, to *T. spiralis* in infected animals. The suppression of IgE antibody to *T. spiralis* by anti-IgE was specific for the IgE isotype. Peritoneal mast cells from the suppressed animals did not release serotonin following stimulation by anti-IgE or *T. spiralis* extract but did release serotonin when incubated with the calcium ionophore A23187. The magnitude of the eosinophil response to *T. spiralis* infection in the peripheral blood and around the encysted *T. spiralis* muscle larvae was less in the IgE-suppressed animals. Finally, the number of encysted larvae in the IgE-suppressed rats was significantly greater than in the animals treated with normal serum. The results point to the conclusion that IgE-armed mast cells are stimulated by parasite antigens and attract eosinophils into the lesions where the encysted larvae are presumably destroyed.

In other experiments Brown et al. (12) have studied resistance to a larval tick, *Amblyomma americanum*. When guinea pigs are exposed to the tick, they become immune in that few ticks are able to attack and feed. When such immune animals are challenged by exposure to the tick, a cutaneous reaction develops in which basophils (68% of total white blood cells), eosinophils (25%), and mononuclear cells (6%) are present at the site of tick feeding. When these immune animals are treated with antiserum to the basophil, their resistance to tick challenge is abolished. The antibasophil-serum-treated animals also lacked bone marrow and blood basophils, and they failed to develop a cutaneous basophil response at the site of tick challenge. The antibasophil serum had no effect on peripheral blood eosinophils, but the eosinophils at the challenge sites were reduced; this observation suggests that basophils may participate in eosinophil recruitment to tick feeding sites. When the immune guinea pigs were treated with antiserum to the eosinophil, their resistance was also reduced, although less completely than in the case with antibasophil serum. Antieosinophil serum reduced the numbers of eosinophils in the blood and at the tick feeding sites, but it had no effect on circulating basophils or on the accumulation of basophils at feeding sites. Guinea pigs treated with normal rabbit serum or rabbit antiguinea pig albumin as controls showed no reduction in resistance or cell counts. These data point to a cooperation between the basophil and the eosinophil such that basophils, presumably as a consequence of degranulation and release of eosinophil chemotactic factors, attract eosinophils to the lesions. The effects of the antisera on tick immunity point to the possibility that both the basophil and the eosinophil participate in damaging the tick.

Thus, one can postulate the existence of a system consisting of homocytotropic antibody, mediator-containing cells, and eosinophils which functions in resistance to parasites and also contributes to hypersensitivity reactions. Presumably, the system evolved to deal with ecto- and endoparasites, and in the improved hygenic conditions of certain environments, such as in the developed countries of Europe and North America where parasitism is often quite rare, one sees only the hypersensitivity side of the coin. Atopy as manifested by an ability to make IgE antibodies can then be regarded as a genetic marker for resistance to parasites, a capability of some advantage during earlier times.

ACKNOWLEDGMENTS

Supported by grants from the National Institute of Allergy and Infectious Diseases, AI 9728, AI 15231, and AI 07047, and from the Mayo Foundation.

REFERENCES

1. Ackerman, S. J., Gleich, G. J., Weller, P. F., and Ottesen, E. A. (1981): Eosinophilia and elevated serum levels of eosinophil major basic protein and Charcot-Leyden crystal protein (lysophospholipase) after treatment of patients with Bancroft's filariasis. *J. Immunol.*, 127:1093-1098.
2. Ackerman, S. J., Loegering, D. A., and Gleich, G. J. (1980): The human eosinophil Charcot-Leyden crystal protein: Biochemical characteristics and measurement by radioimmunoassay. *J. Immunol.*, 125:2118-2126.
3. Ackerman, S. J., Loegering, D. A., Wassom, D. L., and Gleich, G. J. (1981): Elevated levels of human eosinophil Charcot-Leyden crystal protein (lysophospholipase) in sera of patients wtih eosinophilia. *Fed. Proc.*, 40:1068 (Abstract).

4. Archer, G. T., Air, G., Jackas, M., and Morell, D. B. (1965): Studies on rat eosinophil peroxidase. *Biochem. Biophys. Acta*, 99:96–101.
5. Archer, G. T., and Blackwood, A. (1965): Formation of Charcot-Leyden crystals in human eosinophils and basophils and study of the composition of the isolated crystal. *J. Exp. Med.*, 122:173–180.
6. Archer, G. T., and Hirsch, J. G. (1963): Isolation of granules from eosinophil leukocytes and study of their enzyme content. *J. Exp. Med.*, 118:277–286.
7. Baehmer, R. L., and Johnston, R. B., Jr. (1971): Metabolic and bactericidal activities of human eosinophils. *Br. J. Haematol.*, 20:277–285.
8. Bainton, D. F., and Farquhar, G. M. (1970): Segregation and packaging of granule enzymes in eosinophilic leukocytes. *J. Cell Biol.*, 45:54–73.
9. Beeson, P. B., and Bass, D. A. (1977): The eosinophil. In: *Major Problems in Internal Medicine*, edited by L. H. Smith, Jr., pp. 39–42. W. B. Saunders Co., Philadelphia.
10. Benvenisti, D. S., and Ultmann, J. E. (1969): Eosinophilic leukemia. Report of five cases and review of the literature. *Ann. Intern. Med.*, 71:731–745.
11. Bilding, M. E., and Klebanoff, S. J. (1970): Peroxidase-mediated virucidal systems. *Science*, 167:195–196.
12. Brown, S. J., Galli, S. J., Gleich, G. J., Dvorak, H. F., and Askenase, P. W. (1981): Anti-basophil or anti-eosinophil serum reverses immune cutaneous resistance to ectoparasites (ticks) in guinea pigs. *Fed. Proc.*, 40:1073 (abstract).
13. Buddecke, E., Essellier, A. F., and Morti, H. R. (1956): Uber die chemische Natur der Charcot-Leydenschen Kristalle. *Hoppe Seylers Z. Physiol. Chem.*, 305:203–206.
14. Bujak, J. S., and Root, R. K. (1974): The role of peroxidase in the bactericidal activity of human blood eosinophils. *Blood*, 43:727–736.
15. Butterworth, A. E., Vadas, M. A., Wassom, D. L., Dessein, A., Hogan, M., Sherry, B., Gleich, G. J., and David, J. R. (1979): Interactions between human eosinophils and schistosomules of *Schistosoma mansoni*. II. The mechanisms of irreversible eosinophil adherence. *J. Exp. Med.*, 150:1456–1471.
16. Butterworth, A. E., Wassom, D. L., Gleich, G. J., Loegering, D. A., and David, J. R. (1979): Damage to schistosomula of *Schistosoma mansoni* induced directly by eosinophil major basic protein. *J. Immunol.*, 122:221–229.
17. Cardell, B. S., and Pearson, B. R. S. (1979): Death in asthmatics. *Thorax*, 14:341–352.
18. Chusid, M. J., Dale, D. D., West, B. C., and Wolff, S. M. (1975): The hypereosinophilic syndrome: analysis of fourteen cases with review of the literature. *Medicine*, 54:1–27.
19. Cotran, R. S., and Litt, M. (1969): The entity of granule-associated peroxidase into the phagocytic vacuoles of eosinophils. *J. Exp. Med.*, 129:1291–1299.
20. Cutz, E., Levison, H., and Coopers, D. M. (1978): Ultrastructure of the airways in children with asthma. *Histopathology*, 2:407–421.
21. Dahl, R., and Venge, P. (1978): Blood leukocyte and eosinophil cationic protein: in vivo study of the influence of beta-2-adrenergic drugs and steroid administration. *Scand. J. Resp. Dis.*, 59:319–322.
22. Dahl, R., and Venge, P. (1979): Enhancement of wokinase-induced plasminogen activation by the cationic protein of human eosinophil granulocytes. *Thromb. Res.*, 14:599–608.
23. Dahl, R., Venge, P., and Olsson, I. (1978): Blood eosinophil leukocytes and eosinophil cationic protein: diurnal variation in normal subjects and patients with bronchial asthma. *Scand. J. Resp. Dis.*, 59:323–325.
24. Dahl, R., Venge, P., and Olsson, I. (1978): Variations of blood eosinophils and eosinophil cationic protein in serum in patients with bronchial asthma: studies during inhalation challenge test. *Allergy*, 33:211–215.
25. Dessein, A. J., Parker, W. L., James, S. L., and David, J. R. (1981): IgE antibody and resistance to infection. I. Selective suppression of the IgE antibody response in rats diminishes the resistance and the eosinophil response to *Trichinella spiralis* infection. *J. Exp. Med.*, 153:423–436.
26. Dresser, R. K., Himmelhock, S. R., Evans, W. H., Januska, M., Mage, M., and Shelton, E. (1972): Guinea pig heterophil and eosinophil peroxidase. *Arch. Biochem. Biophys.*, 148:452–465.
27. Dunnill, M. S. (1971): The pathology of asthma. In: *The Identification of Asthma*, edited by R. Porter and J. Birch, pp. 35–46. Ciba Foundation Symposium, London, Churchill-Livingstone.
28. Durack, D. T., Ackerman, S. J., Loegering, D. A., and Gleich, G. J. (1981): Purification of human eosinophil-derived neurotoxin. *Proc. Natl. Acad. Sci.*, U.S.A., 78:5165-5169.

29. Durack, D. T., Sumi, S. M., and Klebanoff, S. J. (1979): Neurotoxicity of human eosinophils. *Proc. Natl. Acad. Sci. U. S. A.*, 76:1443–1447.
30. Enomoto, I., and Kitani, T. (1966): Electron microscopic studies on peroxidase and acid phosphatase reaction in human leukocytes in normal and leukemic cells and on phagocytosis. *Acta Haematol. Jpn.*, 29:554–570.
31. Filley, W. V., Kephart, G. M., and Gleich, G. J. (1981): Localization of the eosinophil granule major basic protein in the bronchi of patients with asthma. *J. Allergy Clin. Immunol.*, 67(Suppl 1):54 (abstract).
32. Frigas, E., Loegering, D. A., and Gleich, G. J. (1980): Cytotoxic effects of guinea pig eosinophil major basic protein on tracheal epithelium. *Lab. Invest.*, 42:35–43.
33. Frigas, E., Loegering, D. A., Solley, G. O., Farrow, G. M., and Gleich, G. J. (1981): Elevated levels of the eosinophil granule major basic protein in the sputum of patients with bronchial asthma. *Mayo Clin. Proc.*, 56:345-353.
34. Glauert, A. M., Butterworth, A. E., Sturrock, R. F., et al. (1978): The mechanism of antibody-dependent, eosinophil-mediated damage to schistosomula of *Schistosoma mansoni* in vitro: a study by phase-contrast and electron microscopy. *J. Cell. Sci.*, 34:173–192.
35. Gleich, G. J., Frigas, E., Loegering, D. A., Wassom, D. L., and Steinmuller, D. (1979): Cytotoxic properties of eosinophil major basic protein. *J. Immunol.*, 123:2925–2927.
36. Gleich, G. J., and Loegering, D. A. (1973): Selective stimulation and purification of eosinophils and neutrophils from guinea pig peritoneal fluids. *J. Lab. Clin. Med.*, 82:522–528.
37. Gleich, G. J., Loegering, D. A., Kueppers, F., Bajaj, S. P., and Mann, K. G. (1974): Physiochemical and biological properties of the major basic protein from guinea pig eosinophil granules. *J. Exp. Med.*, 140:313–332.
38. Gleich, G. J., Loegering, D. A., and Maldonado, J. E. (1973): Identification of a major basic protein in guinea pig eosinophil granules. *J. Exp. Med.*, 137:1459–1471.
39. Gleich, G. J., Loegering, D. A., Mann, K. G., and Maldonado, J. E. (1976): Comparative properties of the Charcot-Leyden crystal protein and the major basic protein from human eosinophils. *J. Clin. Invest.*, 57:633–640.
40. Gleich, G. J., Olson, G. M., and Herlich, H. (1979): The effect of antiserum to eosinophils on susceptibility and acquired immunity of the guinea pig to *Trichostrongylus colubriformis*. *Immunology*, 37:873–880.
41. Gleich, G. J., Olson, G. M., and Loegering, D. A. (1979): The effect of ablation of eosinophils on immediate-type hypersensitivity reactions. *Immunology*, 38:343–353.
42. Goetzl, E. J., Wasserman, S. I., and Austen, K. F. (1975): Eosinophil polymorphonuclear function in immediate-type hypersensitivity. *Arch. Pathol.*, 99:1–4.
43. Gordon, M. H. (1933): Remarks on Hodgkin's disease. A pathogenic agent in the glands and its application in diagnosis. *Br. Med. J.*, 1:641–647.
44. Grove, D. I., Mahmoud, A. A. F., and Warren, K. S. (1977): Eosinophils in resistance to *Trichinella spiralis*. *J. Exp. Med.*, 145:755–759.
45. Hallgren, R., Venge, P., Cullhed, I., and Olsson, I. (1979): Blood eosinophils and eosinophil cationic protein after acute myocardial infarction or corticosteroid administration. *Br. J. Haematol.*, 42:147–154.
46. Henderson, W. R., Chi, E. Y., and Klebanoff, S. J. (1980): Eosinophil peroxidase-induced mast cell secretion. *J. Exp. Med.*, 152:265–279.
47. Henderson, W. R., Jong, E. C., and Klebanoff, S. J. (1980): Binding of eosinophil peroxidase to mast cell granules with retention of peroxidatic activity. *J. Immunol.*, 124:1383–1388.
48. Hilding, A. C. (1943): The relation of ciliary insufficiency to death from asthma and other respiratory diseases. *Ann. Otol. Rhinol. Laryngol.*, 52:5–19.
49. Hornung, M. (1962): Preservation, recrystallization and preliminary biochemical characterization of Charcot-Leyden crystals. *Proc. Soc. Exp. Biol. Med.*, 110:119–124.
50. Jacobs, A. A., Loew, I. E., Paul, B. B., Strauss, R. R., and Sbarra, A. T. (1972): Mycoplasmicidal activity of peroxidase-H_2O_2-halide system. *Immunology*, 51:127–131.
51. Johansson, S. G. O., Bennich, H. H., and Berg, T. (1972): The clinical significance of IgE. *Prog. Clin. Immunol.*, 1:157–181.
52. Jong, E. C., Henderson, W. R., and Klebanoff, S. J. (1980): Bactericidal activity of eosinophil peroxidase. *J. Immunol.*, 124:1378–1382.
53. Jong, E. C., Mahmoud, A. A. F., and Klebanoff, S. J. (1981): Peroxidase-mediated toxicity to schistosomules of *Schistosoma mansoni*. *J. Immunol.*, 126:468–471.

54. Kater, L. A., Goetzl, E. J., and Austen, K. F. (1980): Isolation of human eosinophil phospholipase D. *J. Clin. Invest.*, 58:1173–1180.
55. Kazura, J. W. (1980): Protective role of eosinophils. In: *The Eosinophil in Health and Disease*, edited by A. A. F. Mahmoud and K. F. Austen, pp. 231–251. Grune & Stratton, New York.
56. Kelenyi, G., Zombai, E., and Nemeth, A. (1965): Histochemische und elektronenmikroskopische Beobachtungen an der spezifischen Granulation der eosinophilen Granulozyten. *Acta Histochem.*, 22:77–89.
57. Kierszenbaum, F., Ackerman, S. J., and Gleich, G. J. (1981): Destruction of bloodstream forms of *Trypanosoma cruzi* by eosinophil major basic protein. *Am. J. Trop. Med. Hyg.*, 30:775-779.
58. King, L. S. (1939): Encephalopathy following injections of bone marrow extract. *J. Exp. Med.*, 70:303–304.
59. Klebanoff, S. J. (1967): Iodination of bacteria: a bactericidal mechanism. *J. Exp. Med.*, 126:1063–1078.
60. Klebanoff, S. J., Durack, D. T., Rosen, H., and Clark, R. A. (1977): Functional studies on human peritoneal eosinophils. *Infect. Immunol.*, 17:167–173.
61. Klebanoff, S. J., Jong, E. C., and Henderson, W. R., Jr. (1980): The eosinophil peroxidase: purification and biological properties. In: *The Eosinophil in Health and Disease*, edited by A. A. F. Mahmoud and K. F. Austen, pp. 99–114. Grune & Stratton, New York.
62. Lehrer, R. I. (1969): Antifungal effects of peroxidase systems. *J. Bacteriol.*, 99:361–365.
63. Lewis, D. M., Lewis, J. C., Loegering, D. A., and Gleich, G. J. (1978): Localization of the guinea pig eosinophil major basic protein to the core of the granule. *Cell Biol.*, 77:702–713.
64. Lewis, D. M., Loegering, D. A., and Gleich, G. J. (1976): Antiserum to the major basic protein of guinea pig eosinophil granules. *Immunochemistry*, 13:743–746.
65. Lewis, D. M., Loegering, D. A., and Gleich, G. J. (1976): Isolation and partial characterization of a major basic protein from rat eosinophil granules. *Proc. Soc. Exp. Biol. Med.*, 152:512–515.
66. Lindor, L. J., Loegering, D. A., Wassom, D. L., and Gleich, G. J. (1981): Recovery of eosinophils from the peritoneal cavity of the guinea pig. *J. Immunol. Methods*, 41:125–134.
67. Litt, M. (1960): Studies in experimental eosinophilia. I. Repeated quantitation of peritoneal eosinophils in guinea pigs by a method of peritoneal lavage. *Blood*, 16:1318–1329.
68. Mahmoud, A. A. F., Warren, K. S., and Peters, P. A. (1975): A role for the eosinophil in acquired resistance to *Schistosoma mansoni* infection as determined by antieosinophil serum. *J. Exp. Med.*, 142:805–813.
69. McLaren, D. J., Ramalho-Pinto, F. J., and Smithers, S. R. (1978): Ultrastructural evidence for complement and antibody-dependent damage to schistosomula of *Schistosoma mansoni* by rat eosinophils *in vitro. Parasitology*, 77:313–324.
70. McNaught, J. B. (1938): The Gordon's test for Hodgkin's disease. *J. A. M. A.*, 111:1280–1284.
71. Mezey, R. J., Cohn, M. A., Fernandez, R. J., Januszkiewicz, A. J., and Wanner, A. (1978): Mucociliary transport in allergic patients with antigen-induced bronchospasm. *Am. Rev. Resp. Dis.*, 118:677–684.
72. Mickenberg, I. D., Poot, R. K., and Wolff, S. M. (1972): Bactericidal and metabolic activities of the human eosinophil. *Blood*, 39:67–80.
73. Migler, R., DeChatelet, L. R., and Bass, D. A. (1978): Human eosinophilic peroxidase: role in bactericidal activity. *Blood*, 51:445–456.
74. Miller, F., de Harven, E., and Palade, G. E. (1962): The structure of the leukocyte granules in rodents and man. *J. Cell Biol.*, 31:349–362.
75. Naylor, B. (1962): The shedding of the mucosa of the bronchial tree in asthma. *Thorax*, 17:69–72.
76. Olds, G. R., and Mahmoud, A. A. F. (1980): Role of host granulomatous response in murine schistosomiasis mansoni. *J. Clin. Invest.*, 66:1191–1199.
77. Olsson, I., and Venge, P. (1974): Cationic proteins of human granulocytes. II. Separation of the cationic proteins of the granules of leukemic myeloid cells. *Blood*, 44:235–246.
78. Olsson, I., Venge, P., Spitznagel, J. K., and Lehrer, R. I. (1977): Arginine-rich cationic proteins of human eosinophil granules. *Lab. Invest.*, 36:493–500.
79. Ottesen, E. A., and Cohen, S. G. (1978): The eosinophil, eosinophilia, and eosinophil-related disorders. In: *Allergy, Principles and Practice*, edited by E. Middleton, Jr., C. E. Reed, and E. F. Ellis, pp. 584–632. C. V. Mosby Co., St. Louis.
80. Ottolenghi, A. (1969): The relationship between eosinophilic leukocytes and phospholipase B activity in some rat tissues. *Lipids*, 5:531–588.

81. Ottolenghi, A., Pickett, J. P., and Greene, W. B. (1967): Histochemical demonstration of phospholipase B (lysolecithinase) activity in rat tissues. *J. Histochem. Cytochem.*, 14:907–914.
82. Parrillo, J. E., and Fauci, A. S. (1978): Human eosinophils, purification, and cytotoxic capability of eosinophils from patients with the hypereosinophilic syndrome. *Blood*, 51:457–473.
83. Pineda, A. A., Brzica, S. M., Jr., and Taswell, H. F. (1977): Continuous- and semi-continuous-flow blood centrifugation systems: therapeutic applications, with plasma-, platelet-, lympha- and eosinapheresis. *Transfusion*, 17:407–416.
84. Pincus, S. H. (1978): Production of eosinophil-rich guinea pig peritoneal exudates. *Blood*, 52:127–134.
85. Rytomaa, T. (1960): Organ distributions and histochemical properties of eosinophil granulocytes in the rat. *Acta Pathol. Microbiol. Scand.*, 50(Suppl 140):1–118.
86. Rytomaa, T., and Teir, H. (1961): Relationship between tissue eosinophils and peroxidase activity. *Nature (London)*, 192:271–272.
87. Santa Cruz, R., Landa, J., Hirsch, J., and Sackner, M. A. (1974): Tracheal mucous velocity in normal man and patients with obstructive lung disease; effect of terbutaline. *Am. Rev. Resp. Dis.*, 109:458–463.
88. Schwartz, A. M., Lapham, L. W., and Van den Noort, S. (1966): Cytologic and cytochemical studies of neuroglia. IV. Experimentally induced protoplasmic astrocytosis in Bergman glia of cerebellum. *Neurology*, 16:1118–1126.
89. Seiler, G., Westerman, R. A., and Wilson, J. A. (1969): The role of specific eosinophil granules in eosinophil-induced experimental encephalitis. *Neurology*, 19:478–488.
90. Snead, O. C., and Kalavsky, S. M. (1976): Cerebrospinal fluid eosinophilia. A manifestation of a disorder resembling multiple sclerosis in childhood. *J. Pediatr.*, 89:83–84.
91. Tada, T., and Ishizaka, K. (1970): Distribution of IgE forming cells in lymphoid tissues of the human and monkey. *J. Immunol.*, 104:377–387.
92. Terplan, K., Kraus, R., and Barnes, S. (1957): Eosinophilic meningo-encephalitis, with predominantly cerebellar changes caused by Trichinella infection. *J. Mt. Sinai Hosp.*, 24:1293–1309.
93. Turner, J. C., Jackson, H., Jr., and Parker, F., Jr. (1938): The etiologic relation of the eosinophil to the Gordon phenomenon in Hodgkin's disease. *Am. J. Med. Sci.*, 195:27–33.
94. Udell, I., Gleich, G. J., Allansmith, M. R., Ackerman, S. J., and Abelson, M. B. (1981): Elevated levels of eosinophil granule major basic protein in tears. *Am. J. Ophthal. (in press)*.
95. Unditz, E., Lang, M., and Van Oyi, E. (1956): La reaction proxydasique des eosinophiles: comme moyen de toxonomie. *Le Sang*, 27:513–515.
96. Vadas, M. A., Butterworth, A. E., Sherry, B., Dessein, A., Hogan, M., Bout, D., and David, J. R. (1980): Interactions between human eosinophils and schistosomules of Schistosoma mansoni. II. Stable and irreversible antibody-dependent eosinophil adherence. *J. Immunol.*, 124:1441–1448.
97. Vadas, M. A., David, J. R., Butterworth, A. E., Pisani, N. T., and Siongok, T. A. (1979): A new method for the purification of human eosinophils and neutrophils, and a comparison of the abilities of these cells to damage schistosomula of Schistosoma mansoni. *J. Immunol.*, 122:1228–1236.
98. Van Arsdel, P. P., Jr., and Beall, G. N. (1960): The metabolism and functions of histamine. *Arch. Intern. Med.*, 106:714–733.
99. Venge, P., Dahl, R., and Hallgren, R. (1979): Enhancement of Factor XII dependent reactions by eosinophil cationic protein. *Thromb. Res.*, 14:641–649.
100. Venge, P., Dahl, R., Hallgren, R., and Olsson, I. (1980): Cationic proteins of human eosinophils and their role in the inflammatory reaction. In: *The Eosinophil in Health and Disease*, edited by A. A. F. Mahmoud and K. F. Austen, pp. 131–144. Grune & Stratton, New York.
101. Venge, P., Roxin, L. E., and Olsson, I. (1977): Radioimmunoassay of human cationic protein. *Br. J. Haematol.*, 37:331–335.
102. Venge, P., Zetterstrom, O., Dahl, R., Roxin, L. E., and Olsson, I. (1977): Low levels of eosinophil cationic proteins in patients with asthma. *Lancet*, 2:373–375.
103. Vercauteren, R., and Blonde, B. (1954): The cytochemistry of peroxidase in horse leukocytes. *Enzymologia*, 16:371–383.
104. Vercauteren, R., and Peeters, G. (1952): On the presence of an antihistaminicum in isolated eosinophil granules. *Arch. Int. Pharmacodyn. Ther.*, 89:10–14.
105. Wasserman, S. I., Goetzl, E. J., and Austen, K. F. (1975): Inactivation of the slow reacting substance of anaphylaxis by human eosinophil arylsulfatase. *J. Immunol.*, 114:645–649.

106. Wassom, D. L., and Gleich, G. J. (1979): Damage to *Trichinella spiralis* newborn larvae by eosinophil major basic protein. *Am. J. Trop. Med. Hyg.*, 28:860–863.
107. Wassom, D. L., Loegering, D. A., and Gleich, G. J. (1979): Measurement of guinea pig eosinophil major basic protein by radioimmunoassay. *Mol. Immunol.*, 16:711–719.
108. Wassom, D. L., Loegering, D. A., Solley, G. O., Moore, S. B., Schooley, R. T., Fauci, A. S., and Gleich, G. J. (1981): Elevated levels of the eosinophil granule major basic protein in patients with eosinophilia. *J. Clin. Invest.*, 67:651–661.
109. Watanabe, K., Hasegawa, M., Saito, Y., and Takayama, S. (1977): Eosinophilic leukocytes in nasal allergy-movement of enzymes. *Clin. Allergy*, 7:263–271.
110. Weller, P. F., Goetzl, E. J., and Austen, K. F. (1980): Identification of human eosinophil lyso-phospholipase as the constituent of Charcot-Leyden crystals. *Proc. Natl. Acad. Sci. U.S.A.*, 77:7440–7443.
111. Weller, P. F., Wasserman, S. I., and Austen, K. F. (1981): Selected enzymes preferentially present in the eosinophil. In: *The Eosinophil in Health and Disease*, edited by A. A. F. Mahmoud and K. F. Austen, pp. 115–128. Grune & Stratton, New York.
112. Wever, R., Hamers, M. N., Wiesing, R. S., and Roos, D. (1980): Characterization of the peroxidase in human eosinophils. *Eur. J. Biochem.*, 108:491–495.
113. Wilhelm, J. A., Spelsberg, T. C., and Hnilica, L. S. (1971): Nuclear proteins in genetic restriction. I. The histones. *Subcell Biochem.*, 1:39–65.
114. Wintraub, B. U., Dvorak, A. M., Mihm, M. C., Jr., and Gleich, G. J. (1981): Bullous pemphigoid: cytotoxic eosinophil degranulation and release of eosinophil major basic protein. *Clin. Res.*, 29:618A.
115. Yamada, E., and Yamauchi, R. (1966): Some observations on the cytochemistry and morphogenesis of the granulocytes in the rat bone marrow as revealed by electron microscopy. *Acta Haematol. Jpn.*, 29:530–541.
116. Yii, C-Y. (1976): Clinical observations on eosinophilic meningitis and meningoencephalitis caused by *Angiostrongylus cantonensis* in Taiwan. *Am. J. Trop. Med. Hyg.*, 25:233–249.
117. Zeiger, R. S., and Colten, H. R. (1977): Histaminase release from human eosinophils. *J. Immunol.*, 118:540–543.

Subject Index